Liver
Disorders
SOURCEBOOK

Health Reference Series

First Edition

Liver
Disorders
SOURCEBOOK

*Basic Consumer Health Information
about the Liver and How It Works; Liver
Diseases, Including Cancer, Cirrhosis,
Hepatitis, and Toxic and Drug Related
Diseases; Tips for Maintaining a Healthy
Liver; Laboratory Tests, Radiology Tests, and
Facts about Liver Transplantation; Along
with a Section on Support Groups, a
Glossary, and Resource Listings*

Edited by
Joyce Brennfleck Shannon

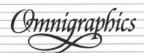

Omnigraphics

615 Griswold • Detroit, MI 48226

Bibliographic Note

Because this page cannot legibly accommodate all the copyright notices, the Bibliographic Note portion of the Preface constitutes an extension of the copyright notice.

Beginning with books published in 1999, each new volume of the *Health Reference Series* will be individually titled and called a "First Edition." Subsequent updates will carry sequential edition numbers. To help avoid confusion and to provide maximum flexibility in our ability to respond to informational needs, the practice of consecutively numbering each volume will be discontinued.

Edited by Joyce Brennfleck Shannon

Health Reference Series

Karen Bellenir, *Series Editor*
Peter D. Dresser, *Managing Editor*
Joan Margeson, *Research Associate*
Dawn Matthews, *Verification Assistant*
Margaret Mary Missar, *Research Coordinator*
Jenifer Swanson, *Research Associate*

Omnigraphics, Inc.

Matthew P. Barbour, *Vice President, Operations*
Laurie Lanzen Harris, *Vice President, Editorial Director*
Kevin Hayes, *Production Coordinator*
Thomas J. Murphy, *Vice President, Finance and Comptroller*
Peter E. Ruffner, *Senior Vice President*
Jane J. Steele, *Marketing Consultant*

Frederick G. Ruffner, Jr., Publisher

© 2000, Omnigraphics, Inc.

Library of Congress Cataloging-in-Publication Data

Mental health disorders sourcebook : basic consumer health information about anxiety disorders, depression, and other mood disorders . . . / edited by Karen Bellenir. — 2nd ed.
    p. cm. — (Health reference series)
Includes bibliographical references and index.
ISBN 0-7808-0240-3 (alk. paper)
    1. Mental illness. 2. Psychiatry. I. Bellenir, Karen.
II. Health reference series (Unnumbered)
RC454.4 .M458 1999
616.89—dc21   99-049596

∞

This book is printed on acid-free paper meeting the ANSI Z39.48 Standard. The infinity symbol that appears above indicates that the paper in this book meets that standard.

Printed in the United States

Table of Contents

Part X: Additional Help and Information

Preface

About This Book

The liver is the largest organ in the body. It plays a vital role in regulating such complex life processes as:

- converting food into chemicals necessary for life and growth

- manufacturing and exporting important substances used by the rest of the body

- processing drugs absorbed from the digestive tract into forms that are easier for the body to use

- detoxifying and excreting substances that otherwise would be poisonous.

As the body's refining and detoxifying factory, the liver can become an overworked organ. Liver damage and disease rates are increasing. For example, an estimated 140,000 Americans become infected with the hepatitis B virus each year, and 1-1.25 million people are chronically infected. Even though an injured liver can regenerate if ten percent of it is functioning, many diseases damage the entire organ. When liver failure occurs, transplantation is the only treatment option available. In 1985, 602 liver transplants were performed in the U.S. The number had increased to 4,058 by 1996. Currently 12,987 individuals are waiting for a liver transplant.

This *Sourcebook* provides basic health care information about liver functions, guidelines for liver health, and tests which assess liver distress. It also presents the symptoms, treatments, and preventive measures available for liver cancer, hepatitis A, B, C, D, and E, genetically based liver diseases, and other liver diseases. The transplantation process is explained. A glossary, a directory of organizations and support groups with up-to-date contact information, including websites and e-mail addresses, and a listing of transplant centers conclude the volume.

How to Use This Book

This book is divided into parts and chapters. Parts focus on broad areas of interest. Chapters are devoted to single topics within a part.

Part I: Liver Mechanics and Maintenance provides the details of essential liver functions, its role in digestion, and diet guidelines for maintaining a healthy liver.

Part II: Medical Tests describes the procedures used to assess liver functions and to determine the cause of liver distress. This part includes information on blood studies, known as liver function tests, radiology tests, and liver biopsies.

Part III: Liver Distress looks at conditions which can cause the liver to be stressed, injured, or scarred including cirrhosis, viruses, parasites, pregnancy, and newborn jaundice.

Part IV: The Effects of Drugs on the Liver emphasizes how drugs can alter the activity of liver enzyme systems with destructive results, including alcohol-induced liver disease, harmful effects of medicines, acetaminophen overdose dangers, and the need for cautious use of herbs and other alternative therapies.

Part V: Liver Cancer gives an overview of the diagnosis, staging, and treatment options for childhood and adult liver cancer.

Part VI: Hepatitis presents information about the hepatitis virus— the nation's most common blood-borne infection—and other causes of liver inflammation, including autoimmune disease and occupational hazards.

Part VII: Genetically Based Liver Disease describes symptoms and treatment options for inherited diseases and syndromes which damage the liver or cause liver malfunction.

Part VIII: Other Diseases of the Liver presents symptoms, diagnosis, and treatment of liver diseases caused by bile duct obstruction or destruction, clotting of the hepatic vein, congenital abnormalities, excessive build-up of fat in the liver, or enzyme deficiencies.

Part IX: Liver Transplantation gives an overview of the transplant process, including transplant preparation, finances, organ donation, candidate selection, and such supportive services as transportation and the bioartificial liver.

Part X: Additional Help and Information provides a glossary, a listing of contact information for patient organizations and support groups, and a directory of transplant centers.

Bibliographic Note

This volume contains documents and excerpts from publications issued by the following U.S. government agencies: Centers for Disease Control and Prevention (CDC), Food and Drug Administration (FDA), Department of Health and Human Services (DHHS), Health Resources and Services Administration (HRSA), National Institute on Alcohol Abuse and Alcoholism (NIAAA), National Cancer Institute (NCI), National Center for Infectious Diseases (NCID), National Center for Research Resources (NCRR), National Institute of Dental Research (NIDR), National Institute of Diabetes and Digestive and Kidney Diseases (NIDDK), National Institute of General Medical Sciences (NIGMS), National Institute of Neurological Disorders and Stroke (NINDS), and the Occupational Safety and Health Administration (OSHA).

In addition, this volume contains copyrighted documents from the following organizations and individuals: AirLifeLine National Office; American Hemochromatosis Society, Inc.; American Institute of Ultrasound in Medicine; American Liver Foundation; Steven H. Brick, M.D.; Chek Med Systems, Inc.; Hepatitis B Foundation; Hepatitis Foundation International; Immunization Action Coalition; The Nemours Foundation; Oxalosis and Hyperoxaluria Foundation; The PBC Foundation; The Personal Communications Industry Association; Primary Biliary Cirrhosis Support Group; United Network for Organ

Sharing; University of Pittsburgh, and Howard Worman, M.D. A copyrighted article from *The Liver Circulation Newsletter* is also included.

Full citation information is provided on the first page of each chapter. Every effort has been made to secure all necessary rights to reprint the copyrighted material. If any omissions have been made, please contact Omnigraphics to make corrections for future editions.

Acknowledgements

Special thanks to the many organizations, agencies, and individuals who have contributed materials for this *Sourcebook* and to Karen Bellenir, Maria Franklin, Joan Margeson, and Dawn Matthews for their assistance. This book is dedicated to those individuals and their families who know the day to day struggle of living with liver disease.

Note from the Editor

This book is part of Omnigraphics' *Health Reference Series*. The series provides basic information about a broad range of medical concerns. It is not intended to serve as a tool for diagnosing illness, in prescribing treatments, or as a substitute for the physician/patient relationship. All persons concerned about medical symptoms or the possibility of disease are encouraged to seek professional care from an appropriate health care provider.

Our Advisory Board

The *Health Reference Series* is reviewed by an Advisory Board comprised of librarians from public, academic, and medical libraries. We would like to thank the following board members for providing guidance to the development of this series:

Nancy Bulgarelli, William Beaumont Hospital Library, Royal Oak, MI

Karen Imarasio, Bloomfield Township Public Library, Bloomfield Township, MI

Karen Morgan, Mardigian Library, University of Michigan-Dearborn, Dearborn, MI

Rosemary Orlando, St. Clair Shores Public Library, St. Clair Shores, MI

Health Reference Series *Update Policy*

The inaugural book in the *Health Reference Series* was the first edition of *Cancer Sourcebook* published in 1992. Since then, the Series has been enthusiastically received by librarians and in the medical community. In order to maintain the standard of providing high-quality health information for the lay person the editorial staff at Omnigraphics felt it was necessary to implement a policy of updating volumes when warranted.

Medical researchers have been making tremendous strides, and the challenge to stay current with the most recent advances is one our editors take seriously. Each decision to update a volume will be made on an individual basis. Some of the considerations will include how much new information is available and the feedback we receive from people who use the books. If there's a topic you would like to see added to the update list, or an area of medical concern you feel has not been adequately addressed, please write to:

Editor
Health Reference Series
Omnigraphics, Inc.
615 Griswold
Detroit, MI 48226

The commitment to providing on-going coverage of important medical developments has also led to some technical changes in the *Health Reference Series*. Beginning with books published in 1999, each new volume will be individually titled and called a "First Edition." Subsequent updates will carry sequential edition numbers. To help avoid confusion and to provide maximum flexibility in our ability to respond to informational needs, the practice of consecutively numbering each volume will be discontinued.

Part One

Liver Mechanics and Maintenance

Chapter 1

A Guide to the Liver

How Can You Love Me If You Don't Know Me?

Hi...I'm Your Liver. Let Me Tell You How Much I Love You.

- I store the iron reserves you need, as well as a lot of vitamins and other minerals.

  Without me you wouldn't have the strength to carry on!

- I make bile to help digest your food.

  Without me you'd waste away to nothing!

- I detoxify poisonous chemicals you give me, and that includes alcohol, beer, wine, prescribed drugs, and over-the-counter drugs as well as illegal substances.

  Without me, your "bad" habits would kill you!

- I store energy, like a battery, by stockpiling sugar (carbohydrates, glucose, and fat) until you need it.

  Without me the sugar level in your blood would fall dramatically and you'd go into a coma!

Reprinted with permission from the American Liver Foundation, 1-800-GO-Liver, "Your Liver Loves You," © 1997, and "Your Liver, A Vital Organ," © 1997.

3

Let's face it! You couldn't have gotten out of bed this morning if I weren't on the job.

- I make the blood that got your system going even before you were born.

    Without me you wouldn't be here!

- I manufacture new proteins that your body needs to stay healthy and grow.

    Without me you wouldn't grow properly!

- I remove poisons from the air, exhaust, smoke, and chemicals you breathe.

    Without me you'd be poisoned by pollutants!

- I make clotting factors that stop the bleeding when you nick yourself shaving or paring an apple.

    Without me you'd bleed to death!

- I help defend you against the "germ warfare" going on in your body all the time. I take those cold germs, flu bugs and other germs you encounter, and knock them dead—or at least weaken them.

    Without me you'd be a sitting duck
    for every infection known to man.

That's How Much I Love You—But Do You Love Me?

Let me tell you some easy ways to love your liver:

1. Don't drown me in beer, alcohol or wine!

    Even one drink is too much for some people and could scar me for life.

2. Watch those drugs!

    All drugs are chemicals, and when you mix them up without a doctor's advice you could create something poisonous that could damage me badly.

I scar easily...and those scars, called "cirrhosis" are permanent.

Medicine is sometimes necessary. But taking pills when they aren't necessary is a bad habit. All those chemicals can really hurt a liver.

3. Be careful with aerosol sprays!

    Remember, I also have to detoxify what you breathe. So when you go on a cleaning binge with aerosol cleaners, make sure the room is ventilated, or wear a mask. That goes double for bug sprays, mildew sprays, paint sprays, and all those other chemical sprays you use. Be careful what you breathe!

4. Watch what gets on your skin!

    Those insecticides you put on trees and shrubs not only kill bugs they can get to me right through your skin and destroy my cells, too. Remember they're all chemicals. So cover your skin with gloves, long sleeves, and a hat and mask every time insecticides are in the air or if you're handling them.

5. A hug is better than a kiss or other intimate contact...because certain kinds of hepatitis are contagious.

    Hepatitis viruses live in body fluids, blood, saliva, and seminal fluid. Most often I kill off the virus...but sometimes hepatitis viruses get the best of me. So if you catch hepatitis, we'll both be in trouble.

6. Don't eat too many fatty foods!

    I make the cholesterol your body needs, and I try to make the right amount. Give me a break. Eat a good, well balanced nourishing diet. If you eat the right stuff for me, I'll really do my stuff for you!

Warning

I can't, and won't, tell you I'm in trouble until I'm almost at the end of my rope—and yours.

Remember: I am not a complainer. Overloading me with drugs, alcohol, and other junk can destroy me! This may be the only warning you will ever get.

Take My Advice, Please!

- Check me out with your doctor.

- Blood screening tests can identify some trouble. So ask to be tested.

- If I'm soft and smooth, that's good. If I'm hard and bumpy, that could mean trouble.

- If your doctor suspects trouble, ultrasound and CAT scans can look into it.

- Sometimes a needle biopsy is needed to find out how many scars you've given me. Nobody likes needles, so don't let me get into such bad shape.

- My life, and yours, depends on how you treat me.

Now you know how much I care for you. Please treat me with tender loving care.

Your silent partner and Ever-Loving Liver.

Experts estimate that more than half of all liver diseases could be prevented if people acted upon the knowledge we already have. Each year more than 25 million Americans are afflicted with liver and gall bladder diseases and more than 27,000 die of cirrhosis. There are few effective treatments for most life-threatening liver diseases, except for liver transplants. Research has recently opened up exciting new paths for investigation, but much more remains to be done to find cures for more than 100 different liver diseases. Meanwhile, patients and their families must cope with medical, financial, and emotional problems.

Your Liver, A Vital Organ

Your liver, the largest organ in your body, plays a vital role in regulating life processes. This complex organ performs many functions essential to life. You simply cannot live without it.

The Location of the Liver

The liver, located behind the lower ribs on the right side of your abdomen, weighs about 3 pounds, and is roughly the size of a football.

Functions of Your Liver

This vital organ performs many complex functions. Some of these are:

1. To convert food into chemicals necessary for life and growth;

2. To manufacture and export important substances used by the rest of the body;

3. To process drugs absorbed from the digestive tract into forms that are easier for the body to use; and

4. To detoxify and excrete substances that otherwise would be poisonous.

Your liver plays a key role in converting food into essential chemicals of life. All of the blood that leaves the stomach and intestines must pass through the liver before reaching the rest of the body. The liver is thus strategically placed to process nutrients and drugs absorbed from the digestive tract into forms that are easier for the rest of the body to use. In essence, the liver can be thought of as the body's refinery.

Furthermore, your liver plays a principal role in removing from the blood ingested and internally produced toxic substances. The liver converts them to substances that can be easily eliminated from the body. It also makes bile, a greenish-brown fluid which is essential for digestion. Bile is stored in the gallbladder which, after eating, contracts and discharges bile into the intestine, where it aids digestion.

Many drugs taken to treat diseases are also chemically modified by the liver. These changes govern the drug's activity in the body.

Your liver helps you by:

• Producing quick energy when it is needed;

• Manufacturing new body proteins;

• Preventing shortages in body fuel by storing certain vitamins, minerals, and sugars;

• Regulating transport of fat stores;

• Regulating blood clotting;

• Aiding in the digestive process by producing bile;

• Controlling the production and excretion of cholesterol;

7

- Neutralizing and destroying poisonous substances;

- Metabolizing alcohol;

- Monitoring and maintaining the proper level of many chemicals and drugs in the blood;

- Cleansing the blood and discharging waste products into the bile;

- Maintaining hormone balance;

- Serving as the main organ of blood formation before birth;

- Helping the body resist infection by producing immune factors and by removing bacteria from the bloodstream;

- Regenerating its own damaged tissue; and

- Storing iron.

Liver Diseases

There are many types of liver diseases, but among the most important are:

- Viral hepatitis;
- Cirrhosis;
- Liver disorders in children;
- Gallstones;
- Alcohol related liver disorders; and
- Cancer of the liver.

Symptoms and Signs of Liver Disease

1. **Abnormally yellow discoloration of the skin and eyes.** This is called jaundice which is often the first and sometimes the only sign of liver disease.

2. **Dark Urine.**

3. **Gray, yellow, or light-colored stools.**

4. **Nausea, vomiting, and/or loss of appetite.**

5. **Vomiting of blood, bloody or black stools.** Intestinal bleeding can occur when liver diseases obstruct blood flow through the liver. The bleeding may result in vomiting of blood or bloody stools.

6. **Abdominal swelling.** Liver disease may cause ascites, an accumulation of fluid in the abdominal cavity.

7. **Prolonged generalized itching.**

8. **Unusual change of weight.** An increase or decrease of more than 5% within two months.

9. **Abdominal pain.**

10. **Sleep disturbances, mental confusion, and coma** are present in severe liver disease. These result from an accumulation of toxic substances in the body which impair brain function.

11. **Fatigue or loss of stamina.**

12. **Loss of sexual drive or performance.**

If any of these signs or symptoms appear, consult your physician immediately.

Prevention

- Don't drink more than two alcoholic drinks a day.
- Be cautious about mixing several drugs; in particular, alcohol and many "over-the-counter" and prescription medicines do not mix well.
- Avoid taking medicines unnecessarily. Also avoid exposure to industrial chemicals whenever possible.
- Maintain a healthful, balanced diet.
- Consult your physician if you observe any signs or symptoms of liver disease.

A Brief Overview of Liver Diseases

Gallstones

Gallstones are formed when the cholesterol and/or pigment in bile crystallize in the gallbladder forming stones that vary in size from small pebbles to as large as golf balls. Sometimes gallstones get stuck in the bile ducts leading from the gallbladder to the duodenum (i.e., the first part of the small intestine). The gallbladder and bile ducts then try to push the stones out by muscular contractions. This can cause attacks of excruciating abdominal pain. Blockage of the ducts by stones also prevents flow of bile into the intestines. Bile then backs up into the bloodstream, causing jaundice.

Gallstones are more common in people over 40, especially in women and the obese.

Each year, 400,000-500,000 surgical operations to remove the gallbladder are performed in the United States.

Drugs are now available to dissolve cholesterol gallstones in selected patients and give hope for fewer surgeries in the future.

Viral Hepatitis

Hepatitis (meaning an inflammation of the liver) is caused by several different viruses. Hepatitis A is spread through contaminated water and food and is excreted in the stools. Hepatitis B is acquired from transfusions or other blood products. It can be transmitted through minute cuts, abrasions, or by such simple acts as kissing, tooth brushing, ear piercing, tattooing, dental work, or during sexual contact. It can be transmitted from a pregnant woman to her baby. Hepatitis C, formerly called non-A, non-B hepatitis, is primarily spread through infected blood. It causes cirrhosis in 50% of the cases.

The liver often becomes tender and enlarged, and the patient usually exhibits symptoms including fever, weakness, nausea, vomiting, jaundice, and aversion to food. The virus may be present in the bloodstream, intestines, feces, saliva, and in other body secretions.

Hepatitis is common in the United States and some forms of it can be extremely infectious. Most people recover from viral forms of the disease without treatment, but some die and others may develop a chronic, disabling illness.

In the United States there are more than four million "carriers" of hepatitis, people who are not ill themselves, but may pass hepatitis on to others.

A vaccine for hepatitis B has been shown to be safe and effective in the prevention of infection if given before exposure. It is recommended for all infants, those who come into contact with blood in their work, and for anyone with more than one sex partner. Treatments with interferon are effective in some cases of hepatitis B and C.

A vaccine for hepatitis A has been approved. It is effective in protecting over 90% of those who are vaccinated for at least six to 12 months and perhaps longer.

Alcohol-related Liver Disorders

There are three separate liver disorders related to alcohol: fatty liver, alcoholic hepatitis, and alcoholic cirrhosis.

Fatty liver, the most common alcohol-related liver disorder, causes enlargement of the liver and right upper abdominal discomfort. The swollen liver is often tender or painful. Severe fatty liver may cause temporary jaundice and abnormalities of liver function. Abstinence from alcohol can effect complete reversal and cure without leaving residual cirrhosis.

Alcoholic hepatitis is an acute illness often characterized by nausea, vomiting, right upper and middle abdominal pain, fever, jaundice, enlarged and tender liver, and an elevation of the white blood cell count. Sometimes alcoholic hepatitis may be present without symptoms. As with fatty liver, treatment is primarily supportive and preventive.

Any disease which is brought on by alcohol abuse cannot be reversed until alcohol intake is stopped. Once alcoholic hepatitis develops, progression to cirrhosis will occur if alcohol consumption continues.

Alcoholic cirrhosis occurs in 10% to 15% of people who consume large amounts of alcohol over a prolonged period of time. However, there is considerable variation in the degree of susceptibility of people to given amounts of alcohol, and further research is needed to determine why some individuals are more vulnerable to alcohol than others.

Cirrhosis

Each year over 25,000 Americans die from cirrhosis, the seventh leading cause of death in the United States. In fact, between the ages of 25 and 44, it is the fourth disease-related cause of death.

Cirrhosis of the liver is a degenerative disease where liver cells are damaged and replaced by scar formation. As scar tissue progressively accumulates, blood flow through the liver is diminished, causing even more liver cells to die. Loss of liver function results in gastrointestinal disturbances, emaciation, enlargement of the liver and spleen, jaundice, and accumulation of fluid in the abdomen and other tissues of the body. Obstruction of the venous circulation often causes massive vomiting of blood.

Anything which results in severe liver injury can cause cirrhosis. Over half of the deaths from cirrhosis of the liver are caused by alcohol abuse, hepatitis, and other viruses. Some chemicals, many poisons, too much iron or copper, severe reaction to drugs, and obstruction of the bile duct can also cause cirrhosis.

Some types of cirrhosis can be treated, but often there is no cure. At this point, treatment is mostly supportive and may include a strict diet, diuretics, vitamins, and abstinence from alcohol. However, there has been much progress in managing the major complications of cirrhosis such as fluid retention in the abdomen, bleeding, and changes in mental function.

Liver Disorders in Children

Tens of thousands of American children—from newborn infants to adolescents—get liver diseases, and hundreds die from them every year. There are more than 100 different types of liver diseases that have been identified in infants and children.

The more common of these diseases are:

Biliary atresia—the absence or inadequate size of bile ducts from the liver to the intestine. Unable to excrete bile, the infant usually dies from cirrhosis and bleeding by 2 years of age. A surgical operation may relieve obstruction in a small percentage of cases.

Chronic active hepatitis gradually destroys and replaces the normal liver cells with scar tissue through an unknown process which resembles an allergy to the child's own liver tissue.

Galactosemia is an inherited disease in which an enzyme needed to digest milk sugar is missing, causing the milk sugar to build up in the liver and other organs, leading to cirrhosis of the liver, cataracts of the eyes, and brain damage. Unless the baby is taken off milk and given an artificial formula that has no milk sugar, the child will die.

In Wilson's Disease, large amounts of copper build up in the liver due to an inherited abnormality, causing cirrhosis of the liver and brain damage.

Reye's Syndrome an acute, rare fatal disorder in which fat accumulates in the liver and the child goes into a deep coma.

Cirrhosis can be caused by any extensive injury to the liver including most of the disorders described above.

Cancer of the Liver

The most common form of cancer of the liver is the spread of cancer from other organ systems to the liver.

Not much is known about cancer which originates in the liver except that it is associated with viral hepatitis and certain parasites, drugs, and environmental toxins. Each year, 1,000 Americans die of primary liver cancer. Chronic carriers of the hepatitis B or C viruses are at increased risk to develop liver cancer.

Hope For Tomorrow Through Research

Liver diseases appear to be on the increase. Part of this increase may be due to our frequent contact with chemicals and environmental pollutants. The amount of medicine consumed has increased greatly with resulting dangers to the liver.

The liver, the detoxifying factory in the body, has become an increasingly overworked organ.

The present investment in liver research is scant in relation to the magnitude, severity and destructiveness of these diseases.

Liver diseases are poorly understood. An adequate investment in effective liver research has the potential of saving billions of dollars and preventing untold human suffering.

Experts estimate that more than half of all liver diseases could be prevented if people acted upon the knowledge we already have.

Each year more than 25 million Americans are afflicted with liver and gallbladder diseases and more than 43,000 die of liver disease each year. There are few effective treatments for most life-threatening liver diseases, except for liver transplants. Research has recently opened up exciting new paths for investigation, but much more remains to be done to find cures for more than 100 different liver diseases.

Meanwhile, patients and their families must cope with medical, financial and emotional problems.

For More Information

American Liver Foundation
75 Maiden Lane, Suite 603
New York, NY 10038

1-800-GO-LIVER (465-4837)
1-888-4-HEP-ABC (443-7222)
Fax: 212-483-8179
E-mail: webmail@liverfoundation.org
URL: http://www.liverfoundation.org

The information contained in this chapter is provided for information only. This information does not constitute medical advice and it should not be relied upon as such. The American Liver Foundation (ALF) does not engage in the practice of medicine. ALF, under no circumstances, recommends particular treatments for specific individuals, and in all cases recommends that you consult your physician before pursuing any course of treatment.

Chapter 2

Your Liver and Your Digestive System: How They Work

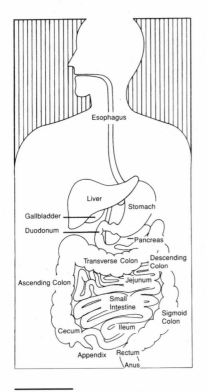

Figure labels: Esophagus, Liver, Stomach, Gallbladder, Duodonum, Pancreas, Transverse Colon, Descending Colon, Ascending Colon, Jejunum, Small Intestine, Sigmoid Colon, Cecum, Ileum, Appendix, Rectum, Anus

The digestive system is a series of hollow organs joined in a long, twisting tube from the mouth to the anus (see figure 2.1). Inside this tube is a lining called the mucosa. In the mouth, stomach, and small intestine, the mucosa contains tiny glands that produce juices to help digest food.

There are also two solid digestive organs, the liver and the pancreas, which produce juices that reach the intestine through small tubes. In addition, parts of other organ systems (for instance, nerves and blood) play a major role in the digestive system.

Figure 2.1. *The Digestive System*

"Your Digestive System and How It Works," National Institute of Diabetes and Digestive and Kidney Diseases (NIDDK), NIH Publication No. 97-2681, August 1992. E-text updated January 12, 1999.

Why Is Digestion Important?

When we eat such things as bread, meat, and vegetables, they are not in a form that the body can use as nourishment. Our food and drink must be changed into smaller molecules of nutrients before they can be absorbed into the blood and carried to cells throughout the body. Digestion is the process by which food and drink are broken down into their smallest parts so that the body can use them to build and nourish cells and to provide energy.

How Is Food Digested?

Digestion involves the mixing of food, its movement through the digestive tract, and chemical breakdown of the large molecules of food into smaller molecules. Digestion begins in the mouth, when we chew and swallow, and is completed in the small intestine. The chemical process varies somewhat for different kinds of food.

Movement of Food Through the System

The large, hollow organs of the digestive system contain muscle that enables their walls to move. The movement of organ walls can propel food and liquid and also can mix the contents within each organ. Typical movement of the esophagus, stomach, and intestine is called peristalsis. The action of peristalsis looks like an ocean wave moving through the muscle. The muscle of the organ produces a narrowing and then propels the narrowed portion slowly down the length of the organ. These waves of narrowing push the food and fluid in front of them through each hollow organ.

The first major muscle movement occurs when food or liquid is swallowed. Although we are able to start swallowing by choice, once the swallow begins, it becomes involuntary and proceeds under the control of the nerves.

The esophagus is the organ into which the swallowed food is pushed. It connects the throat above with the stomach below. At the junction of the esophagus and stomach, there is a ring-like valve closing the passage between the two organs. However, as the food approaches the closed ring, the surrounding muscles relax and allow the food to pass.

The food then enters the stomach, which has three mechanical tasks to do. First, the stomach must store the swallowed food and liquid. This requires the muscle of the upper part of the stomach to relax and accept large volumes of swallowed material. The second job is to mix up the food, liquid, and digestive juice produced by the stomach. The lower part of the stomach mixes these materials by its muscle action. The third task of the stomach is to empty its contents slowly into the small intestine.

Several factors affect emptying of the stomach, including the nature of the food (mainly its fat and protein content) and the degree of muscle action of the emptying stomach and the next organ to receive the stomach contents (the small intestine). As the food is digested in the small intestine and dissolved into the juices from the pancreas, liver, and intestine, the contents of the intestine are mixed and pushed forward to allow further digestion.

Finally, all of the digested nutrients are absorbed through the intestinal walls. The waste products of this process include undigested parts of the food, known as fiber, and older cells that have been shed from the mucosa. These materials are propelled into the colon, where they remain, usually for a day or two, until the feces are expelled by a bowel movement.

Production of Digestive Juices

Glands of the digestive system are crucial to the process of digestion. They produce both the juices that break down the food and the hormones that help to control the process.

The glands that act first are in the mouth—the salivary glands. Saliva produced by these glands contains an enzyme that begins to digest the starch from food into smaller molecules.

The next set of digestive glands is in the stomach lining. They produce stomach acid and an enzyme that digests protein. One of the unsolved puzzles of the digestive system is why the acid juice of the stomach does not dissolve the tissue of the stomach itself. In most people, the stomach mucosa is able to resist the juice, although food and other tissues of the body cannot.

After the stomach empties the food and its juice into the small intestine, the juices of two other digestive organs mix with the food to continue the process of digestion. One of these organs is the pancreas. It produces a juice that contains a wide array of enzymes to break down the carbohydrates, fat, and protein in our food. Other enzymes that are active in the process come from glands in the wall of the intestine or even a part of that wall.

The liver produces yet another digestive juice—bile. The bile is stored between meals in the gallbladder. At mealtime, it is squeezed out of the gallbladder into the bile ducts to reach the intestine and mix with the fat in our food. The bile acids dissolve the fat into the watery contents of the intestine, much like detergents that dissolve grease from a frying pan. After the fat is dissolved, it is digested by enzymes from the pancreas and the lining of the intestine.

Absorption and Transport of Nutrients

Digested molecules of food, as well as water and minerals from the diet, are absorbed from the cavity of the upper small intestine. The absorbed materials cross the mucosa into the blood, mainly, and are carried off in the bloodstream to other parts of the body for storage or further chemical change. As noted above, this part of the process varies with different types of nutrients.

Carbohydrates: An average American adult eats about half a pound of carbohydrate each day. Some of our most common foods contain mostly carbohydrates. Examples are bread, potatoes, pastries, candy, rice, spaghetti, fruits, and vegetables. Many of these foods contain both starch, which can be digested, and fiber, which the body cannot digest.

The digestible carbohydrates are broken into simpler molecules by enzymes in the saliva, in juice produced by the pancreas, and in the lining of the small intestine. Starch is digested in two steps: First, an enzyme in the saliva and pancreatic juice breaks the starch into molecules called maltose; then an enzyme in the lining of the small intestine (maltase) splits the maltose into glucose molecules that can be absorbed into the blood. Glucose is carried through the bloodstream to the liver, where it is stored or used to provide energy for the work of the body.

Table sugar is another carbohydrate that must be digested to be useful. An enzyme in the lining of the small intestine digests table sugar into glucose and fructose, each of which can be absorbed from the intestinal cavity into the blood. Milk contains yet another type of sugar, lactose, which is changed into absorbable molecules by an enzyme called lactase, also found in the intestinal lining.

Protein: Foods such as meat, eggs, and beans consist of giant molecules of protein that must be digested by enzymes before they can be used to build and repair body tissues. An enzyme in the juice of the stomach starts the digestion of swallowed protein. Further digestion of the protein is completed in the small intestine. Here, several enzymes from the pancreatic juice and the lining of the intestine carry out the breakdown of huge protein molecules into small molecules called amino acids. These small molecules can be absorbed from the hollow of the small intestine into the blood and then be carried to all parts of the body to build the walls and other parts of cells.

Fats: Fat molecules are a rich source of energy for the body. The first step in digestion of a fat such as butter is to dissolve it into the watery content of the intestinal cavity. The bile acids produced by the liver act as natural detergents to dissolve fat in water and allow the enzymes to break the large fat molecules into smaller molecules, some of which are fatty acids and cholesterol. The bile acids combine with the fatty acids and cholesterol and help these molecules to move into the cells of the mucosa. In these cells the small molecules are formed back into large molecules, most of which pass into vessels (called lymphatics) near the intestine. These small vessels carry the reformed fat to the veins of the chest, and the blood carries the fat to storage depots in different parts of the body.

Vitamins: Another vital part of our food that is absorbed from the small intestine is the class of chemicals we call vitamins. There are two different types of vitamins, classified by the fluid in which they can be dissolved: water-soluble vitamins (all the B vitamins and vitamin C) and fat-soluble vitamins (vitamins A, D, and K).

Water and Salt: Most of the material absorbed from the cavity of the small intestine is water in which salt is dissolved. The salt and water come from the food and liquid we swallow and the juices secreted by the many digestive glands. In a healthy adult, more than a gallon of water containing over an ounce of salt is absorbed from the intestine every 24 hours.

How Is the Digestive Process Controlled?

Hormone Regulators

A fascinating feature of the digestive system is that it contains its own regulators. The major hormones that control the functions of the digestive system are produced and released by cells in the mucosa of the stomach and small intestine. These hormones are released into the blood of the digestive tract, travel back to the heart and through the arteries, and return to the digestive system, where they stimulate digestive juices and cause organ movement. The hormones that control digestion are gastrin, secretin, and cholecystokinin (CCK):

- Gastrin causes the stomach to produce an acid for dissolving and digesting some foods. It is also necessary for the normal growth of the lining of the stomach, small intestine, and colon.

- Secretin causes the pancreas to send out a digestive juice that is rich in bicarbonate. It stimulates the stomach to produce pepsin, an enzyme that digests protein, and it also stimulates the liver to produce bile.

- CCK causes the pancreas to grow and to produce the enzymes of pancreatic juice, and it causes the gallbladder to empty.

Nerve Regulators

Two types of nerves help to control the action of the digestive system. Extrinsic (outside) nerves come to the digestive organs from the unconscious part of the brain or from the spinal cord. They release a chemical called acetylcholine and another called adrenaline. Acetylcholine causes the muscle of the digestive organs to squeeze with more force and increase the "push" of food and juice through the digestive tract. Acetylcholine also causes the stomach and pancreas to produce more digestive juice. Adrenaline relaxes the muscle of the stomach and intestine and decreases the flow of blood to these organs.

Even more important, though, are the intrinsic (inside) nerves, which make up a very dense network embedded in the walls of the esophagus, stomach, small intestine, and colon. The intrinsic nerves are triggered to act when the walls of the hollow organs are stretched by food. They release many different substances that speed up or delay the movement of food and the production of juices by the digestive organs.

Additonal Readings

Facts and Fallacies About Digestive Diseases, 1991. This fact sheet discusses commonly held beliefs about digestive diseases. Available from the National Digestive Diseases Information Clearinghouse, 2 Information Way, Bethesda, MD 20892-3570. (301) 654-3810.

Larson DE, Editor-in-chief. *Mayo Clinic Family Health Book*. New York: William Morrow and Company, Inc., 1990. General medical guide with section on the digestive system and how it works. Available in libraries and bookstores.

Tapley DF, et al., eds. *The Columbia University College of Physicians and Surgeons, Complete Home Medical Guide*, revised edition. New York: Crown Publishers, Inc., 1990. General medical guide with section on the digestive system and how it works. Available in libraries and bookstores.

Additional Information

National Digestive Diseases Information Clearinghouse
2 Information Way
Bethesda, MD 20892-3570
E-mail: nddic@info.niddk.nih.gov

The National Digestive Diseases Information Clearinghouse (NDDIC) is a service of the National Institute of Diabetes and Digestive and Kidney Diseases (NIDDK). The NIDDK is part of the National Institutes of Health under the U.S. Public Health Service. Established in 1980, the clearinghouse provides information about digestive diseases to people with digestive disorders and to their families, health care professionals, and the public. NDDIC answers inquiries; develops, reviews, and distributes publications; and works closely with professional and patient organizations and Government agencies to coordinate resources about digestive diseases.

Chapter 3

50 Ways to Love Your Liver

1. Avoid taking unnecessary medications. (Too many chemicals can harm me.)

2. Don't mix medicines without the advice of a doctor. (You could create something poisonous that could damage me badly)

3. Street drugs cause serious damage and scar me permanently.

4. Don't drown me in beer, liquor or wine. (If you drink alcohol, have two or fewer drinks per day.)

5. Never mix alcohol with other drugs and medications.

6. Be careful when using aerosol cleaners. I have to detoxify what you breathe in, so when you go on a cleaning binge, make sure the room is well ventilated, or wear a mask.

7. Bug sprays, paint sprays, and all those other chemical sprays you use can harm me too. Be careful what you breathe.

8. Watch what gets on your skin! (Those insecticides you put on trees and shrubs to kill bugs can get to me right through your skin and destroy some cells.) Remember, they're serious chemicals.

Reprinted with permission of the American Liver Foundation, 1-800-GO-LIVER, © 1997.

Hepatitis B & C—Contagious Viral Infections That Cause Chronic Liver Disease

9. Use caution and common sense regarding intimate contact. (Hepatitis viruses live in body fluids, including blood and seminal fluid.)

10. The hepatitis B virus also lives in saliva and, unlike the AIDS virus, can be transmitted through this fluid with relative ease. If you were stuck with a needle used by a person with AIDS, you'd have a one in 2,000 chance of picking up the AIDS virus. But if that person had hepatitis B, your chances of picking up the virus increase to one in four!

11. Hepatitis C, spread primarily through direct blood contact, can be transmitted through contaminated needles used in tattooing, body piercing, or IV drug injection.

12. Untreated, chronic hepatitis B and C can cause cirrhosis and liver cancer and is the most frequent reason for liver transplants.

13. Many infected people do not have symptoms until liver damage occurs, sometimes many years later.

14. Teach your children what a syringe looks like and tell them to leave it alone.

15. Never, ever, touch a discarded syringe or needle.

An Insidious Disease

Over 5 million Americans have hepatitis B or C, resulting in an estimated 13,000 to 15,000 deaths annually. Yet many people do not know they are infected until serious liver damage occurs because they have few, if any, symptoms. Who's at greater risk of contracting hepatitis B or C? How do you find out if you're a carrier? Here are the answers.

16. If you or your family has immigrated from Africa, Southeast Asia, Mediterranean countries, or the Caribbean, where hepatitis B affects up to 15% of the population, you should have a blood test to determine if you are a carrier. Your doctor can arrange this for you.

17. If you received a blood transfusion prior to 1990, you may have hepatitis C. As many as 300,000 people may have been infected in this way before the test for hepatitis C was developed.

Who Else Should Be Tested for Hepatitis B and C?

18. Users of intravenous drugs, particularly those who share their needles.

19. Men or women who have multiple sexual partners.

20. Health care (including ambulance) workers.

21. Staff of institutions for people with developmental disabilities.

22. Firefighters, police officers, mortuary attendants, and day-care workers.

23. If anyone in your family or a sexual partner tests positive for the hepatitis B virus, ask your doctor to test you for the virus. If the test is negative, your doctor will vaccinate you against the virus. A simple series of three vaccinations over six months will protect you against the virus for many years.

If You Test Positive for Hepatitis B or C...

24. Consult your doctor. He or she will determine whether you have liver disease and if you need referral to a specialist.

25. If you have hepatitis B, have your family tested. Those who have never contracted hepatitis B should be vaccinated.

26. Ask your doctor to screen for liver cancer in order to detect tumors while they are still small and treatable.

27. If you are a pregnant, hepatitis B-infected mother, you can pass the infection to your infant around the time of birth. More than 90% of this form of transmission can be prevented by vaccination of the baby.

Eat for Health!

Since everything we eat must pass through the liver, special attention to nutrition and diet can help keep your liver healthy. Here are some tips on eating for health—healthy liver, healthy you!

28. Eat a well-balanced, nutritionally adequate diet. If you enjoy foods from each of the four food groups, you will probably obtain the nutrients you need.

29. Cut down on the amount of deep-fried and fatty foods you and your family consume. Doctors believe that the risk of gallbladder disorders (including gallstones, a liver-related disease) can be reduced by avoiding high fat and cholesterol foods.

30. Minimize your consumption of smoked, cured, and salted foods. Taste your food before adding salt! Or try alternative seasonings in your cooking such as lemon juice, onion, vinegar, garlic, pepper, mustard, cloves, sage, or thyme.

    Meat, Fish, Poultry and Alternatives Provide:

    - protein
    - vitamin A
    - iron
    - vitamin B12
    - niacin
    - fiber
    - thiamin

    Bread and Cereals Provide:

    - carbohydrate
    - niacin
    - thiamin
    - iron
    - riboflavin
    - fiber

    Fruits and Vegetables Provide:

    - vitamin A
    - vitamin C
    - iron
    - fiber
    - folacin

    Milk and Milk Products Provide:

    - calcium
    - riboflavin
    - niacin
    - folacin
    - vitamin A
    - vitamin B12
    - vitamin D

31. Increase your intake of high-fiber foods such as fresh fruits and vegetables, whole grain breads, rice, and cereals. A high-fiber diet is especially helpful in keeping your liver healthy.

32. Rich desserts, snacks, and drinks are high in calories because of the amount of sweetening (and often fat) they contain. Why not munch on some fruit instead?

33. Keep your weight close to ideal. Medical researchers have established a direct correlation between obesity and the development of gallbladder disorders.

34. If you are dieting to lose weight, make sure that you are still getting all the vitamins and minerals your body—and liver—need to function properly.

35. A regular exercise routine, two or three days a week, will help keep your liver healthy, too.

Trouble Signs...

Here are some signs of liver trouble. If you experience any of these symptoms, please contact your doctor:

36. Yellow discoloration of the skin or eyes.

37. Abdominal swelling or severe abdominal pain.

38. Prolonged itching of the skin.

39. Very dark urine or pale stools, or the passage of bloody or tar-like stools.

40. Chronic fatigue, nausea or loss of appetite.

A word from your liver: "I can't and won't tell you I'm in trouble until I'm almost at the end of my rope... and yours. Learn to listen to your body—I may be telling you something."

What To Do If You Have Liver Disease...

41. Follow your doctor's advice on food, exercise, and other lifestyle guidelines. Learn about liver disease and understand how your diet helps you. Learn what and how much you can eat and drink.

42. Contact the American Liver Foundation for a listing of chapters near you (available in chapter 60 of this book). Join the chapter—talking to other people who are also affected by liver disease will help.

43.   Invite family and close friends to attend chapter meetings or any learning sessions your local chapter may hold.

The Limitations of Transplants

While transplants are not the answer for eliminating liver disease (We need to find cures!), transplants are the only hope for survival many liver disease patients have. Unfortunately, there just are not enough organ donors to meet the demand.

44.   Consider donating your organs in the event of your death. You can sign the organ donor card on your driver's license if your state has such a program or obtain an organ donor card from the American Liver Foundation. Be sure to discuss your wishes with your family and your family doctor.

The American Liver Foundation

Your contribution to the American Liver Foundation will allow them to:

- provide financial support for medical research in liver disease and liver function;

- provide educational programs for the medical profession, patients, and the general public; and

- provide support groups for patients and families affected by liver diseases.

Consider How to Help Continue this Important Work!

45.   Support the American Liver Foundation with a tax-deductible donation. Whatever you can afford to give would be greatly appreciated.

46.   Consider leaving a gift to the American Liver Foundation in your will. Contact the ALF national office for a free pamphlet on the planned giving program.

47.   You may also wish to name the American Liver Foundation as the beneficiary of a life insurance policy. Contact their office for more information.

48.   If you can spare just a few hours a week, consider becoming a volunteer for the American Liver Foundation. The ALF office can tell you about all the ways in which you can help.

Finally...

49.   See your doctor for a check-up on a regular basis. Remember, prevention is always the best medicine.

50.   Take care of yourself in everything you do. Be a healthy "live"r—keep a healthy liver.

For Additional Information

American Liver Foundation
75 Maiden Lane, Suite 603
New York, NY 10038
1-800-GO LIVER (465-4837)
Fax: 212-483-8179
E-mail: webmail@liverfoundation.org
URL: http://www.liverfoundation.org

The American Liver Foundation is a national voluntary health organization dedicated to preventing, treating, and curing hepatitis and other liver and gallbladder diseases through research and education.

Note: The information contained in this chapter is provided for information only. This information does not constitute medical advice and it should not be relied upon as such. The American Liver Foundation (ALF) does not engage in the practice of medicine. ALF, under no circumstances, recommends particular treatments for specific individuals, and in all cases recommends that you consult your physician before pursuing any course of treatment.

Chapter 4

Eating to Health

Diet and Your Liver

What Does Nutrition Have to Do with Your Liver?

Nutrition and the liver are interrelated in many ways. Some functions are well understood; others are not. Since everything we eat, breathe, and absorb through our skin must be refined and detoxified by the liver, special attention to nutrition and diet can help keep the liver healthy. In a number of different kinds of liver disease, nutrition takes on considerably more importance.

Why Is the Liver Important?

The liver is the largest organ in the body and it plays a vital role, performing many complex functions which are essential for life. Your liver serves as your body's internal chemical power plant. While there are still many things we do not understand about the liver, we do know that it is impossible to live without it, and the health of the liver is a major factor in the quality of one's life.

Some important functions of the liver are:

- to convert the food we eat into stored energy, and chemicals necessary for life and growth;

Reprinted with permission "The Pyramid Diet," © Chek Med Systems, Inc., and "Diet and Your Liver," © 1997, American Liver Foundation 1-800-GO-LIVER, reprinted with permission.

- to act as a filter to remove alcohol and toxic substances from the blood and convert them to substances that can be excreted from the body;

- to process drugs and medications absorbed from the digestive system, enabling the body to use them effectively and ultimately dispose of them;

- to manufacture and export important body chemicals used by the body. One of these is bile, a greenish-yellow substance essential for the digestion of fats in the small intestine.

Why Is the Liver so Important in Nutrition?

85-90% of the blood that leaves the stomach and intestines carries important nutrients to the liver where they are converted into substances the body can use.

The liver performs many unique and important metabolic tasks as it processes carbohydrates, proteins, fats, and minerals to be used in maintaining normal body functions.

Carbohydrates, or sugars, are stored as glycogen in the liver and are released as energy between meals or when the body's energy demands are high. In this way, the liver helps to regulate the blood sugar level, and to prevent a condition called hypoglycemia, or low blood sugar. This enables us to keep an even level of energy throughout the day. Without this balance, we would need to eat constantly to keep up our energy. Proteins reach the liver in their simpler form called amino acids. Once in the liver, they are either released to the muscles as energy, stored for later use, or converted to urea for excretion in the urine. Certain proteins are converted into ammonia, a toxic metabolic product, by bacteria in the intestine or during the breakdown of body protein. The ammonia must be broken down by the liver and made into urea which is then excreted by the kidneys. The liver also has the unique ability to convert certain amino acids into sugar for quick energy.

Fats cannot be digested without bile, which is made in the liver, stored in the gallbladder, and released as needed into the small intestine. Bile (specific bile "acids") acts somewhat like a detergent, breaking apart the fat into tiny droplets so that it can be acted upon by intestinal enzymes and absorbed. Bile is also essential for the absorption of vitamins A, D, E, and K, the fat soluble vitamins. After digestion, bile acids are reabsorbed by the intestine, returned to the liver, and recycled as bile once again.

Can Poor Nutrition Cause Liver Disease?

There are many kinds of liver disease, and the causes of most of them are not known. Poor nutrition is not generally a cause, with the exception of alcoholic liver disease and liver disease found among starving populations. It is much more likely that poor nutrition is the result of chronic liver disease, and not the cause.

On the other hand, good nutrition—a balanced diet with adequate calories, proteins, fats, and carbohydrates—can actually help the damaged liver to regenerate new liver cells. In fact, in some liver diseases, nutrition becomes an essential form of treatment. Patients are strongly advised not to take megavitamin therapy or to use nutritional products bought in special stores or by catalogue without consulting a doctor.

How Does Liver Disease Affect Nutrition?

Many chronic liver diseases are associated with malnutrition. One of the most common of these is cirrhosis. Cirrhosis refers to the replacement of damaged liver cells by fibrous scar tissue which disrupts the liver's important functions. Cirrhosis occurs as a result of excessive alcohol intake (most common), common viral hepatitis, obstruction of the bile ducts, and exposure to certain drugs or toxic substances.

People with cirrhosis often experience loss of appetite, nausea, vomiting, and weight loss, giving them an emaciated appearance. Diet alone does not contribute to the development of this liver disease. People who are well nourished, for example, but drink large amounts of alcohol, are also susceptible to alcoholic disease.

Adults with cirrhosis require a balanced diet rich in protein, providing 2,000 to 3,000 calories a day to allow the liver cells to regenerate. However, too much protein will result in an increased amount of ammonia in the blood; too little protein can reduce healing of the liver. Doctors must carefully prescribe the correct amount of protein for a person with cirrhosis. In addition, the physician can use two medications (lactulose and neomycin) to control blood ammonia levels.

What Other Nutritional Problems Are Caused by Cirrhosis?

When the scarring of cirrhosis interferes with the flow of blood from the stomach and intestines to the liver, a condition called portal hypertension may develop. This simply means that there is back pressure in the veins entering the liver. Surgical "shunting", or rerouting of blood away from the liver and into the general circulation can relieve this pressure, but it often causes a new set of problems. Because the shunted blood has bypassed the liver, it contains high levels of amino acids, ammonia, and possibly toxins. When these compounds reach the brain, they cause a condition called hepatic encephalopathy, which means "liver caused mental impairment." Patients become confused and some temporary loss of memory occurs.

Can Nutrition Be Used to Treat Hepatic Encephalopathy?

Restricting the amount of protein in the diet will generally lower the levels of amino acids and ammonia in the bloodstream and brain. Most physicians advise their patients with this condition to eat only about 40 grams of protein a day, and will prescribe lactulose or neomycin to lower amino acid production. Non-meat proteins, such as those found in vegetables and milk, are also recommended. Certain amino acids are used in treatment, since they are considered less likely to cause mental impairment. A dietary supplement rich in these amino acids is used at many liver treatment centers.

Food to avoid: Shell fish if uncooked can be very dangerous to take in patients with cirrhosis. Either avoid or be careful. *Vibro vulnificus*, a bacteria can be contracted by eating raw oysters.

Can Diet Help in Treating Other Complications of Cirrhosis?

There are a number of complications of cirrhosis which can be helped through a modified diet. Persons with cirrhosis often experience an uncomfortable buildup of fluid in the abdomen (ascites) or a swelling of the feet, legs, or back (edema). Both conditions are a result of portal hypertension (increased pressure in the veins entering the liver). Since sodium (salt) encourages the body to retain water, patients with fluid retention can cut their sodium intake by avoiding such foods as canned soups and vegetables, cold cuts, dairy products, and condiments like mayonnaise and ketchup. In fact, most prepared foods contain liberal amounts of sodium, while fresh foods contain almost no sodium at all. The best-tasting salt substitute is lemon juice.

In general, a reduction in meat protein which is the most toxic protein to the brain and substituting vegetable protein is advised when cirrhosis is present.

Are There Other Liver Diseases Where Specific Changes in Diet Can Help?

Nutrition and a modified diet have been found to have a significant effect on a number of other liver diseases. Some types of liver disease, for example, cause a backup of bile in the liver which is called cholestasis. This means that bile cannot flow into the small intestine to aid in the digestion of fats. When this happens, fat is not absorbed but instead is excreted in large amounts in the feces, which become noticeably pale-colored and foul-smelling. This condition is known as steatorrhea. This loss of fat calories may also cause weight loss.

Special fat substitutes, such as medium chain triglycerides (MCT oil) and safflower oil can help alleviate this condition because they are less dependent on bile for intestinal absorption. They can be used like other oils in cooking, baking, and salad dressings.

Patients with **steatorrhea** may also have difficulty absorbing fat soluble vitamins A, D, E, and K. However, water soluble vitamins are absorbed normally. Supplementing the diet with fat soluble vitamins is possible, though it should only be carried out under the guidance of a physician. Vitamin A in excess over what is needed is very toxic to the liver. Zinc deficiency may occur in some patients with liver disease. Ask your doctor to check for this.

Wilson's disease, in which large amounts of copper may build up in the body, is another liver ailment where diet can help. People with Wilson's disease should avoid eating chocolate, nuts, shellfish, and mushrooms, all copper-containing foods. Medical treatment to remove excess copper from the body involves use of the drug penicillamine.

Hemochromatosis is a disease in which large amounts of iron are transported from the intestine and accumulate in the liver. Persons with this condition must avoid iron injections, all iron-containing foods, and are advised not to use iron cooking utensils. Aside from these precautions, those with hemochromatosis may follow a normal diet.

What Is Fatty Liver and Is It Caused by Eating Too Much Fat?

Fatty liver is not a disease but a pathological finding. A more appropriate term is "fatty infiltration of the liver." It is not caused by excessive eating of fats.

35

Nutritional causes of fat in the liver include: starvation, obesity, protein malnutrition, and intestinal bypass operation for obesity. Fat enters the liver through diet and from fat stored in the fatty tissue. Under normal conditions, fat from the diet is usually metabolized by the liver and other tissues. If the amount exceeds what is required by the body, it is stored in the fatty tissue. If fatty tissue is caused by diabetes, insulin will treat the problem. Fatty liver resulting from poor nutrition should be treated with a well-balanced diet of carbohydrates, proteins, and fats as specified by the physician.

Fatty liver can also be caused by certain chemical or drug compounds, and endocrine disorders. In these cases, the treatment would be directly related to the cause.

Two ways to avoid fatty liver:

- limit alcohol intake (alcohol can decrease the rate of metabolism and secretion of fat, leading to fatty liver);

- watch the diet (starvation and protein malnutrition can result in fat buildup in the liver). Most cases of fatty liver are due to obesity. Gradual weight reduction over time will reduce enlargement of the liver due to fat and associated liver test abnormalities.

What Lies Ahead?

The relationship between nutrition and the liver is under investigation. To what extent good nutrition and dietary practices can control or perhaps even prevent liver disease can only be surmised at this time. Further research in this area could prove very beneficial and is being supported by the American Liver Foundation.

The Pyramid Diet

A healthy diet plays a major role in keeping the body fit and preventing illness. Based on medical research, a regular diet has been developed that arranges food groups into a food guide pyramid. This pyramid symbol makes it easy for individuals to choose what to eat, how much to eat, and how to avoid harmful excesses like too much fat, cholesterol, sugar, sodium, and alcohol.

Nutrition

Scientists have identified more than 40 nutrients—proteins, vitamins, minerals, and fiber—that the body needs for energy and good health. Based on this information, the National Research Council has established the Recommended Dietary Allowance (RDA) of nutrients required for good health. These nutrients should come from a variety of foods, not from just a few highly fortified foods or supplements. Following the pyramid diet provides the RDA for healthy people two years of age and over. This diet is not for people who need special diets designed for certain medical conditions.

The Pyramid

The pyramid is a symbol of stability, good design and structure. It contains a large sturdy base upon which to build. Each level of the pyramid then supports the smaller level above it. Except for the peak, all levels must remain intact to preserve the integrity of the structure. This is exactly how a healthy diet should be designed. The food

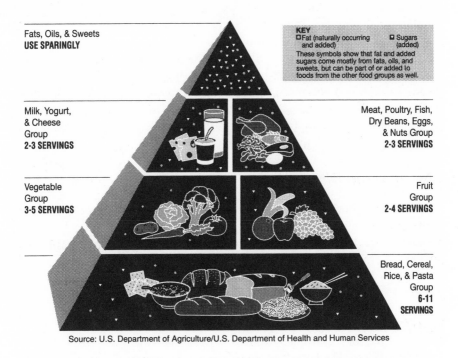

Source: U.S. Department of Agriculture/U.S. Department of Health and Human Services

Figure 4.1. *Food Guide Pyramid (U.S. Department of Agriculture)*

groups are arranged on the pyramid according to the number of servings required from each to construct a healthy diet. For example, the largest number of servings each day should come from the bottom level, the bread or grain group. A smaller number of fruit and vegetable servings are required, so those groups are on the next level, and so on. However, no food group is more important than another. A variety of foods from all levels is needed each day for good health. Of course, much of the peak may be removed without affecting the stability of the diet.

Base Level

Breads, cereals, rice, and pasta come from grains. They provide the body's largest portion of energy. Six to eleven servings should come from this group each day. These grain foods also contain fiber (the indigestible part of plants). There are two types of fiber, and both are needed for good health. Insoluble fiber, such as wheat bran, does not dissolve in water, so it helps the body to regulate bowel function by adding bulk. Soluble fiber is the type found in many fruits. It does dissolve in water and forms a sticky gel in the digestive tract. This soluble fiber gel probably helps to reduce cholesterol levels by binding with it and sweeping it out of the intestines. There is also evidence that increasing fiber in the diet reduces the risk of developing certain cancers. This is why it is recommended that people eat 20 to 30 grams of fiber a day, which should include both soluble and insoluble fibers.

Choose foods from the grain group that are low in fats and sugars—breads, English muffins, bagels, rice, or pasta. Avoid cakes, cookies, croissants, or pastries. These are usually made with processed flours (grains that have had the fiber removed), and they contain large amounts of fat and sugar. Also, avoid placing cream or cheese sauces on pasta and rice because they add fat calories.

Level Two

Fruits and vegetables are together on this level because they are low in fat and provide vitamins, minerals, and fiber. Because different fruits and vegetables provide different nutrients, a variety should be chosen throughout the day. Be sure to have two to four servings of fruit and slightly more servings of vegetables (three to five) each day.

Citrus fruits, melons, and berries are especially rich in vitamin C. Whole fresh fruits contain much less sugar than those canned or frozen in heavy syrup. Whole fruits contain more fiber than is found in fruit juice, but if choosing fruit juice, make sure it is 100% fruit juice. Grape and orange sodas are not fruit juice. Punches and fruit "drinks" contain only a little fruit juice and a large amount of added sugar.

Choose a wide variety of vegetables to get a balance of the nutrients they provide. Select dark green leafy vegetables over light green. Romaine lettuce, for example, has about six times as much vitamin C and eight times as much beta carotene as iceberg lettuce. Legumes (peas and beans) are good sources of fiber and provide lowfat protein that can be used in place of meat. Eat vegetables raw when possible; however, cooked vegetables are also nutritious. It is how they are cooked that is important. To maintain eye and taste appeal and to preserve nutrients, do not over-cook. Sometimes the method of preparation helps to preserve or enhance nutrients. For example, vitamin C-rich vegetables lose half of the vitamin when boiled, but only 15% when microwaved. Remember, variety is the key.

Level Three

The Milk, Yogurt, and Cheese Group and the Meat, Fish, Poultry, Eggs, and Dry Beans Group are good sources of protein, calcium, iron, and zinc. These nutrients are required for growth and normal development of the body. Whole Milk, yogurt, and cheese are the best sources of calcium, but they can also be high in fat. Aged or natural cheeses and ice cream can be very high in fat. Choose lowfat varieties such as skim or 1% fat milk, lowfat yogurt, "part skim" or lowfat cheeses, and ice milk or frozen yogurt. Most people should have at least two servings a day from this group. However, teenagers, young adults under 25, women who are pregnant or breast-feeding, and postmenopausal women should have 3 servings each day.

Choose two to three servings a day of meat, poultry, fish, or alternatives (dry beans, eggs, or nuts). Choose lean cuts of meat, and trim away visible fat and skin. Broil, roast, or bake instead of pan frying. Three ounces of cooked meat, poultry, or fish is about the size of a deck of cards. One-half cup of cooked dry beans, 1 egg, or 2 tablespoons of peanut butter equals one ounce of meat. Dry beans are an excellent alternative to meat because they are a good source of high quality protein, are low in fat and high in fiber. Go easy on eggs because they are high in cholesterol. Use only one yolk per person in egg dishes, and substitute egg whites if more eggs are called for. Nuts and seeds are good sources of calcium and zinc, but they are high in fat and should be eaten in moderation.

Observe the 3/4 plate rule to help control portion sizes, cut down on fat, and get the proper mix of nutrients. This means that 3/4 of the dinner plate should be filled with grains, vegetables, legumes, and fruit. Only 1/4 should be meat, fish, or chicken.

The Peak of the Pyramid

Added fats, oils, and concentrated sweets form the peak of the pyramid. If they were eliminated, the remaining choices would still form a completely nutritious diet. While the majority of fats, oils, and concentrated sweets are located within the peak, a few are scattered throughout the other layers of the pyramid. This is because some choices in the other food groups naturally contain fat and/or sugars. Keep this important fact in mind—that up to half the amount of fat eaten during the day will come from the other food groups, even when lowfat choices are made.

Special Considerations

1. **Fats:** A certain amount of fat is needed in a healthy diet to supply energy and a few nutrients. However, fats are a high calorie source of energy, and too much fat in the diet can increase the risk of heart disease and certain cancers. Fat is measured in grams. One teaspoon of fat equals four grams. There are different kinds of fat in foods, and some types are worse than others.

   - Saturated fats are found in dairy products made with whole milk and in meat. Some meats contain a greater quantity of saturated fats than others: beef more than chicken. Saturated fats are solid at room temperature. Some vegetable fats such as coconut, cocoa butter (found in chocolate), palm and palm kernel oils are also saturated. Eating too much saturated fat raises blood cholesterol, increasing the risk of heart disease.

   - Unsaturated fats, found mostly in plants, are liquid at room temperature. Polyunsaturated fats are found in safflower, sunflower, corn, soybean, and cottonseed oils, and in some fish. Unsaturated fats are less likely to cause heart disease. In fact, monounsaturated fats, found in olive, peanut, and canola oils, appear to lower cholesterol.

- Hydrogenated oils is a term often found in food labels. Through a manufacturing process, normally liquid vegetable oils can be made to stay solid at room temperature. Therefore, they act as saturated fats and should be avoided in the diet.

- Avoid using saturated fats, margarines, gravies, and high fat salad dressings in preparing naturally lowfat foods. For example, one baked potato has 120 calories and only a trace of fat, but the same potato made into french fries has 225 calories and 11 grams of fat!

- The number of fat grams allowed per day depends on a person's caloric requirements. Fat intake should be limited to approximately 30% of daily calories. Saturated fat should be limited to 10% of daily calories, or about 1/3 of the total fat intake. Remember that about half of this fat will come from other food groups, and this should be included when calculating the total fat intake. Determine the number of calories needed each day, and then use the chart below as a guide to determine the number of fat grams permitted.

- Those people who like to do their own math can determine their fat intake requirements by using the following formula.

  A. Multiply the total day's calories by 0.30 to get calories from fat per day.

      Example: 2200 calories multiplied by 0.30 = 660 calories from fat.

  B. Each gram of fat has nine calories, so divide the calories from fat per day by 9 to get grams of fat permitted each day.

      Example: 660 calories from fat divided by 9 = 73 grams of fat allowed per day.

  C. If the total fat intake on this diet is 73 grams for the day, no more than 24 grams (about one-third of the total fat intake) should be in saturated fats.

2. **Cholesterol:** This waxy, fat-like substance is needed for important functions in the body. As is often the case, however, too much of a good thing can be bad. Too much cholesterol in the blood can increase the risk of heart disease. Where does cholesterol come from? Foods from animal sources contain cholesterol because animals produce cholesterol in their bodies. The human body also makes its own cholesterol. In fact, it produces all that it needs, and doesn't require any from the diet. That is why many health authorities recommend limiting foods from animal sources in the diet. Some animal foods are higher in cholesterol than others: egg yolks and organ meats such as liver or sweetbreads. It is recommended that dietary cholesterol be limited to an average of 300 milligrams (mg) or less a day. It is not necessary to stop eating high cholesterol foods completely. Balance is the key; if high cholesterol foods are eaten one day, eat low cholesterol foods the next. Three to four egg yolks a week are generally permissible, including those used in preparing foods such as baked goods and custards. Remember that foods from plants do not contain cholesterol.

3. **Sugars:** Choosing a diet low in sugar is important. Sugars found naturally in fruits and milk are not a problem. It is the adding of sugar to foods in processing, preparing, or at the table that increases calories without providing nutrients. Sugars include white sugar, brown sugar, raw sugar, corn syrup, honey, and molasses. Foods like soft drinks, candy, ice cream, jams, jellies, chocolate milk, and fruits canned in heavy syrups are high in sugar and should by limited in the diet. Use the guide below to avoid getting too many calories from added sugar.

4. **Salt and sodium:** Most people eat more of it than they need. Sodium is an essential element for the body, but eating too much of it can cause health problems. Sodium is found naturally in many foods, but much of the excess in our diets comes from salt added while cooking, in food processing, or at the table. Table salt is about one-half sodium. One teaspoon of salt provides about 2000 mg of sodium. Most health authorities say that sodium intake should be less than 3000 mg a day, so it is important to avoid adding too much salt to foods. Always check food labels for sodium content. It is a good idea to purchase foods with less than 300 mg of sodium per serving.

5. **Learn to read food labels.** Federal regulations require standardized labels on food packages to provide reliable information and to help consumers make healthier food choices. The regulations require full ingredient listing and standardized serving sizes. Health claims and descriptions such as "light" or "low fat" are required to meet certain guidelines.

6. **Ingredients must be listed in order, by quantity,** from the largest to the smallest. For example, if a can of soup contains more water than anything else, water is listed first. Certain nutrients are shown as a percentage of Daily Value. These values were established based on daily calorie requirements. Using an example from this label, on a diet of 2000 calories per day, the daily value of total fat (100%) should equal no more than 65 grams. A serving of this product contains 4 g of fat, about 6% of the daily value.

7. **Always check the serving size.** The values listed are for one serving. This label lists the serving size as one cup, with a total of two servings in the container. A person eating the entire container would be getting 12% of the daily value of fat.

8. **Drinking excessive alcohol is the cause of many health problems.** Some medical studies indicate that a glass of red wine each day may produce benefits for the cardiovascular system. However, if you are a non-drinker, do not begin to use alcohol just for this uncertain benefit. If you do drink alcoholic beverages, do so in moderation. Alcohol adds calories, and little or no nutrients.

How Does the Pyramid Work for Different Individuals?

A person eating the proper number of selections and a variety of foods from each level of the pyramid will be getting the correct proportions of carbohydrate, protein, and fat for a healthy diet. Remember that fat in the diet should not equal more than 30% of total calories. What about the other 70%?

All healthy adults need from 10% to 20% of the total daily calories in protein. However, athletes may need slightly more during periods of intense training. When more protein is eaten than the body needs, the excess is stored as fat. When choosing protein foods, remember that they do not have to come only from animal sources. Certain vegetables and grains also contain protein and are lower in saturated fats.

The remainder of the diet (50% to 60%) should come from carbohydrates. A person eating less than 30% of calories from fat should make up the difference in carbohydrates, not in proteins. These ranges are meant as a guide and may vary depending on individual requirements.

Notice that each food group on the pyramid shows a range of servings. The number of servings needed per day depends on the number of calories needed. A calorie is a unit of measure that explains how much energy various foods supply to the body. The number of calories needed to supply enough energy each day depends on a person's age, gender, size, and activity level. Use table 4.4 as a guide.

It is simple to adjust the pyramid diet for weight gain or weight loss. To lose weight, obviously it is necessary to reduce food or calorie intake. Reduce the number of servings in each food group by one or more, being careful to maintain the balance. Do not go below the lowest number of servings required per food group. If more weight reduction is needed reduce fats and sugars further, and increase physical activity. To gain weight, increase the number of servings proportionately in all food groups.

For young children, the calorie requirements can vary. Some preschool children need the same variety of foods as older family members, but may need fewer than 1600 calories. In this case they can simply eat smaller servings to maintain variety. A child's weight and height are the best guides to follow. An overweight child is getting too many calories. It is best to check with the child's physician to determine individual requirements.

Women who are pregnant or breast-feeding may need more calories or selections from certain food groups, and should consult their physicians. Finally, for any questions or individual guidance on using the food pyramid, check with a physician or a registered dietitian.

Table 4.1. Some Food Sources of Fiber

Insoluble Fiber	Soluble Fiber
Whole grains; including wheat, rye, brown rice, bran, and cereals	Citrus fruits
Cabbage, Brussels sprouts, broccoli, and cauliflower	Strawberries
Root vegetables	Oatmeal
Dried peas and beans	Dried beans and other legumes
Apples	Apples

Table 4.2. Fat Intake by Daily Calories

Daily Calories	Total Fat (Grams)	Total Saturated Fat (Grams)
1000	33	11
1200	40	13
1500	50	16
2000	66	22
2200	73	24
2500	83	27
2800	93	31

Table 4.3. Amount of Added Sugar by Daily Calorie Intake

Daily Calorie Intake	Limit Added Sugar To
1600 calories	6 teaspoons
2200 calories	12 teaspoons
2800 calories	18 teaspoons

Table 4.4. Food Group and Calorie Recommendations by Age, Gender, and Activity Level.

Food Group and Calorie Level	Sedentary Women and many Older Adults About 1600	Sedentary Men, Teen Girls, Active Women Children About 2200	Active Men and Teen Boys About 2800
Bread Group	6	9	11
Vegetable Group	3	4	5
Fruit Group	2	3	4
Milk Group	2-3	2-3	2-3
Meat Group	2, total of 5 oz.	2, total of 6 oz.	3, total of 7 oz.
Total Fat Grams	53	73	93
Total tsp. Added Sugar	6	12	18

Chapter 5

If You Eat Mushrooms or Raw Oysters—You Need to Know

About 20 million American eat raw oysters. However, for some people, eating raw oysters can cause serious illness or even death. What causes this? How do you know if you are at risk? What can you do about it?

The Cause: Vibrio Vulnificus

Vibrio vulnificus a bacterium that occurs naturally in marine waters and is commonly found in Gulf of Mexico oysters. While not a threat to most healthy people, *Vibrio vulnificus* can cause sudden chills, fever, nausea, vomiting, blood poisoning, and death within two days in people with certain medical conditions. Forty percent of *Vibrio vulnificus* infections from raw oyster consumption are fatal. **The bacteria are not a result of pollution, so, although oysters should always be obtained from reputable sources, eating oysters from "clean" waters or in reputable restaurants with high turnover does not provide protection.** Eating raw oysters with hot sauce or while drinking alcohol does not kill the bacteria, either.

This chapter contains text from "If You Eat Raw Oysters, You Need to Know...," FDA Brochure, July 1995, "Stalking the Wild Mushroom," by Marian Segal, *FDA Consumer* October 1994, and "Foodborne Pathogenic Microorganisms and Natural Toxins Handbook," *Bad Bug Book,* Center for Food Safety & Applied Nutrition (CFSAN), FDA. January 1992, updated March 1999.

The Risk Factors

Certain health conditions put you at risk for serious illness or death from *Vibrio vulnificus* infection. Some of these conditions have no signs or symptoms so you may not know you are at risk. Check with your doctor if you are unsure of your risk.

These conditions include:

- liver disease, either from excessive alcohol intake, viral hepatitis, or other causes
- hemochromatosis, an iron disorder
- diabetes
- stomach problems, including previous stomach surgery and low stomach acid (for example, from antacid use)
- cancer
- immune disorders, including HIV infection
- long-term steroid use (as for asthma and arthritis).

If you are an older adult, you also may be at increased risk because older people more often have these risk conditions than younger people. If you are or think you may be in any of these risk categories, you should not eat raw oysters. However, because fully cooking oysters completely kills the bacteria, you can continue to enjoy oysters in many cooked preparations.

Drinking Alcoholic Beverages Regularly and Liver Disease

If you drink alcoholic beverages regularly, you may be at risk for liver disease, and, as a result, at risk for serious illness or death from raw oysters. Even drinking two to three drinks each day can cause liver disease, which may have no symptoms. Liver disease will put you at increased risk for *Vibrio vulnificus* infection from raw oysters. The risk of death is almost 200 times greater in those with liver disease than those without liver disease.

Oyster Safety: What You Can Do

At Restaurants

Order oysters fully cooked. Some states display notices for those at risk. Use them as reminders of how to avoid illness.

Cooking at Home

In the Shell

- Boil live oysters in boiling water for 3 to 5 minutes after shells open. Use small pots to boil or steam oysters. Do not cook too many oysters in the same pot because the ones in the middle may not get fully cooked. Discard any oysters that do not open during cooking.

- Steam live oysters 4 to 9 minutes in a steamer that's already steaming.

Shucked

- Boil or simmer for at least 3 minutes or until edges curl.

- Fry in oil for at least 3 minutes at 375° F.

- Broil 3 inches from heat for 3 minutes.

- Bake (as in Oysters Rockefeller) for 10 minutes at 450° F.

If you have additional questions call the FDA Seafood Hotline, 1-800-FDA-4010.

Stalking the Wild Mushroom

Poisonous mushrooms can wreak havoc on men, women and children. If ingested, their toxins can cause stomach upset, dizziness, hallucinations, and other neurological symptoms. The more lethal species can cause liver and kidney failure, coma, and even death.

In the United States, Food and Drug Administration biologist John Gecan worries about ignorance when it comes to harvesting wild mushrooms. Many edible mushrooms have toxic "look-alike" species, Gecan says, and untrained pickers often are woefully incompetent to distinguish the bad from the good.

The Unskilled

"People go out and harvest wild mushrooms without the foggiest notion of what they're picking. They may know what mushrooms they're looking for, but they may also mistakenly pick up toxic look-a-likes found in the same place," he says. Gecan, a mushroom expert with the agency's Center for Food Safety and Applied Nutrition, says quite simply: "As a novice, you'd better not go out and pick mushrooms, eat them, and expect to live very long."

FDA regulates commercially grown and harvested mushrooms, which are cultivated in concrete buildings or caves, but there are no systematic controls on individual gatherers harvesting wild species.

Some of the most deadly mushrooms produce toxic amanitins. Among them is the genus Amanita, whose members have telltale common names such as death angel, fool's mushroom, and destroying angel. These, and less deadly species, may end up in gourmet shops, co-ops, supermarkets, and restaurants, mistaken for their nontoxic, edible look-a-likes.

There are two general groups of fleshy fungi—ascomycetes and basidiomycetes—which are differentiated by their spore-bearing reproductive structures. Ascomycetes bear spores enclosed in a sac-like cell called an ascus. They include the cup fungi, false morels, and true morels. Basidiomycetes bear spores on one end of a specialized cell called a basidium. This group is further broken down into subgroups based on their spore-bearing structures and include, among others, the chanterelles, gilled fungi (including the "button" mushrooms commonly seen in supermarkets), and puffballs.

Gecan, whose primary expertise is identifying morels and their look-a-likes, illustrates the complexity of the task. He notes, for example, that the edible bell morel Verpa conica and half-free morel Morchella semilibera, and the poisonous early "false morel" Verpa bohemica all have caps that look like a partially closed parasol with vertical ridges and striations. The three can easily be confused by an inexperienced harvester, as their distinguishing features are not conspicuous.

The edible half-free and bell morels both have eight spores per ascus, but the stem on the half-free attaches halfway up inside the cap, while the stem of the bell morel attaches at the very top of the cap. The stem of the poisonous early false morel also attaches at the very top of the cap, but it has only two to four large spores per ascus.

The Unscrupulous

Unskilled harvesters are not the only problem of the wild mushroom trade; the lucrative market has generated its share of unsavory characters.

"There's such an economic gain to be had here that people are going out knowingly including the toxic Verpa bohemica in their harvest of edible morels. This was a serious contamination problem in morels coming from India in the late 1980s," Gecan says. He tells of an importer who admitted that some harvesters will pick up anything that looks like a morel, adding that some pickers even stuff them with stones to increase the weight.

The wild mushroom business has also spawned violence. Some wild mushrooms sell for $100 or more a pound, Gecan says, and armed robberies are occurring in the Pacific Northwest, where the combination of heavy-covered forests and moist environment yields a plentiful crop.

The Evidence

FDA first became involved with analyzing wild mushrooms when agency field inspectors sent samples to headquarters laboratories following a poisoning outbreak in 1977. Four people suffered abdominal pains, dizziness, vomiting, and fainting after eating "veal morel" at a New York City restaurant. The morels, imported from France and Switzerland, included Gyromitra esculenta mushrooms, which produce the methylhydrazine derivative gyromitrin, a toxin that can sometimes cause death. "It's basically one of the components of rocket fuel," Gecan says.

He explains that "Gyromitra is picked and canned and eaten in France and elsewhere in Europe with no ill effects, because the chefs over there know how to prepare them."

In July 1978, FDA issued an import alert directing sampling of morel shipments from the French and Swiss firms implicated in the 1977 outbreak. In 1980, analysis of samples of French morels collected by FDA's Denver district showed they contained Gyromitra.

In 1987, a food poisoning investigation by FDA's Detroit district led to a shipment of dried "morels" packed by two firms in India. The mushrooms contained Gyromitra as well as another toxic species, Verpa bohemica.

In December 1990, the agency identified Verpa bohemica in samples of two lots of dried "morels" from a third French firm.

The agency's current import alert instructs the districts to sample morels shipped from all the firms implicated in previous poisoning outbreaks and send them to Gecan for identification. Also, morel shipments from other firms—particularly in France, Switzerland and India—must be examined for proper labeling and packaging and, if necessary, sampled. When toxic species are identified, the shipment is refused entry.

The Survey

To determine the extent of the problem of toxic wild mushrooms in the U.S. market, Gecan and his FDA colleague, biologist Stanley Cichowicz, directed a two-year survey of wild mushrooms in commercial distribution. They published their results in the August 1993 *Journal of Food Protection.*

For the survey, 10 FDA districts were directed to collect samples of specific species of canned, dried and fresh imported and domestic mushrooms. About two dozen species were collected at ports of entry and from gourmet shops, supermarkets, health food stores, and other commercial establishments. They included morels, false morels, shiitakes, straw mushrooms, chanterelles, hiratakes, and others, as well as mixed mushrooms.

Of the 344 samples collected, toxic mushrooms were found only in the morels and the mixed mushrooms. Of the 42 morel samples collected, nine contained toxic species. Seven of the nine were from France, the other two from India. Of 13 mixed mushroom samples collected, two—both from France—contained toxic species.

Although all the toxic mushrooms identified in the survey originated overseas, potential problems exist with wild mushrooms harvested here at home as well. Except for Michigan, where wild mushroom growers and harvesters must be licensed, and Illinois, which prohibits the sale of wild-picked mushrooms through wholesale, retail or food service establishments, the states do not regulate the sale of wild mushrooms. And FDA has no regulatory authority for products not sold in interstate commerce.

During the survey, Gecan received a quart canning jar of mushrooms an FDA investigator bought in a Chicago bar. The investigator learned from the bar owner that some local women who had immigrated from Poland had been hired to pick the mushrooms in a Wisconsin woods. The mushrooms were packed in brine in mason jars and sold at local bars.

The mushrooms turned out to be okay, Gecan says, but both the possibility of toxic mushrooms and the brine levels were cause for worry. Improper processing could have caused botulism toxicity.

New World, New Species

Gecan says that immigrants who commonly pick mushrooms in their native lands have particular problems when they continue that tradition here. The mushrooms in this country may look like the ones they or their parents and grandparents picked in the old country. But appearances can be deceiving.

Cichowicz explains that North America has perhaps four times as many mushroom species as Europe, so European immigrants think they're picking the same mushrooms as back home, when actually they're harvesting toxic look-alikes.

Immigrants from other parts of the world have similar problems. Gecan tells of a group of Koreans in the Pacific Northwest who, looking for straw mushrooms, picked death caps instead. "They cleaned them, cooked them, and ate them, and all needed liver transplants," he says.

It gets still more complex, Cichowicz says, because even within different parts of this country, a particular mushroom grown under certain conditions—a certain type of soil or nutrient source—will look one way, whereas the same species grown under different conditions will have a slightly different appearance. He says a species grown east of the Rockies might be edible, whereas west of the Rockies it might not.

The Clubs

Not all wild mushroom harvesters are unskilled or unscrupulous. There are mycology (mushroom) clubs in the United States with extremely knowledgeable members that organize forays and gain continuing experience from their field work. Gecan recommends that interested amateurs contact a club through the North American Mycological Association.

He says, "Experienced collectors should go out in the field, know every mushroom they pick, and if there's a question in their mind, should chuck it away."

The common button mushroom Agaricus bisporus sold in retail markets is commercially grown under controlled conditions and presents no hazard of contamination with toxic mushroom species. But because there are no absolute guarantees that toxic mushrooms won't reach the market, Gecan endorses the maxim "buyer beware." Because of increased demand, retail food stores are offering more and more varieties of wild mushrooms, while their harvesting remains largely unregulated.

That is not to say that Americans need forever forgo the taste delights of wild mushrooms. Gecan says that although toxic morel look-alikes are occasionally found in commercial mushrooms, they are rarely fatal. In addition, individuals have different thresholds for the toxins, so that some people might display only mild symptoms or none at all. Someone who gets sick from eating wild mushrooms should go to a hospital emergency room for treatment.

Mushroom Poisoning, Toadstool Poisoning

Mushroom toxins include Amanitin, Gyromitrin, Orellanine, Muscarine, Ibotenic Acid, Muscimol, Psilocybin, and Coprine

Mushroom poisoning is caused by the consumption of raw or cooked fruiting bodies (mushrooms, toadstools) of a number of species of higher fungi. The term toadstool (from the German Todesstuhl, death's stool) is commonly given to poisonous mushrooms, but for individuals who are not experts in mushroom identification there are generally no easily recognizable differences between poisonous and nonpoisonous species. Old wives' tales notwithstanding, there is no general rule of thumb for distinguishing edible mushrooms and poisonous toadstools. The toxins involved in mushroom poisoning are produced naturally by the fungi themselves, and each individual specimen of a toxic species should be considered equally poisonous. Most mushrooms that cause human poisoning cannot be made nontoxic by cooking, canning, freezing, or any other means of processing. Thus, the only way to avoid poisoning is to avoid consumption of the toxic species. Poisonings in the United States occur most commonly when hunters of wild mushrooms (especially novices) misidentify and consume a toxic species, when recent immigrants collect and consume a poisonous American species that closely resembles an edible wild mushroom from their native land, or when mushrooms that contain psychoactive compounds are intentionally consumed by persons who desire these effects.

Nature of Disease(s)

Mushroom poisonings are generally acute and are manifested by a variety of symptoms and prognoses, depending on the amount and species consumed. Because the chemistry of many of the mushroom toxins (especially the less deadly ones) is still unknown and positive identification of the mushrooms is often difficult or impossible, mushroom poisonings are generally categorized by their physiological effects. There are four categories of mushroom toxins:

- **protoplasmic poisons** (poisons that result in generalized destruction of cells, followed by organ failure);

- **neurotoxins** (compounds that cause neurological symptoms such as profuse sweating, coma, convulsions, hallucinations, excitement, depression, spastic colon);

- **gastrointestinal irritants** (compounds that produce rapid, transient nausea, vomiting, abdominal cramping, and diarrhea); and

- **disulfiram-like toxins**. Mushrooms in this last category are generally nontoxic and produce no symptoms unless alcohol is consumed within 72 hours after eating them, in which case a short-lived acute toxic syndrome is produced.

Normal Course of Disease(s):

The normal course of the disease varies with the dose and the mushroom species eaten. Each poisonous species contains one or more toxic compounds that are unique to few other species. Therefore, cases of mushroom poisonings generally do not resemble each other unless they are caused by the same or very closely related mushroom species. Almost all mushroom poisonings may be grouped in one of the categories outlined above.

Protoplasmic Poisons

Amatoxins:

Several mushroom species, including the Death Cap or Destroying Angel (Amanita phalloides, A. virosa), the Fool's Mushroom (A. verna) and several of their relatives, along with the Autumn Skullcap (Galerina autumnalis) and some of its relatives, produce a family of cyclic octapeptides called amanitins. Poisoning by the amanitins is characterized by a long latent period (range 6-48 hours, average 6-15 hours) during which the patient shows no symptoms. Symptoms appear at the end of the latent period in the form of sudden, severe seizures of abdominal pain, persistent vomiting and watery diarrhea, extreme thirst, and lack of urine production. If this early phase is survived, the patient may appear to recover for a short time, but this period will generally be followed by a rapid and severe loss of strength, prostration, and pain-caused restlessness. Death in 50-90% of the cases from progressive and irreversible liver, kidney, cardiac, and skeletal muscle damage may follow within 48 hours (large dose), but the disease more typically lasts 6 to 8 days in adults and 4 to 6 days in children. Two or three days after the onset of the later phase, jaundice, cyanosis, and coldness of the skin occur. Death usually follows a period of coma and occasionally convulsions. If recovery occurs, it generally requires at least a month and is accompanied by enlargement of the liver. Autopsy will usually reveal fatty degeneration and necrosis of the liver and kidney.

Hydrazines:

Certain species of False Morel (Gyromitra esculenta and G. gigas) contain the protoplasmic poison gyromitrin, a volatile hydrazine derivative. Poisoning by this toxin superficially resembles Amanita poisoning but is less severe. There is generally a latent period of 6-10 hours after ingestion during which no symptoms are evident, followed by sudden onset of abdominal discomfort (a feeling of fullness), severe headache, vomiting, and sometimes diarrhea. The toxin affects primarily the liver, but there are additional disturbances to blood cells and the central nervous system. The mortality rate is relatively low (2-4%). Poisonings with symptoms almost identical to those produced by Gyromitra have also been reported after ingestion of the Early False Morel (Verpa bohemica). The toxin is presumed to be related to gyromitrin but has not yet been identified.

Orellanine:

The final type of protoplasmic poisoning is caused by the Sorrel Webcap mushroom (Cortinarius orellanus) and some of its relatives. This mushroom produces orellanine, which causes a type of poisoning characterized by an extremely long asymptomatic latent period of 3 to 14 days. An intense, burning thirst (polydipsia) and excessive urination (polyuria) are the first symptoms. This may be followed by nausea, headache, muscular pains, chills, spasms, and loss of consciousness. In severe cases, severe renal tubular necrosis and kidney failure may result in death (15%) several weeks after the poisoning. Fatty degeneration of the liver and severe inflammatory changes in the intestine accompany the renal damage, and recovery in less severe cases may require several months.

Diagnosis of Human Illness:

A clinical testing procedure is currently available only for the most serious types of mushroom toxins, the amanitins. The commercially available method uses a 3H-radioimmunoassay (RIA) test kit and can detect sub-nanogram levels of toxin in urine and plasma. Unfortunately, it requires a 2-hour incubation period, and this is an excruciating delay in a type of poisoning which the clinician generally does not see until a day or two has passed. A 125I-based kit which overcomes this problem has recently been reported, but has not yet reached the clinic. A sensitive and rapid HPLC technique has been reported in the literature even more recently, but it has not yet seen clinical application. Since most clinical laboratories in this country do not use even the older RIA technique, diagnosis is based entirely on symptomology and recent dietary history. Despite the fact that cases of mushroom poisoning may be broken down into a relatively small number of categories based on symptomatology, positive botanical identification of the mushroom species consumed remains the only means of unequivocally determining the particular type of intoxication involved, and it is still vitally important to obtain such accurate identification as quickly as possible. Cases involving ingestion of more than one toxic species in which one set of symptoms masks or mimics another set are among many reasons for needing this information. Unfortunately, a number of factors (not discussed here) often make identification of the causative mushroom impossible. In such cases, diagnosis must be based on symptoms alone. In order to rule out other types of food poisoning and to conclude that the mushrooms eaten were the cause of the poisoning, it must be established that everyone who ate the suspect mushrooms became ill and that no one who did not eat the mushrooms became ill. Wild mushrooms eaten raw, cooked, or processed should always be regarded as prime suspects. After ruling out other sources of food poisoning and positively implicating mushrooms as the cause of the illness, diagnosis may proceed in two steps. The first step provides an early indication of the seriousness of the disease and its prognosis.

As described above, the protoplasmic poisons are the most likely to be fatal or to cause irreversible organ damage. In the case of poisoning by the deadly Amanitas, important laboratory indicators of liver (elevated LDH, SGOT, and bilirubin levels) and kidney (elevated uric acid, creatinine, and BUN levels) damage will be present. Unfortunately, in the absence of dietary history, these signs could be mistaken for symptoms of liver or kidney impairment as the result of other causes (e.g., viral hepatitis). It is important that this distinction be made as quickly as possible, because the delayed onset of symptoms will generally mean that the organ has already been damaged. The importance of rapid diagnosis is obvious: victims who are hospitalized and given aggressive support therapy almost immediately after ingestion have a mortality rate of only 10%, whereas those admitted 60 or more hours after ingestion have a 50-90% mortality rate. A recent report indicates that amanitins are observable in urine well before the onset of any symptoms, but that laboratory tests for liver dysfunction do not appear until well after the organ has been damaged.

Associated Foods:

Mushroom poisonings are almost always caused by ingestion of wild mushrooms that have been collected by nonspecialists (although specialists have also been poisoned). Most cases occur when toxic species are confused with edible species, and a useful question to ask of the victims or their mushroom-picking benefactors is the identity of the mushroom they thought they were picking. In the absence of a well-preserved specimen, the answer to this question could narrow the possible suspects considerably. Intoxication has also occurred when reliance was placed on some folk method of distinguishing poisonous and safe species. Outbreaks have occurred after ingestion of fresh, raw mushrooms, stir-fried mushrooms, home-canned mushrooms, mushrooms cooked in tomato sauce (which rendered the sauce itself toxic, even when no mushrooms were consumed), and mushrooms that were blanched and frozen at home. Cases of poisoning by home-canned and frozen mushrooms are especially insidious because a single outbreak may easily become a multiple outbreak when the preserved toadstools are carried to another location and consumed at another time.

Relative Frequency of Disease:

Accurate figures on the relative frequency of mushroom poisonings are difficult to obtain. For the 5-year period between 1976 and 1981, 16 outbreaks involving 44 cases were reported to the Centers for Disease Control in Atlanta (Rattanvilay et al. MMWR 31(21): 287-288, 1982). The number of unreported cases is, of course, unknown. Cases are sporadic and large outbreaks are rare. Poisonings tend to be grouped in the spring and fall when most mushroom species are at the height of their fruiting stage. While the actual incidence appears to be very low, the potential exists for grave problems. Poisonous mushrooms are not limited in distribution as are other poisonous organisms (such as dinoflagellates). Intoxications may occur at any time and place, with dangerous species occurring in habitats ranging from urban lawns to deep woods. As Americans become more adventurous in their mushroom collection and consumption, poisonings are likely to increase.

Target Population:

All humans are susceptible to mushroom toxins. The poisonous species are ubiquitous, and geographical restrictions on types of poisoning that may occur in one location do not exist (except for some of the hallucinogenic LBMs, which occur primarily in the American southwest and southeast). Individual specimens of poisonous mushrooms are also characterized by individual variations in toxin content based on genetics, geographic location, and growing conditions. Intoxications may thus be more or less serious, depending not on the number of mushrooms consumed, but on the dose of toxin delivered. In addition, although most cases of poisoning by higher plants occur in children, toxic mushrooms are consumed most often by adults. Occasional accidental mushroom poisonings of children and pets have been reported, but adults are more likely to actively search for and consume wild mushrooms for culinary purposes. Children are more seriously affected by the normally nonlethal toxins than are adults and are more likely to suffer very serious consequences from ingestion of relatively smaller doses. Adults who consume mushrooms are also more likely to recall what was eaten and when, and are able to describe their symptoms more accurately than are children. Very old, very young, and debilitated persons of both sexes are more likely to become seriously ill from all types of mushroom poisoning, even those types which are generally considered to be mild.

Analysis of Foods for Toxins:

The mushroom toxins can with difficulty be recovered from poisonous fungi, cooking water, stomach contents, serum, and urine. Procedures for extraction and quantitation are generally elaborate and time-consuming, and the patient will in most cases have recovered by the time an analysis is made on the basis of toxin chemistry. The exact chemical natures of most of the toxins that produce milder symptoms are unknown. Chromatographic techniques (TLC, GLC, HPLC) exist for the amanitins, orellanine, muscimol/ibotenic acid, psilocybin, muscarine, and the gyromitrins. The amanitins may also be determined by commercially available 3H-RIA kits. The most reliable means of diagnosing a mushroom poisoning remains botanical identification of the fungus that was eaten. An accurate pre-ingestion determination of species will also prevent accidental poisoning in 100% of cases. Accurate post-ingestion analyses for specific toxins when no botanical identification is possible may be essential only in cases of suspected poisoning by the deadly Amanitas, since prompt and aggressive therapy (including lavage, activated charcoal, and plasmapheresis) can greatly reduce the mortality rate.

Pyrrolizidine Alkaloids Poisoning

Pyrrolizidine alkaloid intoxication is caused by consumption of plant material containing these alkaloids. The plants may be consumed as food, for medicinal purposes, or as contaminants of other agricultural crops. Cereal crops and forage crops are sometimes contaminated with pyrrolizidine-producing weeds, and the alkaloids find their way into flour and other foods, including milk from cows feeding on these plants. Many plants from the Boraginaceae, Compositae, and Leguminosae families contain well over 100 hepatotoxic pyrrolizidine alkaloids.

Normal Course of Disease

Most cases of pyrrolizidine alkaloid toxicity result in moderate to severe liver damage. Gastrointestinal symptoms are usually the first sign of intoxication, and consist predominantly of abdominal pain with vomiting and the development of ascites. Death may ensue from 2 weeks to more than 2 years after poisoning, but patients may recover almost completely if the alkaloid intake is discontinued and the liver damage has not been too severe.

Diagnosis of Human Illness

Evidence of toxicity may not become apparent until sometime after the alkaloid is ingested. The acute illness has been compared to the Budd-Chiari syndrome (thrombosis of hepatic veins, leading to liver enlargement, portal hypertension, and ascites). Early clinical signs include nausea and acute upper gastric pain, acute abdominal distension with prominent dilated veins on the abdominal wall, fever, and biochemical evidence of liver disfunction. Fever and jaundice may be present. In some cases the lungs are affected; pulmonary edema and pleural effusions have been observed. Lung damage may be prominent and has been fatal. Chronic illness from ingestion of small amounts of the alkaloids over a long period proceeds through fibrosis of the liver to cirrhosis, which is indistinguishable from cirrhosis of other etiology.

Associated Foods

The plants most frequently implicated in pyrrolizidine poisoning are members of the Borginaceae, Compositae, and Leguminosae families. Consumption of the alkaloid-containing plants as food, contaminants of food, or as medicinals has occurred.

Relative Frequency of Disease

Reports of acute poisoning in the United States among humans are relatively rare. Most result from the use of medicinal preparations as home remedies. However, intoxications of range animals sometimes occur in areas under drought stress, where plants containing alkaloids are common. Milk from dairy animals can become contaminated with the alkaloids, and alkaloids have been found in the honey collected by bees foraging on toxic plants. Mass human poisonings have occurred in other countries when cereal crops used to prepare food were contaminated with seeds containing pyrrolizidine alkaloid.

Target Population

All humans are believed to be susceptible to the hepatotoxic pyrrolizidine alkaloids. Home remedies and consumption of herbal teas in large quantities can be a risk factor and are the most likely causes of alkaloid poisonings in the United States.

Analysis in Foods

The pyrrolizidine alkaloids can be isolated from the suspect commodity by any of several standard alkaloid extraction procedures. The toxins are identified by thin layer chromatography. The pyrrolizidine ring is first oxidized to a pyrrole followed by spraying with Ehrlich reagent, which gives a characteristic purple spot. Gas-liquid chromatographic and mass spectral methods also are available for identifying the alkaloids.

Selected Outbreaks

There have been relatively few reports of human poisonings in the United States. Worldwide, however, a number of cases have been documented. Most of the intoxications in the USA involved the consumption of herbal preparations either as a tea or as a medicine. The first patient diagnosed in the USA was a female who had used a medicinal tea for 6 months while in Ecuador. She developed typical hepatic veno-occlusive disease, with voluminous ascites, centrilobular congestion of the liver, and increased portal vein pressure. Interestingly, the patient completely recovered within one year after ceasing to consume the tea. Another herbal tea poisoning occurred when Senecio longilobus was mistaken for a harmless plant (called "gordolobo yerba" by Mexican Americans) and used to make herbal cough medicine. Two infants were given this medication for several days. The 2-month-old boy was ill for 2 weeks before being admitted to the hospital and died 6 days later. His condition was first diagnosed as Reye's syndrome, but was changed when jaundice, ascites, and liver necrosis were observed. The second child, a 6-month-old female, had acute hepatocellular disease, ascites, portal hypertension, and a right pleural effusion. The patient improved with treatment; however, after 6 months, a liver biopsy revealed extensive hepatic fibrosis, progressing to cirrhosis over 6 months. Another case of hepatic veno-occlusive disease was described in a 47-year-old nonalcoholic woman who had consumed large quantities of comfrey (Symphytum species) tea and pills for more than one year. Liver damage was still present 20 months after the comfrey consumption ceased.

Part Two

Medical Tests

Chapter 6

Common Laboratory Tests in Liver Disease

The diagnosis of liver diseases depends upon a combination of history, physical examination, laboratory testing, and sometimes radiological studies and biopsy. Only a physician who knows all of these aspects of a specific case can reliably make a diagnosis. Many individuals with liver diseases nonetheless have questions about their laboratory test results and seek information about their significance. The purpose of this chapter is to briefly describe some of the common laboratory tests that may be abnormal in individuals with liver diseases. Patients reading this chapter must keep in mind that abnormalities of these laboratory tests are not diagnostic of specific diseases and that only a qualified physician who knows the entire case can provide a reliable diagnosis.

Alanine Aminotransferase (ALT)

ALT is an enzyme produced in hepatocytes, the major cell type in the liver. ALT is often inaccurately referred to as a liver function test, however, its level in the blood tells little about the function of the liver. The level of ALT in the blood (actually enzyme activity is measured in the clinical laboratory) is increased in conditions in which hepatocytes are damaged or die. As cells are damaged, ALT leaks out into the bloodstream. All types of hepatitis (viral, alcoholic, drug-induced, etc.) cause hepatocyte damage that can lead to elevations in the serum ALT activity. The ALT level is also increased in cases of liver cell death resulting from other causes, such as shock or drug toxicity. The level of ALT may correlate roughly with the degree of cell death or inflammation; however, this is not always the case. An accurate estimate of inflammatory activity or the amount cell death can only be made by liver biopsy. (See also aspartate aminotransferase below.)

Aspartate Aminotransferase (AST)

AST is an enzyme similar to ALT (see above) but less specific for liver disease as it is also produced in muscle and can be elevated in other conditions (for example, early in the course of a heart attack). AST is also inaccurately referred to as a liver function test by many physicians. In many cases of liver inflammation, the ALT and AST activities are elevated roughly in a 1:1 ratio. In some conditions, such as alcoholic hepatitis or shock liver, the elevation in the serum AST level may higher than the elevation in the serum ALT level.

Alkaline Phosphatase

Alkaline phosphatase is an enzyme, or more precisely a family of related enzymes, produced in the bile ducts, intestine, kidney, placenta, and bone. An elevation in the level of serum alkaline phosphatase (actually enzyme activity is measured in the clinical laboratory), especially in the setting of normal or only modestly elevated ALT and AST activities, suggests disease of the bile ducts. Serum alkaline phosphatase activity can be markedly elevated in bile duct obstruction or in bile duct diseases such as primary biliary cirrhosis or primary sclerosing cholangitis. Alkaline phosphatase is also produced in bone and blood activity can also be increased in some bone disorders.

Gamma-glutamyltranspeptidase (GGT)

An enzyme produced in the bile ducts that, like alkaline phosphatase, may be elevated in the serum of patients with bile duct diseases. Elevations in serum GGT, especially along with elevations in alkaline phosphatase, suggest bile duct disease. Measurement of GGT is an extremely sensitive test, however, and it may be elevated in virtually any liver disease and even sometimes in normal individuals. GGT is also induced by many drugs, including alcohol, and its serum activity may be increased in heavy drinkers even in the absence of liver damage or inflammation.

Bilirubin

Bilirubin is the major breakdown product that results from the destruction of old red blood cells (as well as some other sources). It is removed from the blood by the liver, chemically modified by a process called conjugation, secreted into the bile, passed into the intestine and to some extent reabsorbed from the intestine. Bilirubin concentrations are elevated in the blood either by increased production, decreased uptake by the liver, decreased conjugation, decreased secretion from the liver, or blockage of the bile ducts. In cases of increased production, decreased liver uptake, or decreased conjugation, the unconjugated or so-called indirect bilirubin will be primarily elevated. In cases of decreased secretion from the liver or bile duct obstruction, the conjugated or so-called direct bilirubin will be primarily elevated. Many different liver diseases, as well as conditions other than liver diseases (e. g. increased production by enhanced red blood cell destruction), can cause the serum bilirubin concentration to be elevated. Most adult acquired liver diseases cause impairment in bilirubin secretion from liver cells that cause the direct bilirubin to be elevated in the blood. In chronic, acquired liver diseases, the serum bilirubin concentration is usually normal until a significant amount of liver damage has occurred and cirrhosis is present. In acute liver disease, the bilirubin is usually increased relative to the severity of the acute process. In bile duct obstruction, or diseases of the bile ducts such as primary biliary cirrhosis or sclerosing cholangitis, the alkaline phosphatase and GGT activities are often elevated along with the direct bilirubin concentration.

Albumin

Albumin is the major protein that circulates in the bloodstream. Albumin is synthesized by the liver and secreted into the blood. Low serum albumin concentrations indicate poor liver function. The serum albumin concentration is usually normal in chronic liver diseases until cirrhosis and significant liver damage is present. Albumin levels can be low in conditions other than liver diseases including malnutrition, some kidney diseases, and other rarer conditions.

Prothrombin Time (PT)

Many factors necessary for blood clotting are made in the liver. When liver function is severely abnormal, their synthesis and secretion into the blood is decreased. The prothrombin time is a type of blood clotting test performed in the laboratory and it is prolonged when the blood concentrations of some of the clotting factors made by the liver are low. In chronic liver diseases, the prothrombin time is usually not elevated until cirrhosis is present and the liver damage is fairly significant. In acute liver diseases, the prothrombin time can be prolonged with severe liver damage and return to normal as the patient recovers. Prothrombin time can also be prolonged in cases of vitamin K deficiency, by drugs (warfarin, used therapeutically as an anticoagulant, prolongs the prothrombin time), and in non-liver disorders.

Platelet Count

Platelets are the smallest of the blood cells (actually fragments of larger cells known as megakaryocytes) that are involved in clotting. In some individuals with liver disease, the spleen becomes enlarged as blood flow through the liver is impeded. This can lead to platelets being sequestered in the enlarged spleen. In chronic liver diseases, the platelet count usually falls only after cirrhosis has developed. The platelet count can be abnormal in many conditions other than liver diseases.

Serum Protein Electrophoresis

In this test, the major proteins in the serum are separated in an electric field and their concentrations determined. The four major types of serum proteins whose concentrations are measured in this test are albumin, alpha-globulins, beta-globulins, and gamma-globulins. Serum protein electrophoresis is a useful test in patients with liver diseases as it can provide clues to several diagnostic possibilities. In cirrhosis, the albumin may be decreased (see above) and the gamma-globulin elevated. Gamma-globulin can be significantly elevated in some types of autoimmune hepatitis. The alpha-globulins can be low in alpha-1-antitrypsin deficiency.

Chapter 7

Liver Biopsy

The liver is the largest organ in the body. It is found high in the right upper abdomen, behind the ribs. The liver is remarkable, quietly making many proteins, eliminating waste products, and participating in the general metabolism and nutrition of the body. It even has the power to regenerate itself. However, there are many different problems that can occur in the liver and some can cause permanent damage. These conditions include virus infections, reactions to drugs or alcohol, tumors, hereditary conditions, and problems with the body's immune system.

Evaluating a Liver Condition

The physician will always take a medical history and perform a physical exam. Blood studies, known as liver function tests (LFT), give an overview of the health of the liver. If LFT results are persistently abnormal, the physician will then perform additional medical studies to determine the exact cause of the problem.

Finding the cause is important because there are now effective treatments for many liver disorders. Finally, the physician will want to know not only the specific cause of the problem, but also how severe the condition may be. The liver biopsy helps answer these questions.

What Is a Biopsy?

A biopsy is a tiny sample of body tissue—in this case, liver tissue. The tissue is prepared and stained in a laboratory, so the physician

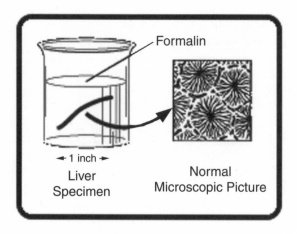

Figure 7.1. *Liver Tissue Preparation*

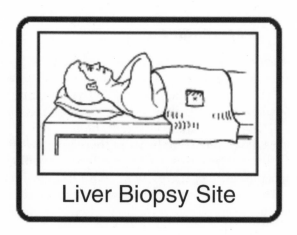

Figure 7.2. *Liver Biopsy*

can view it under a microscope. This usually helps the physician make a specific diagnosis and determine the extent and seriousness of the condition. It is vital information for determining treatment.

The Procedure

The liver biopsy is usually performed on an outpatient basis. A mild sedative may be given to the patient prior to the procedure. Sometimes, an ultrasound or echo machine is used to identify the best location to make the biopsy. Usually, the physician can make this determination simply by examination. The patient lies quietly on the back or slightly to the left side. That area of the skin where the biopsy will be done is carefully cleaned. Then, a local anesthetic agent is used to numb the skin and tissue below. A specially designed thin needle is inserted through the skin. At this point, the physician will tell the patient how to breathe. The needle is advanced into and out of the liver. This takes only 1 or 2 seconds. A slender core of tissue is removed with the needle, and is then processed through the laboratory. The entire procedure from start to finish lasts only 15 to 20 minutes.

Recovery

The patient is kept at rest for several hours following the exam. Medical personnel check the heart rate and blood pressure during this time. There may be some discomfort in the chest or shoulder, however, this is usually temporary. Medication is available for this discomfort, if needed. Before being discharged, the patient is given instructions about returning to normal activities and about eating. Activity is usually restricted for a day or so after the biopsy. However, the procedure does not require a long recovery period.

Complications

In most instances, a liver biopsy is obtained quickly with no problems. As noted, there is occasionally some fleeting discomfort in the right side or shoulder. Internal bleeding can sometimes occur, as can a leak of bile from the liver or gallbladder. These problems are rare and can usually be handled without the need for surgery.

Summary

A liver biopsy is a simple, rapid method of obtaining a sample of liver for analysis. It provides important information for evaluating and treating liver disorders. While some complications can occur, they are unusual. The benefits of the exam always outweigh the risk. Early, specific, and effective therapy can often prevent irreversible liver damage.

This material does not cover all information and is not intended as a substitute for professional care. Please consult with your physician on any matters regarding your health.

Chapter 8

Endoscopic Retrograde Cholangiopancreatography (ERCP)

ERCP stands for endoscopic retrograde cholangiopancreatography. As hard as this is to say, the actual exam is fairly simple. A dye is injected into the bile and pancreatic ducts using a flexible, video endoscope. Then x-rays are taken to outline the bile ducts and pancreas.

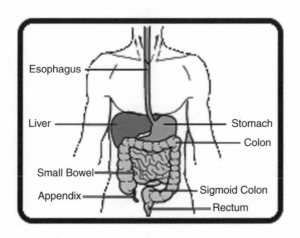

Figure 8.1. *The Digestive System*

The liver produces bile, which flows through the ducts, passes or fills the gallbladder, and then enters the intestine (duodenum) just beyond the stomach. The pancreas, which is six to eight inches long, sits behind the stomach. This organ secretes digestive enzymes that flow into the intestine through the same opening as the bile. Both bile and enzymes are needed to digest food.

Equipment

The flexible endoscope is a remarkable piece of equipment that can be directed and moved around the many bends in the upper gastrointestinal tract. The newer video endoscopes have a tiny, optically sensitive computer chip at the end. Electronic signals are then transmitted up the scope to the computer which then displays the image on a large video screen. An open channel in the scope allows other instruments to be passed through it to perform biopsies, inject solutions, or place stents.

Reasons for the Exam

Due to factors related to diet, environment, and heredity, the bile ducts, gallbladder, and pancreas are the seat of numerous disorders. These can develop into a variety of diseases and/or symptoms. ERCP helps in diagnosing and often in treating the condition.

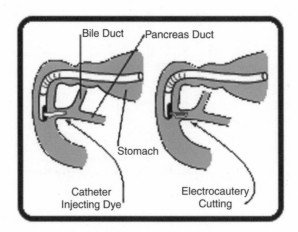

Figure 8.2. *Endoscopic Examination*

ERCP is used for:

- Gallstones, which are trapped in the main bile duct
- Blockage of the bile duct
- Yellow jaundice, which turns the skin yellow and the urine dark
- Undiagnosed upper-abdominal pain
- Cancer of the bile ducts or pancreas
- Pancreatitis (inflammation of the pancreas)

Preparation

The only preparation needed before an ERCP is to not eat or drink for eight hours prior to the procedure. You may be asked to stop certain medications such as aspirin before the procedure. Check with the physician.

The Procedure

An ERCP uses x-ray films and is performed in an x-ray room. The throat is anesthetized with a spray or solution, and the patient is usually mildly sedated. The endoscope is then gently inserted into the upper esophagus. The patient breathes easily throughout the exam, with gagging rarely occurring. A thin tube is inserted through the endoscope to the main bile duct entering the duodenum. Dye is then injected into this bile duct and/or the pancreatic duct and x-ray films are taken. The patient lies on his or her left side and then turns onto the stomach to allow complete visualization of the ducts. If a gallstone is found, steps may be taken to remove it. If the duct has become narrowed, an incision can be made using electrocautery (electrical heat) to relieve the blockage. Additionally, it is possible to widen narrowed ducts and to place small tubing, called stents, in these areas to keep them open. The exam takes from 20 to 40 minutes, after which the patient is taken to the recovery area.

Results

After the exam, the physician explains the results. If the effects of the sedatives are prolonged, the physician may suggest an appointment for a later date when the patient can fully understand the results.

Benefits

An ERCP is performed primarily to identify and/or correct a problem in the bile ducts or pancreas. This means the test enables a diagnosis to be made upon which specific treatment can be given. If a gallstone is found during the exam, it can often be removed, eliminating the need for major surgery. If a blockage in the bile duct causes yellow jaundice or pain, it can be relieved.

Alternative Testing

Alternative tests to ERCP include certain types of x-rays (Computed Tomography: CAT scan, CT) and sonography (ultrasound) to visualize the pancreas and bile ducts. In addition, dye can be injected into the bile ducts by placing a needle through the skin and into the liver. Small tubing can then be threaded into the bile ducts. Study of the blood also can provide some indirect information about the ducts and pancreas.

Side Effects and Risks

A temporary, mild sore throat sometimes occurs after the exam. Serious risks with ERCP, however, are uncommon. One such risk is excessive bleeding, especially when electrocautery is used to open a blocked duct. In rare instances, a perforation or tear in the intestinal wall can occur. Inflammation of the pancreas also can develop. These complications may require hospitalization and, rarely, surgery.

Due to the mild sedation, the patient should not drive or operate machinery for six hours following the exam. For this reason, a driver should accompany the patient to the exam.

Chapter 9

Ultrasound of the Abdomen

What Is Ultrasound?

Ultrasound is like ordinary sound except it has a frequency (or pitch) higher than human beings can hear. When sent into the body from a transducer resting on the patient's skin, the sound is reflected off internal structures. The returning echoes are received by the transducer and converted by an electronic instrument into an image of the internal structures on a viewing screen. These continually changing images can be recorded on videotape or film. Diagnostic ultrasound imaging is commonly called sonography. In an abdominal examination, ultrasound produces images of the major organs including the liver gallbladder, pancreas, spleen, kidneys, and large blood vessels.

Why Should I Have an Ultrasound Exam?

There are many reasons for examining the abdomen with ultrasound. Among the more common reasons:

- To look for causes of upper abdominal pain which may be related to problem in the liver, gallbladder, pancreas, or kidneys,

- To detect gallstones,

This chapter contains text from the following American Institute of Ultrasound in Medicine documents: "Abdomen Ultrasound," © 1992, and "Doppler Ultrasound," © 1992, reviewed 1995, reprinted with permission.

Figure 9.1. *Ultrasound Exam*

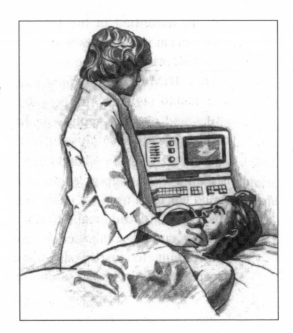

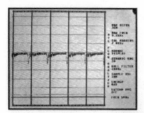

Figure 9.2. Doppler Graph and Image.

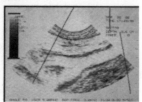

- To determine abnormalities of the liver or spleen,

- To evaluate the kidneys for blockage, or

- To look for enlargements (aneurysms) and other abnormalities of abdominal blood vessels.

Ultrasound will not always be able to provide all the information your doctor requires, in these cases, additional studies may be required.

What Is Doppler?

Doppler ultrasound is a special form of ultrasound. With Doppler ultrasound, it is possible to see the structures inside the body and evaluate blood flow at the same time. In order to do this, the machine uses ultrasound in two ways. One method of evaluation gives information about the structures within the body and the other method tells about blood flow. In the first method, the returning echoes are processed by the machine and a picture is made of the area beneath the scanner. The walls of your blood vessels, for example, are seen this way. On the other hand, if sound waves strike moving objects (like the red blood cells), the frequency of the sound is changed. This process is similar to the change in the pitch of an ambulance siren as it passes the listener. The doctor, vascular technologist, or sonographer performing the scan can display this change in frequency in several ways to evaluate blood flow within the body. An audible sound may be used of the flow may be shown as a graph or color display.

Why Should I Have a Doppler Ultrasound Exam?

A doppler ultrasound exam gives your physician a great deal of information about your blood vessels and about the way blood is passing through them. Doppler ultrasound is particularly well suited to evaluating problems within the veins and arteries. Because we have blood vessels throughout the body, Doppler may be used almost anywhere. One of the most common uses of Doppler ultrasound, however, is in the neck to look at carotid arteries. These vessels supply large amounts of blood to the brain and may become blocked. Blockage can lead to stroke.

In the heart, Doppler can tell about the flow of blood and whether it is directed correctly. In the abdomen, Doppler can help evaluate blood flow to the liver and many other abdominal organs. Doppler also is used to evaluate blood flow in the legs and may be helpful in identifying blockages in the arteries and clots in the veins.

Will It Hurt? Are There Any Special Preparations for the Exam?

There is no pain involved in an ultrasound examination and for most Doppler exams, no preparation is necessary. Your doctor may ask you to refrain from eating the morning of the exam if the scan involves the upper abdomen. A gel is applied to your skin and the instrument is then placed on the area to be examined. This gel may feel cool and, even though it wipes off easily, it is a good idea to wear clothing that is easily washable.

If the gallbladder is to be examined, you should have nothing to eat or drink except water six hours before the exam. This is because most food and drink cause the gallbladder to contract preventing adequate examination with ultrasound.

What Can I Expect during the Exam?

The pictures made by the returning echoes are displayed on one or more small TV screens which are studied by the specialist performing the scan. In addition, returning sound waves which have been reflected by moving blood can be heard by means of speakers in the instrument. The sounds may be similar to the sound of wind blowing through the trees.

How Long Will It Take?

The length of time for the examination will vary depending on the specific reasons for your examination. For some studies, such as examination of the gallbladder for stones, the study may require only 5-15minute. But, for a complete study of all the abdominal organs, 30 minutes or more may be required.

The average Doppler ultrasound exam takes 30-60 minutes. The length of the exam is dependent upon a number of factors including the portion of the body to be examined and the complexity of the anatomy. With atherosclerosis, or hardening of the arteries, the vessels may be very difficult to evaluate and may require more scanning time.

Who Will Perform the Exam?

In most cases, you will be examined by a sonographer specially trained in ultrasound. A series of images will be recorded by the sonograper. These images will then be interpreted by a physician. In some cases, you also will be examined by a physician to confirm or resolve uncertain findings.

Doppler ultrasound may be performed by your physician, a vascular technologist, or a sonographer. The exam will be interpreted by a physician.

Will I Need More Than One Exam?

In many cases, follow-up exams are necessary to evaluate progression of your condition or response to therapy.

Is Ultrasound Safe?

There are no known harmful effects associated with the medical use of sonography. Widespread clinical use of diagnostic ultrasound for many years has not revealed any harm caused. Studies in humans have revealed no direct link between the use of diagnostic ultrasound and any adverse outcomes. Although the possibility exists that biological effects may be identified in the future, current information indicates that the benefits to patients far outweigh the risks, if any.

What Are the Limitations of the Exam?

Because bone weakens sound waves, ultrasound cannot be used to examine the bones surrounding your abdomen, such as your ribs. Also, because sound is weakened as it passed through layers of tissue, results from patients who are obese are not of the same quality as those who are thin. In addition, ultrasound cannot image through gas. Thus, bowel gas may limit visualization of some structures of interest.

How Much Does the Exam Cost?

The price of an ultrasound examination varies widely depending on the reason for the exam and the complexity of the equipment used. Generally, insurance companies will help cover the cost of the examination.

Chapter 10

Computed Tomography (CT) of the Abdomen

In 1972, G.N. Hounsfield, a senior research scientist in Middlesex, England announced the invention of a revolutionary imaging technique that he called computed axial transverse scanning. He presented a cross-sectional image of the head that revealed the internal structures of the brain in a manner previously only seen at surgery or autopsy. Pathologic processes such as blood clots, tumors, and strokes could be easily seen. Structures inside the human body that had never been imaged before could now be visualized.

In the 25 years since Dr. Hounsfield's announcement, his discovery has completely revolutionized the practice of medicine. The name has changed; first to computed axial tomography (CAT), and now to computed tomography (CT). Although the first CT scanners could only image the head, they now have primary roles in diagnosing disorders of the chest, abdomen, and pelvis. The original scanners also took several minutes to acquire a single slice through the brain. The newest scanners can now image the entire body in 1 to 2 minutes.

Equipment

The basic principle behind CT is that the internal structure of an object can be reconstructed from multiple projections of the object. The patient lies on the table within the CT gantry, which is shaped like a giant donut. During each slice acquisition, an x-ray tube circling the

This chapter contains excerpts from "CT How It Works" and "CT of the Abdomen," © 1997, Steven Brick, M.D., reprinted with permission.

patient produces an x-ray beam that passes through the patient and is absorbed by a ring of detectors surrounding the patient. The intensity of the x-ray beam that reaches the detectors is dependent on the absorption characteristics of the tissues it passes through. Since the beam is moving around the patient, each tissue will be exposed from multiple directions. Using a process called Fourier analysis, the computer uses the information obtained from the different amounts of x-ray absorption to reconstruct the density and position of the different structures contained within each slice.

Spiral CT

In standard CT, each revolution of the x-ray tube around the patient produces a single slice that demonstrates the tissue that was traversed by the x-ray beam during that exposure. When imaging the body (i.e. the chest or abdomen), the patient is instructed to hold their breath during the exposure in order to minimize blurring of the image by motion. This exposure usually takes a few seconds. After the exposure, the table moves a small amount so that the next continuous slice of tissue can be exposed. The delay between slices usually takes about 5 to 10 seconds. This process is repeated numerous times until the full extent of the portion of the body being studied is imaged.

The most significant advance in CT technology in the past few years has been the development of spiral (or helical) CT. During spiral CT, the x-ray tube rotates continuously as the patient is smoothly moved through the x-ray scan field. Unlike the separate data sets produced for each individual slice in standard CT, spiral CT produces one continuous volume set of data for the entire region scanned.

Spiral CT has several advantages over standard CT:

- Speed: Since the patient is moving continuously through the scanner, the duration of the exam is markedly shortened. The entire chest or abdomen can be scanned in 30 seconds, usually during a single breath-hold.

- Improved detection of small lesions: In standard CT, the patient holds their breath for a slice acquisition, then breathes, than holds their breath again for the next slice. If they hold their breath slightly differently for each slice, small lesions may fall out of the plane of each contiguous slice and therefore may be missed. Since spiral CT can be performed during a single breath-hold, contiguous slices are truly contiguous. Also, since a volume of data is obtained, the spacing of the acquired slices can be manipulated after the scan is completed. This allows detected lesions to be placed in the middle of the slice, which creates a more accurate image of the lesion.

- Improved contrast enhancement: Intravenous contrast is often injected during the CT scan (see below). Since spiral CT can image a region of interest in such a short period of time, the injection of intravenous contrast can be timed to ensure optimal contrast enhancement and improved evaluation of various organs and blood vessels.

- Image reconstruction and manipulation: The volume of data obtained through spiral CT can be manipulated in many fascinating ways by powerful computers connected to the scanner. The transverse images can be reconstructed in any plane. 3-dimensional images be formed and moved into any position. A surface view of the body can be created, and then skin, muscles, and overlying organs can be stripped away. Contrast enhanced vessels can be isolated and converted into CT angiograms.

Intravenous Contrast

Many patients who undergo CT will receive intravenous contrast. Radiographic intravenous contrast materials all contain iodinated compounds which absorb x-rays. This causes the density of organs or vessels that contain the contrast to increase during the radiographic exam. The contrast used for CT is similar to that used for intravenous pyelography (IVP) and angiography. Intravenous contrast used during CT has two main purposes:

- Vascular enhancement: The enhancement of vessels allow them to be more easily differentiated from adjacent, non-enhancing structures or masses.

- Organ enhancement: Organs such as the liver, pancreas, and kidney will enhance more than tumors in those organs and this makes the tumors easier to identify.

Oral Contrast

Most CT's of the abdomen and pelvis are also performed with oral contrast. This usually consists of a dilute barium solution. Depending

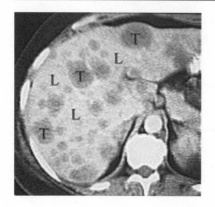

Figure 10.1. In the CT of the liver the multiple liver tumors (T) are easily seen because they enhance less than the surrounding normal liver (L).

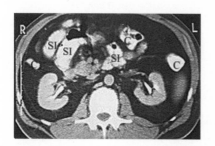

Figure 10.2. This CT of the abdomen shows oral contrast in the small intestine (SI) and colon(C).

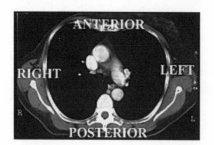

Figure 10.3. This chest CT displays the correct locations on the patient. Anterior refers to the front of the patient, posterior refers to the back.

on the exam, the patient will drink 1 or 2 bottles of the contrast before the study begins. The oral contrast markedly increases the density of the gastrointestinal tract and allows improved differentiation between bowel and tumors, enlarged lymph nodes, and abscesses.

Image Orientation

Most CT's are displayed in the axial, or transverse plane. Imagine the patient is lying on their back, and then sliced by a guillotine. The slice is then viewed as if you are standing at their feet, looking up towards the head.

CT of the Abdomen

The development of Computed Tomography (CT) markedly altered the traditional medical approach to the diagnosis of disorders of the abdomen. CT permitted visualization of the abdominal organs with clarity that had been unimaginable in the past and which has not been surpassed since. This non-invasive test now provides such high resolution and accurate images that "exploratory" surgery is now only very rarely performed. CT now plays a critical role in the diagnosis and management of a wide variety of patients throughout the hospital, including the oncology units, the medical and surgical floors, and the emergency room. The ease of CT also allows patients to undergo extensive diagnostic evaluations without requiring hospitalization. CT of the abdomen also permits evaluation of multiple organ systems with a single test, including the liver and biliary tree, spleen, pancreas, adrenal glands, kidneys, vascular and lymphatic structures, and abdominal cavity.

Liver CT

The liver is the largest organ in the human body. It is responsible for multiple metabolic processes, including synthesis of organic compounds, energy generation and storage, and disposal of toxic substances and waste products. Although relatively insensitive for the detection of diffuse hepatic abnormalities (the term "hepatic" means "relating to the liver") such as hepatitis and cirrhosis, CT is the imaging modality of choice for the detection of tumors and other space-occupying lesions in the liver.

Liver metastases (tumors arising in other organs that have spread to the liver) are found in 25-50% of all cancer patients at autopsy. The

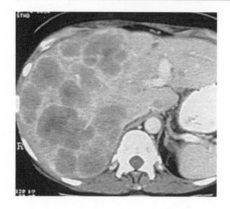

Figure 10.4. Colon Carcinoma Lesions

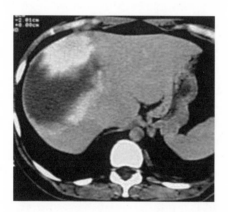

Figure 10.5. Cavernous Hemangioma Initial Study

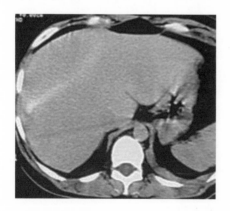

Figure 10.6. Cavernous Hemangioma Delayed Image

most common sites of origin are malignancies of the colon, lung, breast, and pancreas. On an unenhanced CT scan, the density of hepatic metastases can be very similar to the adjacent liver tissue and the lesions can be difficult to detect. Intravenous contrast helps to increase the density differences between the tumor and the normal liver. Although the liver receives 75% of its blood supply from the portal venous system, and 25% form the hepatic artery, most hepatic metastases are supplied by the hepatic arterial circulation. Therefore, following a rapid injection of intravenous contrast, the normal liver will enhance to a greater degree than the metastases and the metastatic lesions will stand out as darker, low density abnormalities. However, some metastases have relatively increased blood flow (renal cell carcinoma, islet cell tumors, melanoma, some breast malignancies) and appear as higher density lesions. One of the advantages of spiral CT is that its speed permits imaging of the liver during both the hepatic arterial and parenchymal phases of contrast enhancement, which improves detection of both types of metastases.

Liver metastases can have a wide variety of sizes and appearances. The lesions in the patient with colon carcinoma are fairly large.

Cavernous hemangioma is the most common benign (non-cancerous) liver tumor. The tumor consists primarily of large vascular channels filled with slow-flowing venous blood. Although patients can very rarely present with abdominal pain, a palpable abdominal mass, or intra-abdominal hemorrhage, this usually only occurs with very large lesions. The vast majority of hemangiomata are discovered incidentally when CT or ultrasound of the abdomen is performed in search of other disease processes. The main significance of these lesions is the need to distinguish them from cancerous liver tumors.

Figures 10.5 and 10.6 illustrate a case that demonstrates the typical CT appearance of a cavernous hemangioma. The initial study obtained after a rapid injection of intravenous contrast (Figure 10.5) demonstrates a large, low density mass with thick peripheral enhancement in the right lobe of the liver. On the delayed image (Figure 10.6), the slow-flowing vascular channels in the tumor have filled with contrast and the tumor becomes almost identical in density to the surrounding liver.

Liver cysts, which are very common, are frequently discovered during CT or ultrasound of the abdomen. They are benign and are of clinical significance only if they become very large and cause symptoms relating to their size. As with cavernous hemangiomata of the liver, their main significance is the need to distinguish them from liver tumors, especially cystic liver metastases.

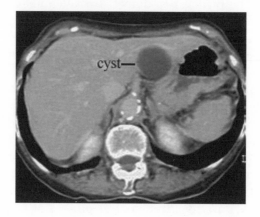

Figure 10.7. *This case shows the usual appearance of a simple hepatic cyst.*

The hepatic cyst is well-defined, with smooth, imperceptible walls and no enhancement. The contents of the cyst are low density, similar to water. Occasionally, differentiation from a cystic tumor can be difficult on CT, and ultrasound or MR can be used for further characterization.

—Steven H. Brick, M.D.

Chapter 11

Cancer Tumor Markers

Tumor markers are substances that can often be detected in higher-than-normal amounts in the blood, urine, or body tissues of some patients with certain types of cancer. Tumor markers are produced either by the tumor itself or by the body in response to the presence of cancer or certain benign (noncancerous) conditions. This chapter describes some tumor markers found in the blood.

Measurements of tumor marker levels can be useful—when used along with x-rays or other tests—in the detection and diagnosis of some types of cancer. However, measurements of tumor marker levels alone are not sufficient to diagnose cancer for the following reasons:

- Tumor marker levels can be elevated in people with benign conditions.

- Tumor marker levels are not elevated in every person with cancer—especially in the early stages of the disease.

- Many tumor markers are not specific to a particular type of cancer; the level of a tumor marker can be raised by more than one type of cancer.

In addition to their role in cancer diagnosis, some tumor marker levels are measured before treatment to help doctors plan appropriate therapy. In some types of cancer, tumor marker levels reflect the

Cancer Facts–Screening, National Cancer Institute (NCI) April 1998.

extent (stage) of the disease and can be useful in predicting how well the disease will respond to treatment. Tumor marker levels may also be measured during treatment to monitor a patient's response to treatment. A decrease or return to normal in the level of a tumor marker may indicate that the cancer has responded favorably to therapy. If the tumor marker level rises, it may indicate that the cancer is growing. Finally, measurements of tumor marker levels may be used after treatment has ended as a part of follow-up care to check for recurrence.

Currently, the main use of tumor markers is to assess a cancer's response to treatment and to check for recurrence. Scientists continue to study these uses of tumor markers as well as their potential role in the early detection and diagnosis of cancer. The patient's doctor can explain the role of tumor markers in detection, diagnosis, or treatment for that person. Described below are some of the most commonly measured tumor markers.

Prostatic Acid Phosphatase

Prostatic acid phosphatase (PAP) is normally present only in small amounts in the blood, but may be found at higher levels in some patients with prostate cancer, especially if the cancer has spread beyond the prostate. However, blood levels may also be elevated in patients who have certain benign prostate conditions or early stage cancer.

Although PAP was originally found to be produced by the prostate, elevated PAP levels have since been associated with testicular cancer, leukemia, and non-Hodgkin's lymphoma, as well as noncancerous conditions such as Gaucher's disease, Paget's disease, osteoporosis, cirrhosis of the liver, pulmonary embolism, and hyperparathyroidism.

CA 125

CA 125 is produced by a variety of cells, but particularly by ovarian cancer cells. Studies have shown that many women with ovarian cancer have elevated CA 125 levels. CA 125 is used primarily in the management of treatment for ovarian cancer.

In women with ovarian cancer being treated with chemotherapy, a falling CA 125 level generally indicates that the cancer is responding to treatment. Increasing CA 125 levels during or after treatment, on the other hand, may suggest that the cancer is not responding to therapy or that some cancer cells remain in the body. Doctors may also use CA 125 levels to monitor patients for recurrence of ovarian cancer.

Not all women with elevated CA 125 levels have ovarian cancer. CA 125 levels may also be elevated by cancers of the uterus, cervix, pancreas, liver, colon, breast, lung, and digestive tract. Noncancerous conditions that can cause elevated CA 125 levels include endometriosis, pelvic inflammatory disease, peritonitis, pancreatitis, liver disease, and any condition that inflames the pleura (the tissue that surrounds the lungs and lines the chest cavity). Menstruation and pregnancy can also cause an increase in CA 125.

Carcinoembryonic Antigen

Carcinoembryonic antigen (CEA) is normally found in small amounts in the blood of most healthy people, but may become elevated in people who have cancer or some benign conditions. The primary use of CEA is in monitoring colorectal cancer, especially when the disease has spread (metastasized). CEA is also used after treatment to check for recurrence of colorectal cancer. However, a wide variety of other cancers can produce elevated levels of this tumor marker, including melanoma; lymphoma; and cancers of the breast, lung, pancreas, stomach, cervix, bladder, kidney, thyroid, liver, and ovary.

Elevated CEA levels can also occur in patients with noncancerous conditions, including inflammatory bowel disease, pancreatitis, and liver disease. Tobacco use can also contribute to higher-than-normal levels of CEA.

Alpha-Fetoprotein

Alpha-fetoprotein (AFP) is normally produced by a developing fetus. AFP levels begin to decrease soon after birth and are usually undetectable in the blood of healthy adults (except during pregnancy). An elevated level of AFP strongly suggests the presence of either primary liver cancer or germ cell cancer (cancer that begins in the cells that give rise to eggs or sperm) of the ovary or testicle. Only rarely do patients with other types of cancer (such as stomach cancer) have elevated levels of AFP. Noncancerous conditions that can cause elevated AFP levels include benign liver conditions, such as cirrhosis or hepatitis; ataxia telangiectasia; Wiscott-Aldrich syndrome; and pregnancy.

Human Chorionic Gonadotropin

Human chorionic gonadotropin (HCG) is normally produced by the placenta during pregnancy. In fact, HCG is sometimes used as a pregnancy test because it increases early within the first trimester. It is also used to screen for choriocarcinoma (a rare cancer of the uterus) in women who are at high risk for the disease, and to monitor the treatment of trophoblastic disease (a rare cancer that develops from an abnormally fertilized egg). Elevated HCG levels may also indicate the presence of cancers of the testis, ovary, liver, stomach, pancreas, and lung. Pregnancy and marijuana use can also cause elevated HCG levels.

CA 19-9

Initially found in colorectal cancer patients, CA 19-9 has also been identified in patients with pancreatic, stomach, and bile duct cancer. Researchers have discovered that, in those who have pancreatic cancer, higher levels of CA 19-9 tend to be associated with more advanced disease. Noncancerous conditions that may elevate CA 19-9 levels include gallstones, pancreatitis, cirrhosis of the liver, and cholecystitis.

CA 15-3

CA 15-3 levels are most useful in following the course of treatment in women diagnosed with breast cancer, especially advanced breast cancer. CA 15-3 levels are rarely elevated in women with early stage breast cancer.

Cancers of the ovary, lung, and prostate may also raise CA 15-3 levels. Elevated levels of CA 15-3 may be associated with noncancerous conditions, such as benign breast or ovarian disease, endometriosis, pelvic inflammatory disease, and hepatitis. Pregnancy and lactation can also cause CA 15-3 levels to rise.

CA 27-29

Similar to the CA 15-3 antigen, CA 27-29 is found in the blood of most breast cancer patients. CA 27-29 levels may be used in conjunction with other procedures (such as mammograms and measurements of other tumor marker levels) to check for recurrence in women previously treated for stage II and stage III breast cancer.

CA 27-29 levels can also be elevated by cancers of the colon, stomach, kidney, lung, ovary, pancreas, uterus, and liver. First trimester pregnancy, endometriosis, ovarian cysts, benign breast disease, kidney disease, and liver disease are noncancerous conditions that can also elevate CA 27-29 levels.

Lactate Dehydrogenase

Lactate dehydrogenase is a protein found throughout the body. Nearly every type of cancer, as well as many other diseases, can cause LDH levels to be elevated. Therefore, this marker cannot be used to diagnose a particular type of cancer.

LDH levels can be used to monitor treatment of some cancers, including testicular cancer, Ewing's sarcoma, non-Hodgkin's lymphoma, and some types of leukemia. Elevated LDH levels can be caused by a number of noncancerous conditions, including heart failure, hypothyroidism, anemia, and lung or liver disease.

Neuron-Specific Enolase

Neuron-specific enolase (NSE) has been detected in patients with neuroblastoma; small cell lung cancer; Wilms' tumor; melanoma; and cancers of the thyroid, kidney, testicle, and pancreas. However, studies of NSE as a tumor marker have concentrated primarily on patients with neuroblastoma and small cell lung cancer. Measurement of NSE level in patients with these two diseases can provide information about the extent of the disease and the patient's prognosis, as well as about the patient's response to treatment.

National Cancer Institute Information Resources

You may want more information for yourself, your family, and your doctor. The following National Cancer Institute (NCI) services are available to help you.

Cancer Information Service (CIS)

Provides accurate, up-to-date information on cancer to patients and their families, health professionals, and the general public. Information specialists translate the latest scientific information into understandable language and respond in English, Spanish, or on TTY equipment.

Toll-free: 1-800-4-CANCER (1-800-422-6237)
TTY: 1-800-332-8615

Internet

These web sites may be useful:

95

http://www.nci.nih.gov/—NCI's primary web site; contains information about the Institute and its programs. Also includes news, upcoming events, educational materials, and publications for patients, the public, and the mass media on http://rex.nci.nih.gov/.

http://cancernet.nci.nih.gov/—CancerNet; contains material for health professionals, patients, and the public, including information from PDQ about cancer treatment, screening, prevention, supportive care, and clinical trials, and CANCERLIT, a bibliographic database.

http://cancertrials.nci.nih.gov/—cancerTrials; NCI's comprehensive clinical trials information center for patients, health professionals, and the public. Includes information on understanding trials, deciding whether to participate in trials, finding specific trials, plus research news and other resources.

E-mail: CancerMail

Includes NCI information about cancer treatment, screening, prevention, and supportive care. To obtain a contents list, send e-mail to cancermail@icicc.nci.nih.gov with the word "help" in the body of the message.

Fax: CancerFax

Includes NCI information about cancer treatment, screening, prevention, and supportive care. To obtain a contents list, dial 301-402-5874 from a fax machine hand set and follow the recorded instructions.

Part Three

Liver Distress

Chapter 12

Cirrhosis

What Is Cirrhosis of the Liver?

The liver weighs about 3 pounds and is the largest organ in the body. It is located in the upper-right side of the abdomen, below the ribs. (See Figure 12.1.) When chronic diseases cause the liver to become permanently injured and scarred, the condition is called cirrhosis.

The scar tissue that forms in cirrhosis harms the structure of the liver, blocking the flow of blood through the organ. The loss of normal liver tissue slows the processing of nutrients,

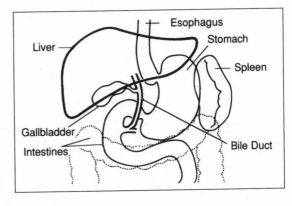

Figure 12.1. Organs of the Digestive System

This chapter contains text from "Cirrhosis: Many Causes," © 1997 reprinted with permission of the American Liver Foundation, 1-800-GO-LIVER, "First Liver Stent Approved," *FDA Consumer* January-February 1996, and "Cirrhosis of the Liver," National Institute of Diabetes and Digestive and Kidney Diseases (NIDDK), NIH Publication No. 98-1134, November 1991, revised 1998.

hormones, drugs, and toxins by the liver. Also slowed is production of proteins and other substances made by the liver.

What Is the Impact of Cirrhosis?

Cirrhosis is the seventh leading cause of death by disease. About 25,000 people die from cirrhosis each year. There also is a great toll in terms of human suffering, hospital costs, and the loss of work by people with cirrhosis.

What Are the Major Causes of Cirrhosis?

Cirrhosis has many causes. In the United States, chronic alcoholism is the most common cause. Cirrhosis also may result from chronic viral hepatitis (types B, C, and D). Liver injury that results in cirrhosis also may be caused by a number of inherited diseases such as cystic fibrosis, alpha-1 antitrypsin deficiency, hemochromatosis, Wilson's disease, galactosemia, and glycogen storage diseases.

Two inherited disorders result in the abnormal storage of metals in the liver leading to tissue damage and cirrhosis. People with Wilson's disease store too much copper in their livers, brains, kidneys, and in the corneas of their eyes. In another disorder, known as hemochromatosis, too much iron is absorbed, and the excess iron is deposited in the liver and in other organs, such as the pancreas, skin, intestinal lining, heart, and endocrine glands.

If a person's bile duct becomes blocked, this also may cause cirrhosis. The bile ducts carry bile formed in the liver to the intestines, where the bile helps in the digestion of fat. In babies, the most common cause of cirrhosis due to blocked bile ducts is a disease called biliary atresia. In this case, the bile ducts are absent or injured, causing the bile to back up in the liver. These babies are jaundiced (their skin is yellowed) after their first month in life. Sometimes they can be helped by surgery in which a new duct is formed to allow bile to drain again from the liver.

In adults, the bile ducts may become inflamed, blocked, and scarred due to another liver disease, primary biliary cirrhosis. Another type of biliary cirrhosis also may occur after a patient has gallbladder surgery in which the bile ducts are injured or tied off.

Other, less common, causes of cirrhosis are severe reactions to prescribed drugs, prolonged exposure to environmental toxins, and repeated bouts of heart failure with liver congestion.

Does Heavy Drinking Always Lead to Cirrhosis?

While almost everyone who drinks excessive amounts of alcohol sustains some liver damage, it does not necessarily develop into cirrhosis. In those individuals who drink one-half to one pint (8 to 16 ounces) of hard liquor per day (or the equivalent in other alcoholic drinks), for 15 years or more, about one-third develop cirrhosis. Another third develop fatty livers, while the remainder have only minor liver problems. In general, the more you drink, the greater the frequency and regularity of excessive intake, the more likely that cirrhosis is to result. A poor diet, long considered to be the main factor in the development of cirrhosis in the alcoholic, is probably only a contributing factor. Alcohol by itself, in large amounts, is a poison that can cause cirrhosis.

Can Social Drinkers Get Cirrhosis?

Some individuals who are "social drinkers," not alcoholics, can develop cirrhosis. Factors affecting the development of cirrhosis include:

- the amount of alcohol consumed
- the regularity of intake
- natural tendency
- perhaps the state of nutrition

It is not known why some individuals are more prone to adverse reactions to alcohol than others. Women are less tolerant of alcohol than men. Researchers believe that this is because men have a greater ability than women to break down the alcohol for elimination. Studies show that a much higher percentage of women, consuming less alcohol than men, go on to cirrhosis.

Does Hepatitis Always Result in Cirrhosis?

Some patients with chronic viral hepatitis develop cirrhosis. There are five known types of viral hepatitis, each caused by a different virus.

- Acute hepatitis A and acute hepatitis E do not lead to chronic hepatitis.

- Acute hepatitis B leads to chronic infection in approximately 5% of adult patients. In a few of these patients, the chronic hepatitis B progresses to cirrhosis.

- Acute hepatitis D infects individuals already infected by hepatitis B.

- Acute hepatitis C becomes chronic in approximately 80% of adults. A minority of these patients (20-30%) will progress to cirrhosis, typically over many years.

What Are the Symptoms of Cirrhosis?

People with cirrhosis often have few symptoms at first. The two major problems that eventually cause symptoms are loss of functioning liver cells and distortion of the liver caused by scarring. The person may experience fatigue, weakness, and exhaustion. Loss of appetite is usual, often with nausea and weight loss.

As liver function declines, less protein is made by the organ. For example, less of the protein albumin is made, which results in water accumulating in the legs (edema) or abdomen (ascites). A decrease in proteins needed for blood clotting makes it easy for the person to bruise or to bleed.

In the later stages of cirrhosis, jaundice (yellow skin) may occur, caused by the buildup of bile pigment that is passed by the liver into the intestines. Some people with cirrhosis experience intense itching due to bile products that are deposited in the skin. Gallstones often form in persons with cirrhosis because not enough bile reaches the gallbladder.

The liver of a person with cirrhosis also has trouble removing toxins, which may build up in the blood. These toxins can dull mental function and lead to personality changes and even coma (encephalopathy). Early signs of toxin accumulation in the brain may include neglect of personal appearance, unresponsiveness, forgetfulness, trouble concentrating, or changes in sleeping habits.

Drugs taken usually are filtered out by the liver, and this cleansing process also is slowed down by cirrhosis. The liver does not remove the drugs from the blood at the usual rate, so the drugs act longer than expected, building up in the body. People with cirrhosis often are very sensitive to medications and their side effects.

A serious problem for people with cirrhosis is pressure on blood vessels that flow through the liver. Normally, blood from the intestines and spleen is pumped to the liver through the portal vein (see Figure 12.2). But in cirrhosis, this normal flow of blood is slowed, building pressure in the portal vein (portal hypertension). This blocks the normal flow of blood, causing the spleen to enlarge. So blood from the intestines tries to find a way around the liver through new vessels.

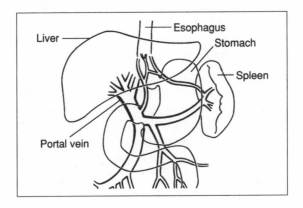

Figure 12.2. *Normal Blood Flow to Liver*

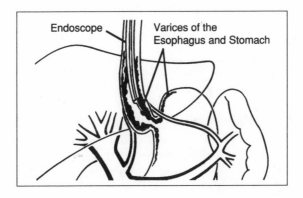

Figure 12.3. *Varices: New Blood Vessels. They have thin walls and carry high pressure.*

Some of these new blood vessels become quite large and are called varices (see Figure 12.3). These vessels may form in the stomach and esophagus (the tube that connects the mouth with the stomach). They have thin walls and carry high pressure. There is great danger that they may break, causing a serious bleeding problem in the upper stomach or esophagus. If this happens, the patient's life is in danger, and the doctor must act quickly to stop the bleeding.

The first implantable liver stent was approved by the Food and Drug Administration (FDA) in September 1995 for preventing recurrent bleeding from esophageal veins in people with cirrhosis. The Wallstent TIPS Endoprosthesis is a flexible metal stent that is threaded into the liver by a catheter through a neck vein. The stent then expands and remains in place so that the blood bypasses circulation through the scarred liver, relieving blood pressure in the liver. If untreated, this pressure can cause bleeding from veins in the esophagus and could result in death.

In a clinical study of 97 patients at eight sites in the United States, the stent successfully diverted blood from the liver in all but one patient. Patients in the study had a significant improvement in survival over that reported with abdominal surgery, and less bleeding after treatment than that reported with alternative medical treatment.

In 1994, liver disease caused more than 119,500 U.S. hospitalizations for conditions including chronic hepatitis and cirrhosis of the liver. An estimated 8,000 to 10,000 patients in the United States may benefit from the stent. It is manufactured by Schneider USA Inc. of Plymouth, Minnesota.

How Is Cirrhosis Diagnosed?

The doctor often can diagnose cirrhosis from the patient's symptoms and from laboratory tests. During a physical exam, for instance, the doctor could notice a change in how your liver feels or how large it is. If the doctor suspects cirrhosis, you will be given blood tests. The purpose of these tests is to find out if liver disease is present. In some cases, other tests that take pictures of the liver are performed such as the computerized axial tomography (CAT) scan, ultrasound, and the radioisotope liver/spleen scan.

The doctor may decide to confirm the diagnosis by putting a needle through the skin (biopsy) to take a sample of tissue from the liver. In some cases, cirrhosis is diagnosed during surgery when the doctor is able to see the entire liver. The liver also can be inspected through a laparoscope, a viewing device that is inserted through a tiny incision in the abdomen.

What Are the Treatments for Cirrhosis?

Treatment of cirrhosis is aimed at stopping or delaying its progress, minimizing the damage to liver cells, and reducing complications. In alcoholic cirrhosis, for instance, the person must stop drinking alcohol to halt progression of the disease. If a person has hepatitis, the doctor may administer steroids or antiviral drugs to reduce liver cell injury.

Medications may be given to control the symptoms of cirrhosis, such as itching. Edema and ascites (fluid retention) are treated by reducing salt in the diet. Drugs called diuretics are used to remove excess fluid and to prevent edema from recurring. Diet and drug therapies can help to improve the altered mental function that cirrhosis can cause. For instance, decreasing dietary protein results in less toxin formation in the digestive tract. Laxatives such as lactulose may be given to help absorb toxins and speed their removal from the intestines.

The two main problems in cirrhosis are liver failure, when liver cells stop working, and the bleeding caused by portal hypertension. The doctor may prescribe blood pressure medication, such as a beta blocker, to treat the portal hypertension. If the patient bleeds from the varices of the stomach or esophagus, the doctor can inject these veins with a sclerosing agent administered through a flexible tube (endoscope) that is inserted through the mouth and esophagus. In critical cases, the patient may be given a liver transplant or another surgery (such as a portacaval shunt) that is sometimes used to relieve the pressure in the portal vein and varices.

Patients with cirrhosis often live healthy lives for many years. Even when complications develop, they usually can be treated. Many patients with cirrhosis have undergone successful liver transplantation.

How Can I Avoid Cirrhosis?

1. **Do not drink to excess.** Avoid the use of alcoholic beverages. Alcohol destroys liver cells. How well damaged cells regenerate varies with each individual. Prior injury to the liver by unknown and unrecognized viruses or chemicals can also affect the regeneration process.

2. **Take precautions when using man-made chemicals.**
The liver must process many chemicals that were not present
in the past. More research is needed to determine the effects on the liver of many of these compounds. When using
chemicals at work, in cleaning your home or working in
your garden:

- be sure there is good ventilation
- follow directions for use of all products
- never mix chemical products
- avoid getting chemicals on the skin, where they can be absorbed, and wash promptly if you do
- avoid inhaling chemicals
- wear protective clothing

3. **Seek medical advice.** Remain under supervision of a physician if you develop viral hepatitis until your recovery is as-
sured.

How Might Cirrhosis Affect Other Diseases I Might Have or Treatment of Them?

The responsibility of the liver for the proper functioning of the
whole body is so great that the chronic disease of the liver may modify
the body's responses to a variety of illnesses. Abnormal function of
the liver in cirrhosis may:

- affect the dose of medicine required in the treatment of other
conditions
- affect the treatment of diabetes
- alter response of the body to infection
- alter tolerance for surgical procedures

Patients with cirrhosis are particularly prone to develop fatal bacterial infections, kidney malfunctions, stomach ulcers, gallstones, a type
of diabetes, and cancer of the liver.

What Are My Prospects for Reasonable Health and Sur-
vival with Treatment?

**Treatment at this stage, with proper adherence to the phy-
sician's recommendations**, leads to improvement in the majority

of cases and the patient is able to pursue a normal life and activities.

When cirrhosis is not discovered until extensive damage has resulted, the outlook may be less favorable for improvement, and complications such as ascites and hemorrhage are more likely to be encountered.

The liver is a large organ and is able to perform its vital functions despite some damage. It also has the ability to repair itself to a limited degree. Cells that die are replaced by new cells. If the cause of cirrhosis can be removed, these factors provide hope for both improvement and carrying on a normal life.

An increasing number of scientific investigators conducting liver research give hope for new breakthroughs in treatment, management and cures for liver diseases in the foreseeable future.

Additional Readings

Biliary Atresia

This brochure presents information on biliary atresia and cirrhosis, including discussions of diagnosis, treatment, and complications. Available from the

American Liver Foundation.
75 Maiden Lane, Suite 603
New York, NY 10038
800-465-4837 (GO-LIVER)
Fax: 212-483-8179
E-mail: webmail@liverfoundation.org
URL: http://www.liverfoundation.org

Cirrhosis

This fact sheet presents general information on cirrhosis of the liver, research, and the work of the American Liver Foundation. Available from the foundation.

Clayman CB, ed. *The American Medical Association Encyclopedia of Medicine*, New York: Random House. 1989. Authoritative reference guide for patients, with sections on cirrhosis, hepatitis, and other disorders affecting the liver. Widely available in libraries and bookstores.

Primary Biliary Cirrhosis

This fact sheet presents information on PBC and cirrhosis, including discussions of diagnosis, treatment, and liver transplantation. Available from the American Liver Foundation.

Rosenfeld I. *Second Opinion: Your Comprehensive Guide to Treatment*, New York: Bantam Books, 1988. General medical guide with sections on cirrhosis and other disorders affecting the liver. Widely available in libraries and bookstores.

Resources

American Liver Foundation
75 Maiden Lane, Suite 603
New York, NY 10038
800-456-4837 (GO-LIVER)
Fax: 212-483-8179
E-mail: webmail@liverfoundation.org
URL: http://www.liverfoundation.org

United Network for Organ Sharing
1100 Boulders Parkway, Suite 500
P.O. Box 13770
Richmond, VA 23225-8770
888-894-6361
URL: http://www.unos.org/frame_Default.asp

National Digestive Diseases Information Clearinghouse
2 Information Way
Bethesda, MD 20892-3570
E-mail: nddic@info.niddk.nih.gov

Chapter 13

Infectious Agents and Parasites

Alveolar Hydatid Disease (AHD)

AHD (al-VEE-oh-ler HIGH-dad-id) disease results from being infected with the larval stage of *Echinococcus multilocularis*, a microscopic tapeworm (1-4 millimeters) found in foxes, coyotes, dogs, and cats. Although human cases are rare, infection in humans causes parasitic tumors to form in the liver, and, less commonly, the lungs, brain, and other organs. If left untreated, infection with AHD can be fatal.

Where Has AHD Been Found?

AHD is found worldwide, mostly in northern latitudes. Cases have been reported in central Europe, Russia, China, Central Asia, Japan, and North America. In North America E. multilocularis is found primarily in the north central region from eastern Montana to central Ohio, as well as Alaska and Canada. Human cases have been reported in Alaska, the province of Manitoba, and Minnesota. Prevalence among wild foxes and coyotes is high, and may reach over 50% in some areas; however, even in these areas, transmission to humans has been low.

This chapter contains text from the following National Center for Infectious Diseases (NCID) documents: "Infectious Agents That Cause or Contribute to Neoplastic Diseases in Humans," November 1998; "Amebiasis Infection" and "Alveolar Hydatid Disease (Echinococcosis)," September 1998; and "Schistosomiasis: Fact Sheet," May 1998.

109

How Does Infection Occur in Foxes, Coyotes, Dogs, and Other Cats?

Wild foxes, coyotes, and cats get infected when they eat *Echinococcus multilocularis* larvae in infected rodents, field mice, or voles. Cats are less susceptible than dogs, but because they probably catch and eat rodents more often, may also become infected. Once the animal becomes infected, the tapeworm matures in its intestine, lays eggs, and the infected animal passes eggs in the stool. These tapeworm eggs, which are directly infectious to other animals, are too tiny to see, and will stick to anything with which they come in contact. Coyotes, foxes, dogs, and cats are not harmed by the tapeworm and do not have symptoms of AHD.

Table 13.1 Infectious Agents That Cause or Contribute to Neoplastic Diseases in Humans

Infectious Agent	Disease
Epstein-Barr virus	Nasopharyngeal carcinoma (undifferentiated) Burkitts's lymphoma Posttransplant lymphoproliferative disease, B-cell lymphoma
Helicobacter pylori	Gastric carcinoma, Mucosa-associated lymphoid tissue lymphoma
Hepatitis B virus	Hepatocellular carcinoma
Hepatitis C virus	Hepatocellar carcinoma
Human herpesvirus-8	Kaposi's sarcoma
Human innumodeficiency virus	Lymphoma
Human papillomavirus	Cervical carcinoma
Human T-cell leukemia virus	Adult T-cell leukemia
Liver flukes	Cholangiocarcinoma
Schistosoma haematobium	Bladder carcinoma

Can Animals Be Tested for E. Multilocularis Tapeworms?

Routine fecal examinations are not sufficient to diagnose *E. multilocularis* infection. Infection with the *E. multilocularis* tapeworm and other tapeworms may occur at the same time. Eggs of the Taenia tapeworm and *E. multilocularis* are similar in shape and size and are very difficult to tell apart. If you live in an area where this parasite occurs or you are concerned about your dog or cat being infected with *E. multilocularis* or other tapeworms, see your vet who can answer your questions and assess the risk of possible infection.

How Can I Be Infected with AHD?

By accidentally swallowing the eggs of the *E. multilocularis* tapeworm. Humans can be exposed to these eggs in two main ways, both of which involve "hand-to-mouth" transfer or contamination:

- By directly ingesting food items contaminated with stool from foxes or coyotes. This might include grass, herbs, greens, or berries gathered from fields.

- By petting or handling household cats and dogs infected with the *E. multilocularis* tapeworm. These pets may shed the tapeworm eggs in their stool, and their fur may be contaminated. Some dogs "scent roll" in foreign material (such as wild animal feces) and may become contaminated this way.

How Likely Am I to Contract AHD?

For 50 years, *E. multilocularis* was confined to the Alaskan coast and Canada. Now, because wild coyotes, foxes, and wolves are being trapped and transported to states where *E. multilocularis* has not previously been found, there is increased risk of spreading the disease to animals and humans. Wild animals carrying the tapeworm could set up the transmission cycle and expose animals not already infected. Many states prohibit this movement of wild animals, but trapping and movement of infected wild canines still occurs. If the transportation and relocation of these animals continues, the risk of human transmission will increase. Although the chances of contracting AHD are low, certain groups may be at greater risk.

You may be at greater risk if you live in an area where AHD is found (see above). People at high risk include trappers, hunters, vets, or others who contact wild foxes, coyotes, or their stool, or household

111

cats and dogs that have the opportunity to eat wild rodents infected with AHD.

What Are the Symptoms of AHD?

AHD is caused by tumor-like or cyst-like tapeworm larvae growing in the body. AHD usually involves the liver, but can spread to other organs of the body. Because the cysts are slow-growing, infection with AHD may not produce any symptoms for many years. Pain or discomfort in the upper abdominal region, weakness, and weight loss may occur as a result of the growing cysts. Symptoms may mimic those of liver cancer and cirrhosis of the liver.

How Can I Find Out if I Have AHD?

See your health care provider if you think you may have been exposed to AHD by one of the ways listed above. He or she can order a blood test for the presence of the parasite or antibodies to *E. multilocularis*.

What Is the Treatment for AHD?

Surgery is the most common form of treatment for AHD, although removal of the cyst is not usually 100 % effective. After surgery, medication may be necessary to keep the cyst from growing back.

How Can I Prevent AHD?

If you live in an area where *E. multilocularis* is found in rodents and wild canines, take the following precautions to avoid infection:

- Don't touch a fox, coyote, or other wild canine, dead or alive, unless you are wearing gloves. Hunters and trappers should use plastic gloves to avoid exposure.

- Don't keep wild animals, especially wild canines, as pets or encourage them to come close to your home.

- Don't allow your cats and dogs to wander freely or to capture and eat rodents.

- If you think that your pet may have eaten rodents, consult your veterinarian about the possible need for preventive treatments.

- After handling pets, always wash your hands with soap and warm water.

- Fence in gardens to keep out wild animals.

- Do not collect or eat wild fruits or vegetables picked directly from the ground. All wild-picked foods should be washed carefully or cooked before eating.

For More Information:

1. Hildreth MB, Johnson MD, Kazacos KR. *Echinococcus multilocularis*: a zoonosis of increasing concern in the United States. *Supplement to the Compendium of Continuing Education for the Practicing Veterinarian* 1991;13: 727-741.

2. Leiby PD, Kritsky DC. *Echinococcus multilocularis*: a possible domestic life cycle in central North America and its public health implications. *J Parasitol* 1972;58: 1213-1215.

3. Schantz PM, Chai J, Craig PS, Eckert J, Jenkins DJ, Macpherson CNL, Thakur A. *Epidemiology and Control*. In: Echinococcosis and Hydatid Disease, R.C.A. Thompson and A.J. Lymbery, eds., London, CAB International, 233-331.

4. Stehr-Green JK, Stehr-Green PA, Schantz PM, Wilson JF, Lanier A. Risk factors for infection with *Echinococcus multilocularis* in Alaska. *Am J Trop Med Hyg* 1988;38: 380-385.

5. WHO. Guidelines for treatment of cystic and alveolar echinococcosis in humans. Bull World Health Organization 1996;74: 231-242.

6. Wilson JF, Rausch RL. Alveolar hydatid disease: a review of clinical features of 33 indigenous cases of *Echinococcus multilocularis* infection in Alaskan Eskimos. *Am J Trop Med Hyg* 1980;29: 1340-1355.

Schistosomiasis (shis-to-so-mi'-uh-sis)

Schistosomiasis (also known as "bilharzia") is a disease caused by parasitic worms. The major types that cause schistosomiasis in humans are *Schistosoma mansoni, S. haematobium*, and *S. japonicum*. The body's reaction to the eggs produced by these worms, and not the worms themselves, causes the symptoms of schistosomiasis. The disease is treatable.

How Is Schistosomiasis Spread?

Persons get schistosomiasis when their skin comes in contact with contaminated fresh water in which certain types of snails are living. Fresh water becomes contaminated by Schistosoma eggs when infected people urinate or defecate in the water. The eggs hatch, and if certain types of snails are present in the water, the parasites grow and develop within the snails. When the parasites leave the snail, they can survive in water for about 48 hours. The parasites penetrate the skin of persons who have contact with this water, such as when they are wading, swimming, bathing, or washing. The parasites penetrate the skin, and, within several weeks, grow inside the blood vessels of the body and produce eggs. Some of these eggs get into the urinary bladder or intestines and are passed into the urine or feces.

What Are the Symptoms of Schistosomiasis?

Within days after becoming infected, some people have a rash or itchy skin, and within a month or two, they may have fever, chills, cough, and muscle aches. Most people, however, have no symptoms at all in this early phase after infection. Usually the eggs of the parasite go to the liver or pass into the intestine or urinary bladder. Rarely, eggs are found in the brain or spinal cord and cause seizures, paralysis, or spinal cord inflammation. After many years of repeated infection, the parasite can damage the liver, intestines, lungs, or urinary bladder. Even without treatment, damage to these organs occurs only rarely in people such as travelers who have relatively short periods of exposure and who avoid reinfection.

Who Is at Risk?

Persons who live in or travel to areas where schistosomiasis occurs and who have skin contact with fresh water (rivers, streams, or lakes) are at risk of getting schistosomiasis. Areas of the world with schistosomiasis include Africa, some countries in Latin America (Brazil, Venezuela, and Surinam), parts of the Caribbean (Saint Lucia, Antigua, Montserrat, Martinique, Guadeloupe, the Dominican Republic, and Puerto Rico), some countries in the Middle East, southern China, the Philippines, and Southeast Asia. In the last few years, CDC has received reports of schistosomiasis in U.S. citizens who went on river rafting trips in Africa, tourists who swam in contaminated waters, and Peace Corps volunteers and other persons who lived and had fresh water contact in areas where schistosomiasis is a problem.

How Can You Prevent Schistosomiasis?

Because there is no easy way to know if water is contaminated, avoid swimming or wading in fresh water when you are in countries where schistosomiasis is known to occur. Swimming in the ocean and in chlorinated swimming pools is generally thought to be safe.

Research is under way to develop a vaccine for humans, but none is available now.

What Should You Do if You Suspect that You Have Schistosomiasis?

See your health care provider. Be sure to give a complete description of the time, place, and length of your exposure to fresh water while in parts of the world where schistosomiasis occurs. You might be asked to undergo stool or urine tests to detect the eggs of the parasite. A blood test developed at CDC is also available. This test may be useful for making the diagnosis, particularly in U.S. travelers returning from areas where schistosomiasis occurs.

What Is the Treatment for Schistosomiasis?

Safe and effective drugs are available for treatment of schistosomiasis. You will be given pills to take for 1-2 days.

For More Information on Schistosomiasis:

CDC. Schistosomiasis in Peace Corps volunteers—Malawi, *MMWR* 1993;42:565-70.

Jordan P. Schistosomiasis. The St. Lucia Project. New York: *Cambridge University Press,* 1985.

Jordan P, Webbe G, Sturrock RF, editors. Human schistosomiasis. Wallingford: *CAB International,* 1993.

Rollinson D. Simpson AJG, editors. The biology of schistosomes from genes to latrines. London: *Academic Press,* 1987.

Tsang VCW, Wilkins PP. Immunodiagnosis of schistosomiasis. Screen with FAST-ELISA and confirm with immunoblot. *Clin Lab Med* 1991;11:1029-39.

World Health Organization. The control of schistosomiasis: Second report of the WHO Expert Committee. *WHO Technical Report Series* 830. Geneva: WHO, 1993.

Amebiasis (Entamoeba Histolytica) Infection

Amebiasis is a disease caused by a one-celled parasite called *Entamoeba histolytica* (ent-a-ME-ba hiss-toe-LI-ti-ka). This parasite is found in the United States and around the world.

What Are the Symptoms of Amebiasis?

Most people who are infected with *E. histolytica* do not become ill or develop only mild intestinal symptoms, which can include abdominal tenderness or discomfort, loose or watery stools, and stomach cramping. Other infectious organisms, such as other parasites or bacteria, can cause similar symptoms.

Amebic dysentery is a severe form of amebiasis associated with stomach pain, bloody stools, and fever. Rarely, *E. histolytica* spreads outside the intestines to the liver and forms an abscess. Even less commonly, it spreads to other parts of the body, such as the lungs or brain.

How Soon After Exposure Do Symptoms of Amebiasis Appear?

Usually 1-4 weeks, but it can be shorter or longer.

How Can I Get Amebiasis?

- By putting anything into your mouth that has touched the stool of a person infected with *E. histolytica*.

- By swallowing something, such as water or food contaminated with *E. histolytica*.

- By touching and bringing to your mouth cysts picked up from surfaces contaminated with *E. histolytica*.

Who Is at Risk for Amebiasis?

Although anyone can get amebiasis, it is most common in people who live in developing countries that have poor sanitary conditions. In the United States, the disease is most often seen in immigrants from developing countries; men who have sex with men; and people who live in institutions that have poor sanitary conditions.

What Should I Do if I Think I Have Amebiasis?

See your health care provider.

How Is Amebiasis Diagnosed?

Your health care provider will ask you to submit stool samples. Because *E. histolytica* can be difficult to diagnose, your health care provider may ask you to submit several stool specimens taken over several days.

A blood test is available, but is only recommended if your health care provider thinks that infection has invaded the wall of the intestines or some other organ of the body, such as the liver. A blood test may be positive if you have had an amebic infection in the past.

How Is Amebiasis Treated?

Several antibiotics are available to treat amebiasis. Treatment must be prescribed by a physician and may require more than one kind of medication.

How Can Amebiasis Be Prevented During Travel in Developing Countries?

• Drink only bottled water, carbonated water, canned or bottled sodas. Boiling water for 1 minute will kill parasites, bacteria, or viruses that may be present. *E. histolytica* is not killed by low doses of chlorine or iodine; do not rely on chemical water purification tablets, such as halide tablets to prevent amebiasis.

• Food should be cooked thoroughly to kill parasites, bacteria, or viruses that may be present. If you plan to eat raw vegetables that may be contaminated, they should first be washed with a strong detergent soap and then soaked in vinegar for 10-15 minutes.

• Do not eat fruit that already has been peeled or cut. Drink only pasteurized milk or dairy products. Avoid eating dairy products or drinking raw milk. They can be contaminated with unclean water.

Should I Be Concerned about Spreading Infection to the Rest of My Household?

No. If the infected person practices adequate personal hygiene, including thorough hand washing with soap and warm water after using the toilet and before handling food, there is little risk of spreading infection.

Chapter 14

Pregnancy and the Liver

How Does Pregnancy Affect the Liver? Are There Changes in Liver Function?

Pregnancy has little effect on a normal liver. There are no significant changes in liver function; however, certain markers of liver function may alter slightly during normal pregnancy. For example, blood levels of the protein albumin will decrease during pregnancy because of dilution of the expectant mother's blood. In addition, the blood test for alkaline phosphatase, usually taken as an indicator of liver disease, will increase during normal pregnancy because of production of this marker by a normal placenta. This small change does not indicate liver disease.

At What Stage of Fetal Development Does a Liver Start Functioning? What Are the Stages of Development for the Child's Liver?

The liver first appears in a developing fetus as early as the third week of pregnancy, although liver function probably does not begin until the sixth to tenth week of pregnancy. Liver function continues to develop over the remainder of pregnancy, but the liver's ability to handle such compounds as bilirubin and bile acids is still not fully mature even at the time of birth. Adult-level liver function probably

Reprinted with permission of the American Liver Foundation, 1-800-GO-LIVER, © 1997.

119

develops by six to twelve months of age. During childhood, liver function is essentially that of the normal adult, except that the liver is appropriately smaller in the young child compared to an adult.

Should Pregnant Women Be Tested for Hepatitis B and C?

It is now recommended that all pregnant women be tested during the last two to three months of pregnancy for the presence of the hepatitis B virus. Babies born to women carrying the hepatitis B virus are at considerable risk of contracting hepatitis B immediately after delivery.

To identify pregnant hepatitis B carriers in time to protect their babies, the U.S. Centers for Disease Control and Prevention (CDC) recommend routine screening of all pregnant women, plus women who have histories of:

- acute or chronic liver disease;

- work or treatment in a kidney dialysis unit;

- work or residence in an institution for the mentally challenged;

- rejection as a blood donor;

- blood transfusions;

- frequent occupational exposure to blood;

- household contact with a hepatitis B carrier or any patient undergoing kidney dialysis;

- multiple episodes of venereal disease;

- intravenous drug abuse.

In general, the baby does not contract hepatitis B in the womb. The placenta usually bars the virus. Transmission does occur through the placenta in about 6% of the cases. The baby usually first encounters the virus upon entering the birth canal. Virus in the blood and vaginal fluids of the mother readily exposes the baby to the disease. All close contact with the mother following birth exposes the baby to virus in the mother's body fluids; saliva, blood, and in the case of nursing infants, breast milk. Prompt administration of hepatitis B immune globulin and hepatitis B vaccine has been shown to effectively protect most babies of hepatitis B carrier mothers.

Estimated number of hepatitis B carriers in U.S. pregnant population:

- Each year in the U.S., an estimated 3,500,000 women give birth. About 250,000 of them are in high-risk groups. Experts estimate that up to 22,000 women who give birth each year are carriers of hepatitis B. Thousands of these women don't know they are carriers. Up to 90% could transmit the virus to their children. Vaccination of the newborns would prevent them from being carriers.

- The CDC currently recommends routine hepatitis B screening of pregnant women, along with the routine screening for German measles and syphilis.

Babies born to women carrying the hepatitis C virus are very unlikely to contract hepatitis C, although transmission can occur. There is no specific preventive treatment available. Therefore, currently, there are no recommendations to test women for hepatitis C.

Should Babies Be Vaccinated for Hepatitis B?

If the mother does not carry the hepatitis B virus but other family members do, then babies and young children should probably be vaccinated as early as possible. It is now recommended that all children ultimately receive vaccination against hepatitis B as well, since it is a preventable infection that may occur at any time.

Can Women Who Are Infected with Viral Hepatitis Become Pregnant?

Yes, especially if their liver has not been seriously damaged.

Can Mothers Who Are Infected with Hepatitis B or C Breast-feed Their Babies?

Mothers who are infected with hepatitis B may breast-feed their babies, especially if the babies have received appropriate vaccination. It is not known whether the hepatitis C virus can be transmitted in breast milk. This, however, seems to be a low risk.

Can a Nursing Mother Take Interferon, the Drug for Hepatitis B or C, or Will It Harm the Baby?

A nursing mother may take interferon for hepatitis B or C. It is not known, however, whether the interferon will have any effects on the nursing baby. Because interferon treatment of chronic hepatitis B or C is elective, it would probably be wise to give a mother interferon either before she becomes pregnant or after she has finished nursing.

Can a Woman with Autoimmune Hepatitis Become Pregnant and Give Birth to a Healthy Baby?

Yes. However, if the autoimmune hepatitis is active, women are much less fertile and are likely to have many complications during pregnancy. Thus, it is recommended that women with autoimmune hepatitis first receive appropriate treatment to obtain control of their disease before they become pregnant. They are frequently treated with prednisone, an anti-inflammatory drug that depresses the immune system, which is considered to be safe during pregnancy. Women with uncontrolled serious autoimmune hepatitis and those who have already developed cirrhosis from autoimmune hepatitis may experience complications of liver disease during pregnancy, and their babies are at higher risk of premature delivery and fetal death. Those babies who are born, however, are normal.

Women with autoimmune hepatitis who require continued use of prednisone to maintain remission may well be able to become pregnant and carry a fetus to term. However, they should continue use of prednisone during pregnancy as the disease may flare up.

Why Do Some Pregnant Women Experience Itching and Jaundice?

During pregnancy some women experience the onset of itching (pruritis) and jaundice, usually related to an impaired bile flow. It arises because of changes in the liver's ability to handle chemicals called bile acids and bilirubin, and to make bile, probably from the effects of large doses of the hormone estrogen (which normally increases during pregnancy). Certain women have an inherited susceptibility to these effects of estrogen. Women who have had impaired bile flow in pregnancy may develop a similar disorder if they take oral contraceptives. For the mother the disorder is mild, although the itching can be very bothersome. In severe cases the fetus may become distressed and there is a risk of premature delivery and a low but increased risk of early fetal death or stillbirths. In general the disease is moderate to mild, and neither the mother nor the baby suffer any lasting consequences.

What Is Wilson's Disease and How Does It Affect Pregnant Women?

Wilson's disease is an inherited defect that results in the body storing too much copper, which then becomes toxic to the liver, brain, and other organs. Women with untreated Wilson's disease have difficulty becoming pregnant, and experience more miscarriages and spontaneous abortions. In addition, in untreated and symptomatic Wilson's disease both mother and fetus are considered at high risk during pregnancy. Women with Wilson's disease that has been well controlled, and in whom body copper levels have been reduced to near normal, regain fertility and may have normal, uneventful pregnancies and healthy babies.

Are There Any Other Liver Diseases That Can Affect Pregnant Women and Their Babies?

In addition to the diseases mentioned, women with less common diseases, such as primary biliary cirrhosis, primary sclerosing cholangitis, and alcoholic liver disease, among others, may consider pregnancy. In general, women in which liver disease has produced severe liver damage (particularly cirrhosis or serious liver dysfunction) are less fertile. These women and their babies are at higher risk of complications during pregnancy. In addition, three rare liver disorders may have serious consequences for pregnant women and their babies. They are intrahepatic cholestasis of pregnancy (impaired bile flow), toxemia-related disease with the HELLP syndrome, and acute fatty liver of pregnancy.

What Is Toxemia (Pre-eclampsia) and How Does It Affect the Liver?

Toxemia (or pre-eclampsia) is a fairly common disorder that occurs late in pregnancy and includes high blood pressure, kidney dysfunction, and the development of leg swelling or edema. In approximately 10% of women with pre-eclampsia, the liver is also affected, with development of blood clots and bleeding into the liver. In mild cases liver function remains normal, although liver blood tests may be abnormal. In severe cases large parts of the liver may be damaged or destroyed, leading to symptoms similar to severe viral hepatitis. In extremely severe cases there may be major bleeding into parts of the liver or abdomen, a life-threatening situation.

What Is the HELLP Syndrome?

The HELLP syndrome is part of the liver disease that affects women with pre-eclampsia. It derives its name from the abbreviations for hemolysis (breakdown of red blood cells), elevated liver tests, and low platelets in the blood. This occurs in approximately 10% of all women with pre-eclampsia, and may be mild (diagnosed through abnormal blood tests) or may develop into severe liver damage. The disease stops immediately after delivery, and the liver generally heals itself within days to weeks. While the disease is ongoing, the mother is at risk of complications of liver damage and bleeding, and the baby is at risk of premature delivery or stillbirth.

Do Oral Contraceptives Have an Adverse Affect on the Liver?

Oral contraceptives have little adverse affect on the liver in most women. They may, however, cause increased growth of an uncommon liver tumor called a liver cell adenoma. Adenomas are benign liver tumors and do not spread outside the liver. Very large adenomas, however, may rupture and bleed. Thus, oral contraceptives probably should not be used by women who have significant adenomas. Oral contraceptives also may cause itching, jaundice, and cholestasis (decreased bile flow) in women with a genetic susceptibility to the effects of estrogens. Although estrogens are normal female sex hormones, at high levels they may interfere with bile formation in some women. If a woman taking an oral contraceptive develops this estrogen-induced cholestasis, the contraceptives should be discontinued. No lasting effect on the liver is anticipated.

Can a Woman Who Has Had a Liver Transplant Become Pregnant?

Women who have had a successful liver transplant with good liver function can become pregnant. Fertility returns within a few months after the transplant, and such women have successfully carried normal pregnancies to term. Only a few women who have had a transplant have gone on to become pregnant, however, so it is not known whether the ability to become pregnant and to carry a normal baby to term is completely normal. In addition, although the drugs used for immunosuppression after liver transplantation are thought to be relatively safe for the developing baby, absolute safety cannot be guaranteed.

Can Someone with Cirrhosis Become Pregnant?

Yes, although it is much more difficult because of markedly decreased fertility. If they do become pregnant, they may give birth to a healthy baby. The mother, however, may experience complications of liver failure during pregnancy, and the baby is at higher risk of premature delivery, spontaneous abortion, miscarriage, and stillbirth. Those children who are born, however, are generally healthy.

Is It Safe for a Pregnant Woman to Drink Moderate Amounts of Alcohol?

No, because it could damage the unborn child. Moderate alcohol consumption (one to two drinks) probably does not affect the liver of an otherwise normal pregnant woman, but even moderate doses may cause damage to the fetus. In addition, for any woman with liver disease, it makes sense to avoid taking in substances such as alcohol that are known to cause liver toxicity in many people.

Chapter 15

Jaundice in Healthy Newborns

A common condition in newborns, jaundice refers to the yellow color of the skin and whites of the eyes caused by excess bilirubin in the blood. Bilirubin is produced by the normal breakdown of red blood cells.

Normally bilirubin passes through the liver and is excreted as bile through the intestines. Jaundice occurs when bilirubin builds up faster than a newborn's liver can break it down and pass it from the body.

Reasons for this include:

- A newborn baby's still-developing liver may not yet be able to remove adequate bilirubin from the blood.

- More bilirubin is being made than the infant's liver can handle.

- Too large an amount of bilirubin is reabsorbed from the intestines before the baby gets rid of it in the stool.

High levels of bilirubin—usually above 20 mg—can cause deafness, cerebral palsy, or brain damage in some babies. In rare cases, jaundice may indicate the presence of hepatitis.

Types of Jaundice

There are several types of newborn jaundice. The following are the most common:

Used with permission © 1999 The Nemours Foundation.

Physiological (normal) jaundice: occurring in more than 50% of newborns, this jaundice is due to the immaturity of the baby's liver, which leads to a slow processing of bilirubin. It generally appears at 2 to 4 days of age and disappears by 1 to 2 weeks of age.

Jaundice of prematurity: This occurs frequently in premature babies since they take longer to adjust to excreting bilirubin effectively.

Breast milk jaundice: in 1% to 2% of breastfed babies, jaundice can be caused by substances produced in their mother's breast milk that can cause the bilirubin level to rise above 20 mg. These substances can prevent the excretion of bilirubin through the intestines. It starts at 4 to 7 days and normally lasts from 3 to 10 weeks.

Blood group incompatibility (Rh or ABO problems): If a baby has a different blood type than the mother, the mother might produce antibodies that destroy the infant's red blood cells. This creates a sudden buildup of bilirubin in the baby's blood. Incompatibility jaundice usually begins during the first day of life. Rh problems once caused the most severe form of jaundice, but now can be prevented with an injection of RhoGAM to the mother within 72 hours after delivery, which prevents her from forming antibodies that might endanger any subsequent babies.

Symptoms and Diagnosis

Jaundice usually appears around the second or third day of life. It begins at the head and progresses downward. A jaundiced baby's skin will appear yellow first on the face, followed by the chest and stomach, and finally, the legs. It can also cause the whites of an infant's eyes to appear yellow.

Since many babies are now released from the hospital at 1 or 2 days of life, parents should keep an eye on their infants to detect jaundice. The American Academy of Pediatrics recommends checking your baby under natural daylight or in a room that has fluorescent lights.

A simple test for jaundice is to gently press your fingertip on the tip of your child's nose or forehead. If the skin shows white (this test works for all races) there is no jaundice; if it shows a yellowish color, you should contact your child's doctor to see if significant jaundice is present.

At the doctor's office, a small sample of your infant's blood can be tested to measure the bilirubin level. The seriousness of the jaundice will vary based on your child's age and the presence of other medical conditions.

When to Call the Doctor

Your child's doctor should be called immediately if jaundice is noted during the first 24 hours of life, the jaundice involves arms or legs, your baby develops a fever over 100 degrees F (37.8 degrees C), or if your child starts to look or act sick. (In children under age 5, temperatures should be taken rectally or aurally.) Call your child's doctor if the color deepens after day 7, the jaundice is not gone after day 15, your baby is not gaining sufficient weight, or if you are concerned about the amount of jaundice in your baby's skin.

Treatments

In mild or moderate levels of jaundice, by 5 to 7 days of age the baby will take care of the excess bilirubin on its own. If high levels of jaundice do not clear up, phototherapy—ultraviolet light that helps rid the body of the bilirubin by altering it or making it easier for your baby's liver to get rid of it—may be prescribed.

More frequent feedings of breast milk or formula to help infants pass the bilirubin in their stools may also be recommended. In rare cases, a blood exchange may be required to give a baby fresh blood and remove the bilirubin.

If your baby develops jaundice that lasts more than a week, your doctor may ask you to temporarily stop breastfeeding. During this time, you can pump your breasts so you can keep producing breast milk and you can start nursing again once the condition has cleared.

If the amount of bilirubin is high, your baby may be readmitted to the hospital for treatment. Once the bilirubin level drops, however, it is unlikely it will increase again.

Part Four

The Effects of Drugs on the Liver

Chapter 16

The Liver's Response to Drugs

How Your Body Responds to Drugs

Once, doctors administered therapeutic agents with little, if any, idea of what happened to them inside the patient. In contrast, today's pharmacologists want to predict exactly how and where a drug will act when given to a particular person. To do this, they must know both the characteristics of the drug molecule and also what chemical alterations it will undergo as it moves through the body.

The ability to predict drug actions came about slowly. Pharmacodynamics (how drugs act on the body) and pharmacokinetics (how the body absorbs, distributes, breaks down, and eliminates drugs) did not emerge as subjects of study until human anatomy and physiology began to be carefully explored.

During the "scientific revolution" of the 15th and 16th centuries, people began to study natural phenomena, including the workings of the human body. Over time, the basic actions of various organ systems— including the circulatory, digestive, respiratory, nervous, and excretory systems—were described and, later, were altered by the use of various chemicals. Eventually, the body came to be regarded as a kind of machine in which food (the body's fuel) is converted through a series of chemical reactions into the energy needed to drive the organ systems.

The study of metabolism—how the body uses and stores its fuel—was well established by the end of the 19th century. Aiding the exploration

Excerpts from *Medicines by Design*, National Institute of General Medical Sciences, NIH Publication No. 93-474, September 1993.

of metabolism were several unifying ideas about the body. One is that the body's basic unit is the cell. Like a miniature body, each cell is surrounded by a skin—the surface membrane—and contains tiny organs, called organelles, that perform specific functions such as the chemical tasks of metabolism.

In this century, a second unifying idea emerged with full force. This is the concept that every cell's activity is directed by a "command center"—the nucleus—in which lie the chromosomes. Chromosomes are made of DNA, the double helix molecule first described by James Watson and Francis Crick in 1953. Some stretches of DNA are genes, which are the coded instructions that a cell used to make proteins. A cell requires various proteins to build and run its organelles, and certain cells also release the proteins they make into the bloodstream to use elsewhere in the body.

Investigations of the circulatory system by many scientists have revealed that blood is a rich melange consisting primarily of oxygen-carrying red blood cells, along with infection-fighting white blood cells and a liquid, called plasma, that carries proteins and hormones such as insulin and estrogen, nutrient molecules of various kinds, and carbon dioxide and other waste products destined for elimination. Many drugs, too, travel in the bloodstream. This presents a challenge to those pharmacologists whose aim is to deliver drugs exclusively to diseased areas.

The knowledge that the blood carries substances to and from all parts of the body, thereby linking widely separated tissues and organs, paved the way for later scientists to propose that the nervous and endocrine (hormonal) systems behave similarly. Physiologists (scientists who study the body's functions) developed the idea that all internal processes are integrated so as to keep the organism in a balanced state (homeostasis).

Your body has many other message carriers that coordinate intercellular activities and respond to incoming information. Drugs can influence these substances as well, often by inhibiting or enhancing their production. A major quest in pharmacolgy has been to find—and exploit—these connections. Usually, a drug's effect is noted first and the way it influences message transmission is discovered later.

Drugs in the Liver

But before pharmacologists can study what effect, if any, a drug has on the body, they must first predict how it will be changed as it passes through the body's chemical processing plant—the liver.

The liver is a site of continuous and frenzied, yet carefully controlled, activity. Everything that enters your bloodstream—whether swallowed, injected, inhaled, absorbed through your skin, or produced by your own cells—is carried to this largest internal organ. There, substances are chemically pummeled, twisted, cut apart, stuck together, and transformed. Thus a drug can enter the liver with one set of properties and leave with quite a different array of characteristics, which may alter its usefulness. The "biotransformations" that take place in the liver are, like metabolic processes throughout the body, performed by the body's busiest proteins, its enzymes.

Every one of your cells has a variety of enzymes, drawn from the body's repertoire of about 100,000. Each enzyme specializes in a particular job. Some break molecules apart, while others link small molecules into long chains. Enzymes are catalysts, which have the special ability to do a chemical task over and over without themselves being permanently changed.

Enzymes act on chemical bonds. It does not matter if the bond is in a food molecule, a drug molecule, or some other kind of molecule. For the most part, liver enzymes make molecules that are either more easily absorbed by other body cells or more easily excreted. Many of the products of enzymatic breakdown, called metabolites, are less chemically active than the molecules from which they are derived. Thus, the liver is properly thought of as a "detoxifying" organ. Over the past several decades, however, pharmacologists have become increasingly aware that drug metabolites can have chemical activities of their own—sometimes as powerful as those of the original drug.

Three other facts make the activities in the liver even more complicated.

1. Drugs can alter the innate activity of liver enzyme systems, often with unpredictable results.

2. Nondrug substances, particularly foods, interact with drugs and liver enzymes and can sometimes cause very unpleasant reactions.

3. Genetically determined variation in liver enzyme activity causes different people to be either "fast" or "slow" metabolizers of certain drugs. For example, Asians tend to metabolize certain blood-pressure-lowering drugs more quickly than do Caucasians. Since less of the active drug gets into the bloodstream, some Asians need a larger-than-standard dose to get a therapeutic result.

Scientists have identified many other drugs including anticancer drugs, muscle relaxants, and antimalarial drugs, whose metabolism is genetically influenced. Better screening techniques are gradually permitting physicians to take these genetic subtleties into account and to identify slow or fast metabolizers before drug treatment begins.

Drug prescription that includes attention to genetic variations illustrates just how far physicians have come since the days when drugs were given with a "fingers crossed" attitude. Although today's drug regimens are both more rational and more likely to bring about a cure than ever before, the quest for new drugs, and new ways to deliver them, is still being vigorously pursued.

Drug Delivery

Ideally, a drug should enter the body slowly and steadily, go directly to the diseased site while bypassing healthy tissue, do its job, and then disappear. Unfortunately, the typical methods of delivering drugs—ingestion or injection—rarely attain this goal.

Drugs that are swallowed may not be able to cross the intestinal membrane and so may never enter the bloodstream. Many therapeutic proteins and enzymes cannot be taken orally because they are rapidly digested. If a drug does enter the blood from the intestine, much of it may be inactivated by enzymes on its first trip through the liver. This "first pass effect" means that several doses of the drug must be administered before a therapeutic level is achieved in the bloodstream. Drug injections are also often unsatisfactory, because they are expensive, difficult for the patient to self-administer, and unpopular if the drug must be taken daily. Both methods of administration also result in fluctuating drug levels in the blood, which besides being inefficient, can also be dangerous, since many modern drugs are more potent than their older counterparts and therefore dosages must be very carefully controlled in order to prevent toxicity.

Delivery dilemmas are being overcome with a variety of ingenious techniques;

- **drug-impregnated skin patches**—bypass the digestive system altogether;

- **nasal delivery systems**—the permeable mucous membrane of the nose can act as a gateway into the circulation for proteins, enzymes, hormones, and other larger molecules;

- **bioerodible implants**—may offer a way to achieve the slow, continuous release of drugs needed to treat chronic problems;

- **patient-activated implants**—experimental, but have the potential for use with drugs that need to be injected at frequent intervals;

- **body-activated pill pumps**—the pill pump is swallowed and, as it passes through the digestive system, water gradually seeps through the coating and dissolves the powder, which leaks out of a tiny laser-drilled hole in the pill. The rate of drug release can be regulated with a fair degree of precision by altering the thickness of the pill's coat;

- **liposomes**—a microscopic bubble of fatty molecules (lipids) surrounding a watery interior into which drugs can be placed. One of the benefits is that the similarity to cell membranes makes them non-toxic. However, liposomes have proven to be difficult to direct to desired sites, other than the liver and spleeen;

- **photodynamic therapy**—the key ingredient is psoralen, a plant-derived chemical with the peculiar property of being inert until exposed to light.

All of these advances in drug development and delivery are reflections of the modern notion that illness, whether inherited or acquired, is the result of molecular malfunction. Today, efforts to treat sickness by focusing therapies precisely on the malfunctioning molecules are increasingly successful. In the future, communicable diseases—including the age-old scourge of the common cold—as well as inherited conditions may be cured, rather than merely. treated, with "drugs" that actually repair cells or protect them from attack.

Chapter 17

Alcohol and the Liver

Alcohol-induced liver disease (ALD) is a major cause of illness and death in the United States. Fatty liver, the most common form of ALD, is reversible with abstinence. More serious ALD includes alcoholic hepatitis, characterized by persistent inflammation of the liver, and cirrhosis, characterized by progressive scarring of liver tissue. Either condition can be fatal, and treatment options are limited. During the past 5 years, research has significantly increased our understanding of the mechanisms by which alcohol consumption damages the liver. This chapter highlights recent research on the mechanisms and treatment of ALD.

The Prevalence of Alcohol-Induced Liver Disease (ALD)

Approximately 10 to 35 percent of heavy drinkers[1] develop alcoholic hepatitis, and 10 to 20 percent develop cirrhosis (1). In the United States, cirrhosis is the seventh leading cause of death among young and middle-age adults. Approximately 10,000 to 24,000 deaths from cirrhosis may be attributable to alcohol consumption each year (2).

The chapter contains text from *Alcohol Alert* No. 42 October 1998 and *Alcohol Alert* No. 35 January 1997, National Institute on Alcohol Abuse and Alcoholism (NIAAA); HHS *News*, October 21, 1998, U.S. Department of Health and Human Services; and "Alcohol and the Liver: Myths vs. Facts," © 1997, reprinted with permission of the American Liver Foundation, 1-800-GO-LIVER.

How Does Alcohol Damage the Liver?

Normal liver function is essential to life. Alcohol-induced liver damage disrupts the body's metabolism, eventually impairing the function of other organs. Multiple physiological mechanisms, discussed in the following sections, interact to influence the progression of ALD. Medications that affect these mechanisms may help prevent some of the medical complications of ALD or reduce the severity of the illness.

Alcohol Metabolism

Metabolism is the body's process of converting ingested substances to other compounds. Metabolism results in some substances becoming more, and some less, toxic than those originally ingested. Metabolism involves a number of processes, one of which is referred to as oxidation. Through oxidation, alcohol is detoxified and removed from the blood, preventing the alcohol from accumulating and destroying cells and organs. A minute amount of alcohol escapes metabolism and is excreted unchanged in the breath and in urine. Until all the alcohol consumed has been metabolized, it is distributed throughout the body, affecting the brain and other tissues. By understanding alcohol metabolism, we can learn how the body can dispose of alcohol and discern some of the factors that influence this process. Studying alcohol metabolism also can help to understand how this process influences the metabolism of food, hormones, and medications.

The Metabolic Process

When alcohol is consumed, it passes from the stomach and intestines into the blood, a process referred to as absorption. Alcohol is then metabolized by enzymes, which are body chemicals that break down other chemicals. In the liver, an enzyme called alcohol dehydrogenase (ADH) mediates the conversion of alcohol to acetaldehyde. Acetaldehyde is rapidly converted to acetate by other enzymes and is eventually metabolized to carbon dioxide and water. Alcohol also is metabolized in the liver by the enzyme cytochrome P450IIE1 (CYP2E1), which may be increased after chronic drinking. Most of the alcohol consumed is metabolized in the liver, but the small quantity that remains unmetabolized permits alcohol concentration to be measured in breath and urine.

The liver can metabolize only a certain amount of alcohol per hour, regardless of the amount that has been consumed. The rate of alcohol metabolism depends, in part, on the amount of metabolizing enzymes in the liver, which varies among individuals and appears to have genetic determinants. In general, after the consumption of one standard drink, the amount of alcohol in the drinker's blood (blood alcohol concentration, or BAC) peaks within 30 to 45 minutes. (A standard drink is defined as 12 ounces of beer, 5 ounces of wine, or 1.5 ounces of 80-proof distilled spirits, all of which contain the same amount of alcohol.) Alcohol is metabolized more slowly than it is absorbed. Since the metabolism of alcohol is slow, consumption needs to be controlled to prevent accumulation in the body and intoxication.

Most of the alcohol a person drinks is eventually broken down by the liver. However, some products generated during alcohol metabolism (e.g., acetaldehyde) are more toxic than alcohol itself. In addition, a group of metabolic products called free radicals can damage liver cells and promote inflammation, impairing vital functions such as energy production. The body's natural defenses against free radicals (e.g., antioxidants) can be inhibited by alcohol consumption, leading to increased liver damage (3).

Factors Influencing Alcohol Absorption and Metabolism

Food. A number of factors influence the absorption process, including the presence of food and the type of food in the gastrointestinal tract when alcohol is consumed. The rate at which alcohol is absorbed depends on how quickly the stomach empties its contents into the intestine. The higher the dietary fat content, the more time this emptying will require and the longer the process of absorption will take. One study found that subjects who drank alcohol after a meal that included fat, protein, and carbohydrates absorbed the alcohol about three times more slowly than when they consumed alcohol on an empty stomach.

Gender. Women absorb and metabolize alcohol differently from men. They have higher BAC's after consuming the same amount of alcohol as men and are more susceptible to alcoholic liver disease, heart muscle damage, and brain damage. The difference in BAC's between women and men has been attributed to women's smaller amount of body water, likened to dropping the same amount of alcohol into a smaller pail of water. An additional factor contributing to the difference in BAC's may be that women have lower activity of the alcohol metabolizing enzyme ADH in the stomach, causing a larger proportion of the ingested alcohol to reach the blood. The combination of these factors may render women more vulnerable than men to alcohol-induced liver and heart damage.

Effects of Alcohol Metabolism

Body Weight. Although alcohol has a relatively high caloric value, 7.1 Calories per gram (as a point of reference, 1 gram of carbohydrate contains 4.5 Calories, and 1 gram of fat contains 9 Calories), alcohol consumption does not necessarily result in increased body weight. An analysis of data collected from the first National Health and Nutrition Examination Survey (NHANES I) found that although drinkers had significantly higher intakes of total calories than nondrinkers, drinkers were not more obese than nondrinkers. In fact, women drinkers had significantly lower body weight than nondrinkers. As alcohol intake among men increased, their body weight decreased. An analysis of data from the second National Health and Nutrition Examination Survey (NHANES II) and other large national studies found similar results for women, although the relationship between drinking and body weight for men is inconsistent. Although moderate doses of alcohol added to the diets of lean men and women do not seem to lead to weight gain, some studies have reported weight gain when alcohol is added to the diets of overweight persons.

When chronic heavy drinkers substitute alcohol for carbohydrates in their diets, they lose weight and weigh less than their nondrinking counterparts. Furthermore, when chronic heavy drinkers add alcohol to an otherwise normal diet, they do not gain weight.

Sex Hormones. Alcohol metabolism alters the balance of reproductive hormones in men and women. In men, alcohol metabolism contributes to testicular injury and impairs testosterone synthesis and sperm production. In a study of normal healthy men who received 220 grams of alcohol daily for 4 weeks, testosterone levels declined after only 5 days and continued to fall throughout the study period. Prolonged testosterone deficiency may contribute to feminization in males, for example, breast enlargement. In addition, alcohol may interfere with normal sperm structure and movement by inhibiting the metabolism of vitamin A, which is essential for sperm development. In women, alcohol metabolism may contribute to increased production of a form of estrogen called estradiol (which contributes to increased bone density and reduced risk of coronary artery disease) and to decreased estradiol metabolism, resulting in elevated estradiol levels. One research review indicates that estradiol levels increased in premenopausal women who consumed slightly more than enough alcohol to reach the legal limit of alcohol (BAC of 0.10 percent) acutely. A study of the effect of alcohol on estradiol levels in postmenopausal women found that in women wearing estradiol skin patches, acute alcohol consumption significantly elevated estradiol levels over the short term.

Medications. Chronic heavy drinking appears to activate the enzyme CYP2E1, which may be responsible for transforming the over-the-counter pain reliever acetaminophen (Tylenol, and many others) into chemicals that can cause liver damage, even when acetaminophen is taken in standard therapeutic doses. A review of studies of liver damage resulting from acetaminophen-alcohol interaction reported that in alcoholics, these effects may occur with as little as 2.6 grams of acetaminophen (four to five "extra-strength" pills) taken over the course of the day in persons consuming varying amounts of alcohol. The damage caused by alcohol-acetaminophen interaction is more likely to occur when acetaminophen is taken after, rather than before, the alcohol has been metabolized. Alcohol consumption affects the metabolism of a wide variety of other medications, increasing the activity of some and diminishing the activity, thereby decreasing the effectiveness, of others.

Scientific Implications

The study of metabolism has both practical and broader scientific implications. On the practical side, information on how the body metabolizes alcohol permits us to calculate, for example, what our blood alcohol concentration (BAC) is likely to be after drinking, including the impact of food and gender differences in the rate of alcohol metabolism on BAC. This information, of course, is important when participating in activities for which concentration is needed, such as driving or operating dangerous machinery.

With respect to its broader scientific application, metabolism, which has long been studied, is emerging with new implications for the study of alcoholism and its medical consequences. For instance, how is metabolism related to the resistance of some individuals to alcoholism? We know that some inherited abnormalities in metabolism (e.g., flushing reaction among some persons of Asian descent) promote resistance to alcoholism. Recent data from two large-scale NIAAA-supported genetics studies suggest that alcohol dehydrogenase genes may be associated with differential resistance and vulnerability to alcohol. These findings are important to the study of why some people develop alcoholism and others do not. Studies of metabolism also can identify alternate paths of alcohol metabolism, which may help explain how alcohol speeds up the elimination of some substances (e.g., barbiturates) and increases the toxicity of others (e.g., acetaminophen). This information will help health care providers in advising patients on alcohol-drug interactions that may decrease the effectiveness of some therapeutic medications or render others harmful.

The Inflammatory Response

Inflammation is the body's response to local tissue damage or infection. Inflammation prevents the spread of injury and mobilizes the defense mechanisms of the immune system. One such defense mechanism is the generation of free radicals that can destroy disease-causing microorganisms. Long-term alcohol consumption prolongs the inflammatory process, leading to excessive production of free radicals, which can destroy healthy liver tissue. Bacteria that live in the human intestine play a key role in the initiation of ALD. Alcohol consumption increases the passage of a noxious bacterial product called endotoxin through the intestinal wall into the bloodstream. Upon reaching the liver, endotoxin activates specialized cells (i.e., Kupffer cells) that monitor the blood for signs of infection. These cells respond to the presence of endotoxin by releasing substances called cytokines that regulate the inflammatory process (4-6).

Cytokines. Cytokines are produced by cells of the liver and immune system in response to infection or cell damage. Alcohol consumption increases cytokine levels, and cytokines in humans produce symptoms similar to those of alcoholic hepatitis (7). Recent studies implicate cytokines in scar formation and in the depletion of oxygen within liver cells, processes that are associated with cirrhosis (7). Each of the disease mechanisms described above contributes to the death of liver cells. The presence of damaged cells triggers the body's defensive responses, including the release of additional cytokines, resulting in a vicious cycle of inflammation, cell death, and scarring.

Scar Formation. Normal scar formation is part of the wound-healing process. Alcohol-induced cell death and inflammation can result in scarring that distorts the liver's internal structure and impairs its function. This scarring is the hallmark of cirrhosis. The process by which cirrhosis develops involves the interaction of certain

144

cytokines and specialized liver cells (i.e., stellate cells). In the normal liver, stellate cells function as storage depots for vitamin A. Upon activation by cytokines, stellate cells proliferate, lose their vitamin A stores, and begin to produce scar tissue. In addition, activated stellate cells constrict blood vessels, impeding the delivery of oxygen to liver cells (6,8).

Acetaldehyde may activate stellate cells directly, promoting liver scarring in the absence of inflammation (9,10). This finding is consistent with the observation that heavy drinkers can develop cirrhosis insidiously, without preexisting hepatitis.

Factors That Influence Vulnerability to ALD

Susceptibility to ALD differs considerably among individuals, so that even among people drinking similar amounts of alcohol, only some develop cirrhosis. Understanding the mechanisms of these differences may help clinicians identify and treat patients at increased risk for advanced liver damage.

Genetic Factors. Structural or functional variability in any of the cell types and biochemical substances discussed above could influence a person's susceptibility to ALD. Researchers are seeking genetic factors that may underlie this variability. Results of this research may provide the basis for future gene-based therapies.

Dietary Factors. Nutritional factors influence the progression of ALD (11). For example, a high-fat, low-carbohydrate diet promotes liver damage in alcohol-fed rats (12,13), and high amounts of polyunsaturated fats may promote the development of cirrhosis in animals (14,15).

Gender. Women develop ALD after consuming lower levels of alcohol over a shorter period of time compared with men (16). In addition, women have a higher incidence of alcoholic hepatitis and a higher mortality rate from cirrhosis than men (17). The mechanisms that underlie gender-related differences are unknown.

Hepatitis C. Many patients with ALD are infected with hepatitis C virus (HCV), which causes a chronic, potentially fatal liver disease (18,19). The presence of HCV may increase a person's susceptibility to ALD and influence the severity of alcoholic cirrhosis. For example, alcohol-dependent patients infected with HCV develop liver injury at a younger age and after consuming a lower cumulative dose of alcohol

145

than do those without HCV (20). Patients with HCV are often treated with an antiviral substance called interferon. However, interferon is less effective in patients with chronic HCV who are heavy drinkers, compared with those who are not (21).

Frequently Asked Questions

How Much Alcohol Can I Safely Drink?

Because some people are much more sensitive to alcohol than others, there is no single right answer that will fit everyone. Generally, doctors recommend that if you drink, don't drink more than two drinks per day.

Are There Dangers from Alcohol Besides the Amount That Is Consumed?

Yes. Even moderate amounts of alcohol can have toxic effects when taken with over-the-counter drugs containing acetaminophen. If you are taking over-the-counter drugs, be especially careful about drinking and don't use an alcoholic beverage to take your medication. Ask your doctor about precautions for prescription drugs.

Can "Social Drinkers" Get Alcoholic Hepatitis?

Unfortunately, yes. Alcoholic hepatitis is frequently discovered in alcoholics, but it also occurs in people who are not alcoholics. People vary greatly in the way their liver reacts to alcohol.

What Kinds of Liver Diseases Are Caused by Too Much Alcohol?

Alcoholic hepatitis is an inflammation of the liver that lasts one to two weeks. Symptoms include loss of appetite, nausea, vomiting, abdominal pain and tenderness, fever, jaundice, and sometimes mental confusion. It is believed to lead to alcoholic cirrhosis over a period of years. Cirrhosis involves permanent damage to the liver cells. "Fatty Liver" is the earliest stage of alcoholic liver disease. If the patient stops drinking at this point, the liver can heal itself.

How Can Alcoholic Hepatitis Be Diagnosed?

Alcoholic hepatitis is not easy to diagnose. Sometimes symptoms are worse for a time after drinking has stopped than they were during the drinking episode. While the disease usually comes on after a period of fairly heavy drinking, it may also be seen in people who are moderate drinkers. Blood tests may help in diagnosis. Proof is established best by liver biopsy. This involves taking a tiny specimen of liver tissue with a needle and examining it under a microscope. The biopsy is usually done under local anesthesia.

Are Men or Women More Likely to Get Alcoholic Hepatitis?

Women appear to be more likely to suffer liver damage from alcohol. Even when a man and woman have the same weight and drink the same amount, the woman generally has a higher concentration of alcohol in the blood because she has relatively more body fat and less water than the man, and her body handles alcohol differently.

Do All Alcoholics Get Alcoholic Hepatitis and Eventually Cirrhosis?

No. Some alcoholics may suffer seriously from the many physical and psychological symptoms of alcoholism but escape serious liver damage. Alcoholic cirrhosis is found among alcoholics about 10-25 percent of the time.

Is Alcoholic Hepatitis Different from "Fatty Liver?"

Yes. Anyone who drinks alcohol heavily, even for a few days, will develop a condition in which liver cells are swollen with fat globules and water. This condition is called "fatty liver." It may also result from diabetes, obesity, certain drugs, or severe protein malnutrition. Fatty liver caused by alcohol is reversible when drinking of alcohol is stopped.

Does Alcoholic Hepatitis Always Lead to Cirrhosis?

No. It usually takes many years for alcoholic hepatitis to produce enough liver damage to result in cirrhosis. If alcoholic hepatitis is detected and treated early, cirrhosis can be prevented.

Is Alcoholic Hepatitis Dangerous?

It may be fatal, especially if the patient has had previous liver damage. Those who have had nutritional deficiencies because of heavy drinking may have other ailments. These medical complications may affect almost every system in the body. It is important to recognize and treat alcoholic cirrhosis early, so that these life-threatening consequences are prevented.

How Can Alcoholic Hepatitis Be Prevented?

The best treatment is to stop drinking. Treatment may also include prescribed medication, good nutrition and rest. The patient may be instructed to avoid various drugs and chemicals.

Since the liver has considerable ability to heal and regenerate, the prognosis for a patient with alcoholic hepatitis is very hopeful—if alcohol drinking is ended forever.

Is Cirrhosis Different from Alcoholic Hepatitis?

Yes. Hepatitis is an inflammation of the liver. In cirrhosis, normal liver cells are damaged and replaced by scar tissue. This scarring keeps the liver from performing many of its vital functions.

What Causes Cirrhosis?

There are many causes for cirrhosis. Long term alcohol abuse is one. Chronic hepatitis is another major cause. In children, the most frequent causes are biliary atresia, a disease that damages the bile ducts, and neonatal hepatitis. Children with these diseases often receive liver transplants.

Many adult patients who require liver transplants suffer from primary biliary cirrhosis. We do not yet know what causes this illness, but it is not in any way related to alcohol consumption.

Cirrhosis can also be caused by hereditary defects in iron or copper metabolism or prolonged exposure to toxins.

Treatment Effectiveness

Abstinence is the cornerstone of ALD therapy. With abstinence, fatty liver, and alcoholic hepatitis are frequently reversible, and survival is improved among patients with ALD, including those with cirrhosis (1). For terminally ill patients, **liver transplantation** remains the only effective treatment. Research has established the effectiveness of liver transplantation in patients with alcoholic cirrhosis (1). More recently, Belle and colleagues (22) summarized follow-up medical data on all persons who received liver transplants in the United States between 1988 and 1995. Deaths among these subjects were not alcohol related. That is, alcohol-dependent patients died from the same conditions that caused deaths among patients without alcoholism (e.g., infection, cancer, or heart disease). Recurrences of liver disease among alcohol-dependent patients are rare (23).

Hepatitis C infection in patients with ALD does not appear to affect survival after liver transplantation, despite the continued presence of the virus in the bloodstream (24).

Medication Interactions. Chronic alcohol consumption may increase the adverse side effects of medications used to treat conditions other than ALD. In particular, excessive use of the widely used pain killer acetaminophen has been associated with liver damage in people drinking heavily (25).

Dr. Michael A. Friedman, Acting FDA Commissioner said, "Consumers need to know that chronic use of alcohol while taking pain relievers or fever reducers can be hazardous to their health. FDA urges people with a history of alcohol use to seek a doctor's advice about their risk of side effects before taking these medications."

The following specific warnings are required for pain relievers and fever reducers as of October 1999:

- Acetaminophen: "Alcohol Warning: If you consume 3 or more alcoholic drinks every day, ask your doctor whether you should take acetaminophen or other pain relievers/fever reducers. Acetaminophen may cause liver damage."

- Aspirin, carbaspirin calcium, choline salicylate, ibuprofen, ketoprofen, magnesiumsalicylate, naproxen sodium, and sodium salicylate: "Alcohol Warning: If you consumer 3 or more alcoholic drinks every day, ask your doctor whether you should take [ingredient] or other pain relievers/fever reducers. [Ingredient] may cause stomach bleeding."

- Combination of acetaminophen with other analgesic/antipyretic ingredients: "Alcohol Warning: If you consumer 3 or more alcoholic drinks every day, ask your doctor whether you should take [ingredients] or other pain relievers/fever reducers. [Ingredients] may cause liver damage and stomach bleeding."

Pain relievers and fever reducers approved for over-the-counter adult use since 1993 have already been required to carry a warning for heavy alcohol users. However, labeling to indicate the specific risk associated with each ingredient has not been required. Products previously required to include an alcohol warning in their labeling include Aleve (naproxyn sodium), Orudis KT and Actron (ketoprofen), Advil Liquigels (solubilized ibuprofen), and Tylenol Extended Release (acetominophen). These products will also be subject to the new rule.

Prospects for Future Treatment

The multiple mechanisms of ALD development provide several potential targets for medical intervention. Some promising lines of inquiry are summarized below.

The role of endotoxin in the inflammatory response suggests the possibility of inhibiting ALD development at its earliest stages. For example, suppression of endotoxin-producing intestinal bacteria reduced signs of liver damage in alcohol-fed rats (4,26).

An adequate daily supply of total carbohydrates is important in treating ALD (13,27). In addition, researchers are investigating certain nutritional supplements for patients with ALD. One such supplement is polyunsaturated lecithin (PUL), a mixture of fatty substances extracted from soybeans. PUL protected against liver scarring in alcohol-fed baboons (9,28). Another dietary factor, S-adenosyl-l-methionine (SAM), can reduce liver cell damage in animals that is induced by alcohol or other toxic substances (29). The safety and effectiveness of these supplements for treating human ALD are under investigation.

Finally, an important goal of ALD research is to develop medications that can moderate the toxic effects of inflammatory cytokines while sparing their essential defensive functions. In one study, administration of antibodies designed to recognize and inactivate key inflammatory cytokines markedly decreased liver injury in rats (30).

Alcohol and the Liver: Research Update—A Commentary by NIAAA Director Enoch Gordis, M.D.

Serious alcoholic liver disease (ALD) is a major public health problem. These conditions—including alcoholic hepatitis and cirrhosis— can be progressive and fatal, especially if the patient continues to consume alcohol. Efforts to decrease the prevalence of ALD have therefore focused on prevention, by attempting to reduce alcohol consumption in the general population and in alcohol-dependent patients.

In recent years, scientists have made significant progress in understanding the biological and environmental factors that combine with the effects of alcohol to damage the liver. For example, many patients with ALD are infected with a nonalcoholic liver disease called hepatitis C. Heavy drinking increases the severity of hepatitis C and complicates its treatment. Researchers are studying the mechanisms by which these diseases interact. This and other studies on ALD may lead to the development of medications to interrupt liver disease processes such as liver inflammation and scarring. Prevention remains the key approach to the problem of ALD, but research provides hope that at least some effects of ALD may be reversible even after the disease has become established.

References

1. National Institute on Alcohol Abuse and Alcoholism. *Alcohol Alert No. 19: Alcohol and the Liver.* PH 329. Rockville, MD: the Institute, 1993.

2. DeBakey, S.F.; Stinson, F.S.; Grant, B.F.; and Dufour, M.C. Surveillance Report #41. *Liver Cirrhosis Mortality in the United States, 1970-93.* Bethesda, MD: National Institute on Alcohol Abuse and Alcoholism, 1996.

3. Kurose, I.; Higuchi, H.; Kato, S.; Miura, S.; and Ishii, H. Ethanol-induced oxidative stress in the liver. *Alcoholism: Clinical and Experimental Research* 20(1):77A-85A, 1996.

4. Nanji, A.A.; Khettry, U.; and Sadrzadeh, S.M.H. Lactobacillus feeding reduces endotoxemia and severity of experimental alcoholic liver (disease). *Proceedings of the Society for Experimental Biology and Medicine* 205(3):243-247, 1994.

5. Thurman, R.G.; Bradford, B.U.; Iimuro, Y.; Knecht, K.T.; Connor, H.D.; Adachi, Y.; Wall, C.; Arteel, G.E.; Raleigh, J.A.; Forman, D.T.; and Mason, R.P. Role of Kupffer cells, endotoxin and free radicals in hepatotoxicity due to prolonged alcohol consumption: Studies in female and male rats. *Journal of Nutrition* 127(S5):903S-906S, 1997.

6. Lands, W.E.M. Cellular signals in alcohol-induced liver injury: A review. *Alcoholism: Clinical and Experimental Research* 19(4):928-938, 1995.

7. McClain, C.J.; Shedlofsky, S.; Barve, S.; and Hill, D.B. Cytokines and alcoholic liver disease. *Alcohol Health & Research World* 21(4):317-320, 1997.

8. Maher, J.J., and Friedman, S.L. Pathogenesis of hepatic fibro-sis. In: Hall, P., ed. *Alcoholic Liver Disease: Pathology and Pathogenesis.* 2d ed. London: Edward Arnold, 1995. pp. 71-88.

9. Lieber, C.S. Hepatic and other medical disorders of alcohol-ism: From pathogenesis to treatment. *Journal of Studies on Alcohol* 59(1):9-25, 1998.

10. Ma, X.; Svegliati-Baroni, G.; Poniachik, J.; Baraona, E.; and Lieber, C.S. Collagen synthesis by liver stellate cells is re-leased from its normal feedback regulation by acetaldehyde-induced modification of the carboxyl-terminal propeptide of procollagen. *Alcoholism: Clinical and Experimental Research* 1(7):1204-1211, 1997.

11. Dannenberg, A.J., and Nanji, A.A. Dietary saturated fatty ac-ids: A novel treatment for alcoholic liver disease. *Alcoholism: Clinical and Experimental Research* 22(3):750-752, 1998.

12. French, S.W.; Morimoto, M.; and Tsukamoto, H. Animal mod-els of alcohol-associated liver injury. In: Hall, P., ed. *Alcoholic Liver Disease: Pathology and Pathogenesis.* 2d ed. London: Edward Arnold, 1995. pp. 279-296.

13. Badger, T.M.; Korourian, S.; Hakkak, R.; Ronis, M.J.J.; Shelnutt, S.R.; Ingelman-Sundberg, M.; and Waldron, J. Car-bohydrate deficiency as a possible factor in ethanol-induced hepatic necrosis. *Alcoholism: Clinical and Experimental Re-search* 22(3):742, 1998.

14. Nanji, A.A., and French, S.W. Dietary factors and alcoholic cirrhosis. *Alcoholism: Clinical and Experimental Research* 10(3):271-273, 1986.

15. Nanji, A.A. Dietary fatty acids and alcoholic liver disease: Pathogenic mechanisms. *Alcoholism: Clinical and Experimen-tal Research* 22(3):747-748, 1998.

16. Gavaler, J.S., and Arria, A.M. Increased susceptibility of women to alcoholic liver disease: Artifactual or real? In: Hall, P., ed. *Alcoholic Liver Disease: Pathology and Pathogenesis.* 2d ed. London: Edward Arnold, 1995. pp. 123-133.

17. Hall, P. Factors influencing individual susceptibility to alco-holic liver disease. In: Hall, P., ed. *Alcoholic Liver Disease:*

Pathology and Pathogenesis. 2d ed. London: Edward Arnold, 1995. pp. 299-316.

18. Tong, M.J.; Blatt, L.M.; McHutchison, J.G.; Co, R.L.; and Conrad, A. Prediction of response during interferon alfa 2b therapy in chronic hepatitis C patients using viral and biochemical characteristics: A comparison. *Hepatology* 26(6):1640-1645, 1997.

19. Grellier, L.F.L., and Dusheiko, G.M. The role of hepatitis C virus in alcoholic liver disease. *Alcohol & Alcoholism* 32(2):103-111, 1997.

20. Maher, J.J. Exploring alcohol's effects on liver function. *Alcohol Health & Research World* 21(1):5-12, 1997.

21. Mochida, S.; Ohnishi, K.; Matsuo, S.; Kakihara, K.; and Fujiwara, K. Effect of alcohol intake on the efficacy of interferon therapy in patients with chronic hepatitis C as evaluated by multivariate logistic regression analysis. *Alcoholism: Clinical and Experimental Research* 20(9):371A-377A, 1996.

22. Belle, S.H.; Beringer, K.C.; and Detre, K.M. Liver transplantation for alcoholic liver disease in the United States: 1988 to 1995. *Liver Transplantation and Surgery* 3(3):212-219, 1997.

23. Lee, R.G. Recurrence of alcoholic liver disease after liver transplantation. *Liver Transplantation and Surgery* 3(3):292-295, 1997.

24. Pera, M.; García-Valdecasas, J.C.; Grande, L.; Rimola, A.; Fuster, J.; Lacy, A.M.; Cifuentes, A.; Cirera, I.; Navasa, M.; and Visa, J. Liver transplantation for alcoholic cirrhosis with anti-HCV antibodies. *Transplant International* 10:289-292, 1997.

25. Whitcomb, D.C. Acetaminophen hepatotoxicity: The rest of the story. *Gastroenterology* 114(5):1105-1106, 1998.

26. Adachi, Y.; Moore, L.E.; Bradford, B.U.; Gao, W.; and Thurman, R.G. Antibiotics prevent liver injury in rats following long-term exposure to ethanol. *Gastroenterology* 108:218-224, 1995.

27. Rao, G.A., and Larkin, E.C. Nutritional factors required for alcoholic liver disease in rats. *Journal of Nutrition* 127(S5):896S-898S, 1997.

28. Lieber, C.S. Pathogenesis and treatment of liver fibrosis in alcoholics: 1996 update. *Digestive Diseases* 15(1-2):42-66, 1997.

29. García-Ruiz, C.; Morales, A.; Colell, A.; Ballesta, A.; Rodés, J.; Kaplowitz, N.; and Fernández-Checa, J.C. Feeding S-adenosyl-l-methionine attenuates both ethanol-induced depletion of mitochondrial glutathione and mitochondrial dysfunction in periportal and perivenous rat hepatocytes. *Hepatology* 21(1):207-214, 1995.

30. Iimuro, Y.; Gallucci, R.M.; Luster, M.I.; Kono, H.; and Thurman, R.G. Antibodies to tumor necrosis factor alfa attenuate hepatic necrosis and inflammation caused by chronic exposure to ethanol in the rat. *Hepatology* 26(6):1530-1537, 1997.

[1]These authors defined "heavy drinking" as the daily consumption of five to six standard drinks, each drink equivalent to approximately 12 ounces of beer, 5 ounces of wine, or 1.5 ounces of distilled spirits.

Chapter 18

Harmful Effects of Medicines, Drugs, and Chemicals

Many medicines taken by mouth may affect the digestive system. These medicines include prescription (those ordered by a doctor and dispensed by a pharmacist) and nonprescription or over-the-counter (OTC) products. A glossary at the end of this chapter describes some common prescription and nonprescription medicines discussed below that may affect the digestive system.

Although these medicines usually are safe and effective, harmful effects may occur in some people. OTC's typically do not cause serious side effects when taken as directed on the product's label. It is important to read the label to find out the ingredients, side effects, warnings, and when to consult a doctor.

Always talk with your doctor before taking a medicine for the first time and before adding any new medicines to those you already are taking. Tell the doctor about all other medicines (prescription and OTC's) you are taking. Certain medicines taken together may inter-

The chapter contains text from "Harmful Effects of Medicines on the Adult Digestive System," National Institute of Diabetes and Digestive and Kidney Diseases (NIDDK), NIH Publication No. 97-3421, September 1992, revised 1997; "Chemical and Drug Induced Liver Injury," © 1997, reprinted with permission of the American Liver Foundation, 1-800-GO-LIVER; "FDA Issues Public Health Advisory on Liver Toxicity Associated with the Antibiotic Trovan," June 9, 1999, FDA Talk Paper; "Liver Injuries Prompt Warning for Diabetes Drug," *FDA Consumer Updates* January-February 1998; "Liver Risk with Long-Term Use of Pain Reliever," *FDA Consumer Updates* May-June 1998; and "Liver Risk Warning Added to Parkinson's Drug," *FDA Consumer Updates* March-April 1999.

act and cause harmful side effects. In addition, tell the doctor about any allergies or sensitivities to foods and medicines and about any medical conditions you may have such as diabetes, kidney disease, or liver disease.

Be sure that you understand all directions for taking the medicine, including dose and schedule, possible interactions with food, alcohol, and other medicines, side effects, and warnings. If you are an older adult read all directions carefully and ask your doctor questions about the medicine. As you get older, you may be more susceptible to drug interactions that cause side effects.

People with a food intolerance such as gluten intolerance should make sure their medicines do not contain fillers or additives with gluten.

Check with your doctor if you have any questions or concerns about your medicines. Follow the doctor's orders carefully, and immediately report any unusual symptoms or the warning signs described below.

The Liver

The liver processes most medicines that enter the bloodstream and governs drug activity throughout the body. Once a drug enters the bloodstream, the liver converts the drug into chemicals the body can use and removes toxic chemicals that other organs cannot tolerate. During this process, these chemicals can attack and injure the liver.

Drug-induced liver injury can resemble the symptoms of any acute or chronic liver disease. The only way a doctor can diagnose drug-induced liver injury is by stopping use of the suspected drug and excluding other liver diseases through diagnostic tests. Rarely, long-term use of a medicine can cause chronic liver damage and scarring (cirrhosis).

Medicines that can cause severe liver injury include large doses of acetaminophen (and even in small doses when taken with alcohol), anticonvulsants such as phenytoin and valproic acid, the antihypertensive methyldopa, the tranquilizer chlorpromazine, antituberculins used to treat tuberculosis such as isoniazid and rifampin, and vitamins such as vitamin A and niacin.

What Chemicals and Drugs Damage the Liver?

Many chemicals that are inhaled or swallowed can damage the liver. Among these are drugs, industrial solvents, and pollutants. Almost every known drug has at one time or another been implicated as a cause of liver damage.

Chemicals which damage the liver fall into two groups:

1. Predictable liver toxins—These damage the liver regularly following exposure to a certain amount of the substance.

2. Unpredictable liver toxins—These cause damage in only a small percentage of people exposed to them.

Why Is the Liver so Susceptible to Injury by Chemicals and Drugs?

The reason seems to be linked to the liver's unique function of processing the chemicals and drugs which enter the blood stream. Many of these chemicals are difficult for the kidneys to excrete out of the body. The liver helps by removing these chemicals from the blood stream and changing them into products that can be readily removed through the bile or urine. In this process, unstable toxic products are sometimes produced. These can attack and injure the liver. Predictable toxic chemical injury usually involves this type of mechanism. Examples are the cleaning solvent, carbon tetrachloride, and the pain medication, acetaminophen. Acetaminophen is present in many over-the-counter and prescription pain killers (e.g. Tylenol, Nyquil, Percocet, Excedrin, Darvocet, Vicodin) and is usually safe when taken as prescribed. When acetaminophen is taken in excessive doses, either at once or over a period of time, severe damage to the liver may occur. Acetaminophen is toxic at lower doses in individuals who are regular, excessive (over two drinks each day) consumers of alcohol, which is also toxic to the liver. In fact, alcohol is by far the most common cause of toxic chemical damage to the liver in our society.

The unpredictable type injury can be produced by many drugs and appears to involve an allergic reaction that is directed at the liver. Many different medicinal drugs (e.g. antibiotics, seizure medications, and anesthetics) can cause this type of reaction in susceptible individuals.

What Are the Symptoms of This Type of Liver Injury?

Symptoms of chemical injury to the liver can resemble any form of acute or chronic liver disease. Acute liver injury can resemble viral hepatitis or blockage of the bile ducts. In other cases, a patient with fever, abdominal pain, and jaundice may have a form of chemical injury that can be confused with conditions such as stones blocking the bile ducts that may require other surgery. Chemicals can also cause chronic liver disease and cirrhosis. Usually, chronic liver disease develops only after long-term use of the drug. Excessive exposure to certain drugs and chemicals may cause tumors of the liver. An important example is the group of drugs known as anabolic steroids, best known for their use in body-building.

Can Illegal Drugs Harm the Liver?

Liver damage is common in people who are regular, illegal drug users. Most instances of liver damage in these individuals result from viral hepatitis caused by sharing contaminated needles and using alcohol. However, certain commonly abused drugs (e.g. cocaine) may be capable of producing liver damage.

How Is the Diagnosis of Chemical Liver Injury Made?

Usually it must be based on circumstantial evidence, as there are no specific tests. In any patient with liver disease, close attention needs to be given to the drugs used and the environmental and occupational exposures. No chemical is too trivial to be considered. Timing may be helpful, since many forms of chemical liver injury will occur days to weeks after the first exposure. However, there are exceptions in which a drug is taken for many months before liver injury or exposure to the toxic substance. In most cases, there will be rapid improvement in days or weeks after removal of the chemical. When drug allergy is involved, giving the patient the drug again will lead to a rapid worsening of the liver disease. This is a conclusive test, but is rarely justified because of the risk to the patient.

Even if chronic liver disease has developed, removal of exposure to the offending chemical or drug can lead to rapid improvement. Usually, no other specific therapy is needed. If there is any concern regarding a particular drug or chemical, a physician or poison control center (located in major hospital centers) should be consulted.

Warning Signs (for Liver Injury)

- Severe fatigue.
- Abdominal pain and swelling.
- Jaundice (yellow eyes and skin, dark urine).
- Fever.
- Nausea or vomiting.

Precautions

- If you have ever had a liver disease or gallstones, you should discuss this with your doctor before taking any medicines that may affect the liver or the gallbladder.

- Take these medicines only in the prescribed or recommended doses.

Glossary of Medicines

The following glossary is a guide to medicines used to treat many medical conditions. The glossary does not include all medicines that may affect the liver. If a medicine you are taking is not listed here, check with your doctor.

Acetaminophen

Acetaminophen relieves fever and pain by blocking pain centers in the central nervous system. Examples of brand names include Tylenol, Panadol, and Datril.

Anticonvulsants

These medicines control epilepsy and other types of seizure disorders. They act by lessening overactive nerve impulses in the brain. Examples of this class of medicines include phenytoin (Dilantin) and valproic acid (Dalpro).

Antihypertensives

Antihypertensives lower high blood pressure. They act by relaxing blood vessels, which makes blood flow more easily. Examples of antihypertensives include methyldopa (Aldomet) and clonidine hydrochloride (Catapres).

Antituberculins

These drugs for tuberculosis limit the growth of bacteria or prevent tuberculosis from developing in people who have a positive tuberculin skin test. Brand names include INH, Dow-Isoniazid, Rifadin, and Rimactane.

Chlorpromazine

This tranquilizer relieves anxiety or agitation. Examples of brand names include Thorazine and Ormazine.

Duract

The drug Duract (bromfenac sodium capsules), a short-term pain reliever, will carry a new warning about the risk of serious liver damage in those who take it for longer than directed.

Duract is specifically indicated for short-term management of acute pain (use for 10 days or less), and is not labeled for long-term use in chronic conditions such as osteoarthritis or rheumatoid arthritis.

Duract's manufacturer, Wyeth-Ayerst Laboratories, Philadelphia, will add a boxed warning to the label emphasizing the importance of taking the drug exactly as directed. The company has sent a letter to doctors alerting them that some patients who have used the drug for longer than 10 days have developed severe hepatitis and liver failure.

Rezulin (troglitazone)

Approved by FDA in January 1997, this drug is used in combination with insulin or sulfonylurea in patients with adult-onset diabetes mellitus whose blood glucose levels are not adequately controlled by these other therapies alone. FDA and the drug's manufacturer, Parke-Davis, recommend checking patients' serum transaminase levels routinely for the first one to two months of Rezulin treatment, every three months for the rest of the first year, and periodically after that. Liver function tests should be done if a patient develops symptoms of liver dysfunction, such as nausea, vomiting, abdominal pain, fatigue, loss of appetite, or dark urine.

Patients should stop taking Rezulin if they develop jaundice or their laboratory tests indicate liver injury.

About 2 percent of patients are expected to have to stop taking Rezulin because of elevated liver enzymes. If the drug is stopped, few, if any, of these patients will develop permanent liver damage.

Tasmar (tolcapone)

FDA and the maker of Tasmar (tolcapone), a drug for treating Parkinson's disease, have warned doctors about three fatal liver injuries associated with the drug and have recommended significant changes in how it is used.

Worldwide, about 60,000 patients have taken Tasmar, a drug approved in 1997 to augment treatment with two other Parkinson's drugs, levadopa and carbidopa. The three deaths amount to a rate of about one reported death for every 20,000 patients using the drug.

In November 1998, Tasmar manufacturer Hoffmann-LaRoche Inc. alerted doctors that the drug's labeling had changed to limit its use to patients who do not have severe movement abnormalities and who do not respond to or who are not appropriate candidates for other available treatments.

The new warning calls for liver monitoring every two weeks, more frequently than previously recommended.

Doctors also should advise patients to monitor themselves for signs of liver disease such as jaundice, fatigue, or loss of appetite. If patients fail to show substantial benefit within the first three weeks of treatment, they should be withdrawn from the drug.

FDA emphasizes that patients should not stop taking Tasmar without first speaking to their doctors. Abrupt withdrawal or reduction in dose can lead to a return of symptoms or other, more serious, complications. All cases of serious liver injury occurring in Parkinson's patients, whether on Tasmar or another drug, should be reported to FDA's MedWatch program, or to Roche Laboratories at 1-800-526-6367.

Trovan (Oral Antibiotic) and Trovan-IV (Alatrofloxacin)

The Food and Drug Administration issued a public health advisory June 9, 1999 to physicians concerning the risks of liver toxicity associated with the use of Trovan (trovafloxacin, an oral antibiotic) and Trovan-IV (alatrofloxacin, the intravenous formulation of the drug). This action follows post-marketing reports of rare but severe liver injuries leading to transplants and deaths.

In issuing this advisory, FDA is informing physicians that Trovan should be reserved for use only in patients who meet all of the following criteria:

• Patients who have at least one of several specified infections such as nosocomial (hospital-acquired) pneumonia or complicated intra-abdominal infections that, in the judgment of the treating physician, is serious and life-or limb-threatening;

• Patients who begin their therapy in in-patient health care facilities (hospitals or long term nursing care facilities);

- And patients for whom the treating physician believes that even given the new safety information, the benefit of the product outweighs the potential risks.

FDA has informed physicians that, in general, therapy with Trovan should not continue for longer than 14 days. Therapy should be discontinued sooner if the patient experiences any clinical signs of liver dysfunction, including fatigue, loss of appetite, yellowing of the skin and eyes, severe stomach pain with nausea and vomiting, or dark urine.

FDA advised physicians that for most patients who meet the treatment criteria, therapy would most likely begin with intravenous Trovan. After clinical stabilization patients may be switched to the oral dosage form. Although oral therapy might be appropriate in some cases as an initial therapy, the agency emphasizes that the oral form of Trovan is not warranted for infections other than those specified.

In addition, the manufacturer has agreed to limit distribution of the product to hospitals and long-term nursing care facilities. The manufacturer will be communicating in the near future with other appropriate pharmacies to provide directions concerning possible return of their present inventories of Trovan.

FDA took this action to reduce the potential risk from Trovan, while at the same time preserving for physicians and patients alike the clinical option of an effective broad-spectrum antibiotic for serious and life-threatening infections. The agency considers this advisory an interim measure until revised labeling for the product can be approved.

No reports of liver failure, liver transplant, or death due to liver problems were reported in the 7,000 patients studied in pre-marketing clinical trials for Trovan. In July 1998, FDA worked with the manufacturer to strengthen the product's labeling concerning liver problems after receiving reports of elevated liver enzymes and symptomatic hepatitis in patients after short-and long-term therapy. Since then, FDA has continued to receive reports of liver toxicity, including reports of a more serious nature.

FDA is aware of 14 cases of acute liver failure that it has concluded are strongly associated with the drug. Six of these patients died: five due to liver failure and one of four additional patients who received liver transplants. Three patients recovered without requiring liver transplants, and for the remaining two patients the final outcome is still pending.

More information about Trovan, including FDA's public health advisory, is available on the World Wide Web at www.fda.gov/cder/

news/trovan/default.htm and from Pfizer, the manufacturer of the drug, at 1-800-438-1985.

The FDA asks that any adverse events associated with Trovan be reported to the agency through MedWatch, FDA's adverse event reporting system. Reports may be submitted to FDA by telephone (800-332-1088), by fax (800-332-0178) or by mail to MedWatch, HF-2, FDA, 5600 Fishers Lane, Rockville, Md. 20857. Reports can also be filed via the internet at www.fda.gov/medwatch. Reports may also be filed directly to the manufacturer.

Vitamins

Vitamins serve as nutritional supplements in people with poor diets, in people recovering from surgery, or in people with special health problems.

- **Niacin** helps the body break down food for energy and is used to treat niacin deficiency and to lower levels of fats and cholesterol.

- **Vitamin A** is necessary for normal growth and for healthy eyes and skin.

- **Vitamin C** is necessary for healthy function of cells.

Additional Readings

AARP Pharmacy Service Prescription Drug Handbook. Glenview, Illinois: Scott, Foreman and Company, 1988.

General reference book for the public by the American Association of Retired Persons that provides information about medicines most frequently prescribed for persons over 50 years of age.

Advice for the Patient: Drug Information in Lay Language, USP DI, 12th edition. Rockville, Maryland: The United States Pharmacopeial Convention, 1992.

Guide for the patient that provides information about medicines by brand and generic names in sections on dosage forms, proper use directions, precautions, and side effects.

Drug Information for the Health Care Professional, USP DI, 12th edition. Rockville, Maryland: The United States Pharmacopeial Convention, 1992.

Guide for health care professionals that provides information about medicines by brand and generic names in sections on pharmacology, indications, precautions, side effects, general dosing, dosage forms, and patient consultation.

Kimmey, MG. Gastroduodenal effects of nonsteroidal anti-inflammatory drugs. *Postgraduate Medicine*, 1989; 85(5): 65-71.

General review article for primary care physicians.

Physicians' Desk Reference, 46th edition. Montvale, New Jersey: Medical Economics Company, Inc., 1992.

Reference book for health care professionals that includes information about 2,800 pharmaceutical products in sections on pharmacology, indications, contraindications, precautions, adverse reactions, and dosage and administration.

Stehlin, D. How to take your medicine: nonsteroidal anti-inflammatory drugs. *FDA Consumer*, 1990; 24(5): 33-35.

General review article for the public.

Additional Resources

National Council on Patient Information and Education
666 11th Street NW.
Suite 810
Washington, DC 20001
(202) 347-6711
E-mail: ncpie@erols.com

Distributes resources to the public and health care professionals about prescription medicines.

The United States Pharmacopeial Convention, Inc.
12601 Twinbrook Parkway
Rockville, MD 20852
(301) 881-0666

Distributes information about drug use and drug standards to health professionals and the public.

The U.S. Government does not endorse or favor any specific commercial product or company. Brand names appearing in this chapter are used only because they are considered essential in the context of the information reported herein.

National Digestive Diseases Information Clearinghouse
2 Information Way
Bethesda, MD 20892-3570
E-mail: nddic@info.niddk.nih.gov

American Liver Foundation
75 Maiden Lane, Suite 603
New York, NY 10038
1-800-GO LIVER (465-4837)

Chapter 19

Acetaminophen Alert

Frequently, parents have a false sense of safety about medications for children purchased without a prescription and sold as a safe alternative to aspirin and other pain relievers. Unintentionally and unknowingly they can harm their own children with over-the-counter medications containing acetaminophen, the active ingredient in Tylenol, Anacin 3, and many other remedies.

The most recent figures from the American Association of Poison Control Centers show 71 serious acetaminophen poisoning incidents among children in 1994, with serious long term or life-threatening results in 10 of them. The Food and Drug Administration reports 13 deaths of children under 13 from acetaminophen poisoning between 1970 and 1991. Acetaminophen can damage the liver and cause it to shut down, leading to permanent disability or death.

When taken as directed, acetaminophen is a safe drug, says Rose Ann Soloway of the Poison Control Centers. However, medications must be given in the exact doses stated, and confusion commonly occurs when people don't realize that the Infant Tylenol, a concentrated liquid, is 3 times stronger than the children's strength, and that one should never be substituted for the other.

This chapter includes © "Caution Critical When Treating Children with Acetaminophen," Hepatitis Foundation International, reprinted with permission, and "Position Statement on Acetaminophen Use and Liver Injury," © 1998, reprinted with permission from the American Liver Foundation, 1-800-GO-LIVER.

It is critically important when using products containing acetaminophen to follow directions carefully. Children are more vulnerable to the serious effects of medications.

Simple steps can be taken to promote safety:

- Always follow instructions exactly. Never double the dose.

- Check the strength to see if you are using a concentrated version.

- Check with other caretakers to be sure the medicine wasn't already given.

- Give medication at times prescribed.

- If you miss a dose, do not double the next dose.

- Always keep all medicines out of the reach of children.

Acetaminophen Use and Liver Injury

The American Liver Foundation believes that warning labels on acetaminophen-containing products should make specific mention of the risk of liver damage. Consumers should be made aware that there are a number of scientific reports that urge that those who regularly consume three or more alcoholic beverages daily should take no more than 2 grams per day of acetaminophen without consulting their physician.

Background

Acetaminophen is generally considered to be safe and effective, but like most drugs, is not entirely without risk. This is particularly true because, unlike most drugs, acetaminophen exhibits a dose-related toxicity and toxic levels may be reached in any individual who takes more than a certain amount. It is recognized that large doses of acetaminophen taken with suicidal intent can lead to liver failure and death. However, recent reports have emphasized the occurrence of unintentional or accidental hepatotoxicity, with liver failure and death in more than 20%, typically occurring in moderate to heavy alcohol users (1,2). In most of these reports the dosage of acetaminophen reported by the patient exceeded the 4gm/24hour limit recommended by the manufacturer, although some patients did report taking doses within this limit. A practical and safe dosage limit for acetaminophen, particularly for the alcohol users, has not been established, but is likely to be lower than previously thought.

The Food and Drug Administration has held hearings to review the risks of over-the-counter analgesic products. With respect to acetaminophen, reports were submitted of cases of hepatotoxicity in liver failure associated with regular alcohol use and high doses of acetaminophen. Other potential risks were identified with other pain relievers, but not directly related to liver failure. Concern was also raised about gastrointestinal bleeding due to non-steroidal anti-inflammatory agents if these were used as substitutes for acetaminophen.

In response to these concerns, McNeil Consumer Products, the manufacturer of Tylenol, one of the most widely used acetaminophen products, has voluntarily added a warning notice on its packages as follows:

"Alcohol warning: For this and all other pain relievers, including aspirin, ibuprofen, ketoprofen, and naproxen sodium. If you generally consume 3 or more alcohol-containing drinks per day you should consult your physician for advice on when and how you should take pain relievers."

This label is now widely used on many, but not all, acetaminophen containing products. The FDA recently published a proposed rule that would require all OTC pain relievers to carry an alcohol warning.

The American Liver Foundation believes that warning labels on acetaminophen-containing products should make specific mention of the risk of liver damage. Consumers should be made aware that there are a number of scientific reports that urge that those who regularly consume three or more alcoholic beverages daily should take no more than 2 grams per day of acetaminophen without consulting their physician.

Risks of Acetaminophen and Alcohol Use

The manufacturer has set the maximum dosage of acetaminophen at 4 grams per day. While acetaminophen is generally a safe and effective drug when taken at recommended doses, several medical authorities recommend that the maximum therapeutic dose be lowered for individuals who drink excessive amounts of alcohol.

Neil Kaplowitz, MD, in his 1996 medical textbook says: "Therefore, chronic alcoholics may develop serious liver injury with therapeutic doses of acetaminophen greater than 2 grams per day"(3). Hyman J. Zimmerman, MD and Willis C. Maddrey. MD, in a review article on this subject concluded: "it is our view that individuals that take more than 60 grams a day of alcohol should take no more than 2 grams per day of acetaminophen" (2). This amount of alcohol would be the equivalent of approximately 6oz of hard liquor, 4 bottles of beer, 19oz of wine, or 12oz of fortified wine each day. Note that the FDA currently, recommends that patients regularly consuming alcohol consult their physician.

Individuals who have been diagnosed with hepatitis and other liver diseases do not appear to be at greater risks for using recommended doses of acetaminophen.

Recommendations for Enhanced Public Awareness

ALF urges manufacturers of acetaminophen to develop, in consultation with FDA, consumer friendly language that warns of the possibility that regular use of alcohol may increase the risk of liver damage from acetaminophen. Warnings should be reasonably visible in readable type on the package, container and in advertising.

Because it is reported that there are over 300 products containing acetaminophen, ALF has a comprehensive list of such products available through ALF's national hotline (1-800-GO LIVER).

ALF urges the implementation of an education campaign with special attention being given to language barriers and socio-economic or educational levels, addressing:

1. General public—a broad-based education campaign stressing proper use of acetaminophen and of the hazards of excessive dosing associated with regular alcohol use should be implemented.

2. Health care professionals (e.g., physicians, pharmacists, nurses)—to improve and/or reinforce their understanding about acetaminophen preparations, the proper use of this drug, the hazards of excessive dosing and groups at greater risk of liver injury.

The Need for Additional Data

Federal agencies (e.g., CDC, NIH, FDA) should initiate additional research to try to define the risk factors, molecular and cellular mechanisms of, and improved prevention and treatments of, acetaminophen toxicity.

ALF will discuss with CDC and/or FDA national surveillance projects and registries for acetaminophen toxicity. ALF agrees with the need for more scientific data to permit determination of when a case of hepatotoxicity is really acetaminophen related.

The role of fasting and other underlying conditions on the susceptibility to acetaminophen liver toxicity in those who regularly consume alcohol needs to be explored.

References

1. Schmidt FV, Rochling FA, Casey DL, Lee WM, Acetaminophen toxicity in an urban county hospital. *N. EngI J Med* 1997; 337: 1112-7.

2. Zimmerman HJ, Maddrey W. Acetaminophen hepatotoxicity with regular intake of alcohol: Analysis of instances of therapeutic misadventure. *Hepatology* 1995; 22: 767-773.

3. Kaplowitz N., Drug metabolism and hepatotoxicity, In Kaplowitz N, ed. Liver and biliary diseases. *Williams and Wilkins*. 1996. pp. 112-120.

The American Liver Foundation acknowledges the following physicians for the assistance they provided in preparing this Position Statement:

Bruce R. Bacon, MD—Saint Louis University School of Medicine

Adrian M. Di Bisceglie MD—Saint Louis University School of Medicine

Neil Kaplowitz, MD—University of Southern California

Craig J McClain, MD—University of Kentucky

William M Lee, MD—University of Texas Southwestern Medical School

Ronald J Sokol, AIM—University of Colorado School of Medicine

John M. Vierling, MD—Cedars-Sinai Medical Center

Paul B. Watkins, MD—University of Michigan Medical Center

Hyman Zimmerman, MD—George Washington University School of Medicine

Additional Information

Hepatitis Foundation International
30 Sunrise Terrace
Cedar Grove, NJ 07009-1423
(800)-891-0707
Fax: (973)-857-5044
E-mail: mail@hepfi.org
URL: http://www.hepfi.org

American Liver Foundation
75 Maiden Lane, Suite 603
New York, NY 10038
1-800-GO LIVER (465-4837)
Fax: 212-483-8179
E-mail: webmail@liverfoundation.org
URL: http://www.liverfoundation.org

Chapter 20

Herbs and Alternatives—
Caution Needed

When traditional medicine fails to provide an answer, more and more distraught patients are turning to alternative medicine. Diet supplements and herbal remedies fill the shelves in supermarkets, pharmacies, health food stores, and offices of herbal practitioners. Testimonials as well as advertisements in health and nutrition magazines promote the use of herbs without explaining the dangers. Just because these are natural preparations from plants that doesn't mean they are safe. Herbal remedies are unregulated by any state or federal agency, and the safety and effectiveness have not been tested.

It has been documented for centuries that some plant substances are toxic to the liver. Doctors are concerned that many herbal related liver injuries go unrecognized because patients are not questioned about their use of herbs and diet supplements. A wide variety of herbal remedies contain multiple ingredients, and the labeled and actual contents of a product may differ. This makes it impossible to identify attack rates for specific herbs.

In a recent article, Dr. Raymond S. Koff questions the role herbal products play in undefined hepatitis and fulminant (sudden and severe) disease. In almost 50% of patients, fulminant disease cannot be related to any identified hepatitis viruses. Liver injury directly related to repeated use of herbal products ranges from mild and limited to extensive disease. Dr. Koff believes that unrecognized herbal use may be the cause of unidentified hepatitis and cirrhosis.

Chaparral has been named as the source of severe hepatitis leading to a liver transplant in a 60 year old woman. She had taken two capsules of chaparral daily for 10 months, and three weeks before being hospitalized increased her dose to six capsules daily. This case showed signs similar to three other cases of chaparral related hepatitis although hers was more severe due to the longer period and the amount she had ingested. Chapparal is prepared by grinding the leaves of the creosote bush, an evergreen desert shrub, and brewing a tea or putting the powder in capsules. It is claimed to have antioxidant properties used to slow the aging process and as a treatment for skin conditions and other disorders.

In addition to chaparral, a Chinese herbal product, JinBuHuan, has been implicated in clinically diagnosed hepatitis in seven patients. Other herbs known to be dangerous to the liver include: germander, comfrey, mistletoe, skullcap, margosa oil, mate tea, Gordolobo yerba tea, and pennyroral (squawmint oil). Dr. Koff stresses that "many more may not yet have been recognized."

Not all herbs are a threat to the liver, but until doctors ask patients about herbal use and have an adequate reporting system, the only way to reduce the risk of damage is to limit use of herbal products. People with hepatitis have an already compromised liver and some herbs may be an added stress increasing damage.

Part Five

Liver Cancer

Chapter 21

Primary Liver Cancer in Adults

Questions and Answers about Liver Cancer

Where Is the Liver and What Is Its Function?

The liver is a large organ located on the right side of the abdomen and is protected by the rib cage. The liver has many functions. It plays a role in converting food into energy. It also filters and stores blood.

What Is Liver Cancer?

Liver cancer is a disease in which liver cells become abnormal, grow out of control, and form a cancerous tumor. This type of cancer is called primary liver cancer. Primary liver cancer is also called malignant hepatoma or hepatocellular carcinoma. Very young children may develop another form of liver cancer known as hepatoblastoma.

Cancer that spreads to the liver from another part of the body (metastatic cancer) is not the same as primary liver cancer. In metastatic cancer cells break away from a primary tumor and travel through the blood or lymphatic system to other parts of the body. The spread of cancerous cells is called metastasis. The cancerous cells may build up in lymph nodes near the primary tumor, or they may travel to distant parts of the body.

This chapter contains text from the following National Cancer Institute publications; Cancer Facts: Fact Sheet 6.28, "Questions and Answers about Liver Cancer," 6/24/97, "Questions and Answers about Metastatic Cancer," 11/12/97, and "Adult Primary Liver Cancer," 6/98.

Metastatic (or secondary) tumors are more likely to grow in some parts of the body than in others. The lymph nodes, brain, lungs, liver, and bones are common sites of metastasis.

How Does a Doctor Know Whether a Cancer Is a Primary or a Secondary Tumor?

The cells in a metastatic tumor resemble those of the primary cancer. When a second cancer is found in a patient who has been treated for cancer in the past, it is more often a metastasis than another primary tumor. By examining the cancerous tissue under a microscope, a pathologist can usually tell whether the type of cell is normally found in the part of the body where the tissue sample was taken. Metastatic cancers may be found at the same time as the primary tumor, or months or years later.

This chapter deals with primary liver cancer in adults. For information on hepatoblastoma refer to chapter 22, Childhood Liver Cancer. For further information about cancer that has spread to the liver from another site, contact the National Cancer Institute's Cancer Information Service (CIS).

What Are the Risk Factors for Liver Cancer?

The development of liver cancer is believed to be related to infection with the hepatitis-B virus (HBV) and hepatitis-C virus (HCV). Scientists estimate that 10 to 20 percent of people infected with HBV will develop cancer of the liver. Evidence of HBV infection is found in nearly one-fourth of Americans with liver cancer. The exact relationship between HCV and cancer of the liver is being studied.

Researchers have found that people with certain other liver diseases have a higher-than-average chance of developing primary liver cancer. For example, 5 to 10 percent of people with cirrhosis of the liver (a progressive disorder that leads to scarring of the liver) will eventually develop liver cancer. Some research suggests that lifestyle factors, such as alcohol consumption and malnutrition, cause both cirrhosis and liver cancer.

Aflatoxins—a group of chemicals produced by a mold that can contaminate certain foods, such as peanuts, corn, grains, and seeds—are carcinogens (cancer-causing agents) for liver cancer.

What Are the Symptoms of Liver Cancer?

Primary liver cancer is difficult to detect at an early stage because its first symptoms are usually vague. As with other types of cancer, this disease can cause a general feeling of poor health. Cancer of the liver can lead to loss of appetite, weight loss, fever, fatigue, and weakness.

As the cancer grows, pain may develop in the upper abdomen on the right side and may extend into the back and shoulder. Some people can feel a mass in the upper abdomen. Liver cancer can also lead to abdominal swelling and a feeling of fullness or bloating. Some people have episodes of fever and nausea, or develop jaundice, a condition in which the skin and the whites of the eyes become yellow and the urine becomes dark.

It is important to note that these symptoms can be caused by primary or metastatic cancer in the liver, by a benign (noncancerous) liver tumor, or by other, less serious conditions. Only a doctor can tell for sure.

How Is Liver Cancer Diagnosed?

To make a diagnosis of liver cancer, the doctor takes a medical history, does a careful physical examination, and orders certain tests.

- Certain blood tests are used to see how well the liver is functioning. Blood tests can also be used to check for tumor markers, substances often found in abnormal amounts in patients with liver cancer. The tumor marker alpha-fetoprotein (AFP) can be useful to help diagnose liver cancer. About 50 to 70 percent of people who have primary liver cancer have elevated levels of AFP. However, other cancers such as germ cell cancer and, in some cases, pancreatic and gastric cancer, also cause elevated AFP levels.

- X-rays of the chest and abdomen, angiograms—x-rays of blood vessels, Computed Tomography (CT) scans—x-rays put together by computer, and Magnetic Resonance Imaging (MRI)—images created by using a magnetic field—may all be part of the diagnostic process.

- Liver scans using radioactive materials can help identify abnormal areas in the liver.

- The presence of liver cancer is confirmed with a biopsy. Tissue from the liver—biopsy specimen—is removed through a needle or during an operation and checked under a microscope for the presence of cancer cells. The doctor may also look at the liver with an instrument called a laparoscope, which is a small tube-shaped instrument with a light on one end. For this procedure, a small cut is made in the abdomen so that the laparoscope can be inserted. The doctor may take a small piece of tissue during the laparoscopy. A pathologist then examines the tissue under the microscope to see if cancer cells are present.

How Is Liver Cancer Treated?

Liver cancer is difficult to control unless the cancer is found when it is very small. However, treatment can relieve symptoms and improve the patient's quality of life. Treatment depends on the stage (extent) of disease, the condition of liver, and the patient's age and general health. The doctor may recommend surgery, chemotherapy (treatment with anticancer drugs), radiation therapy (treatment with high-energy rays), biological therapy (treatment using substances that help the body fight the cancer), or a combination of these treatment methods.

Are Treatment Studies (Clinical Trials) Available for Patients with Liver Cancer?

Treatment studies (clinical trials) are research studies designed to find more effective treatments and better ways to use current treatments. Participation in treatment studies is an option for many patients with liver cancer. In some studies, all patients receive the new treatment. In others, doctors compare different therapies by giving the new treatment to one group of patients and standard therapy to another group. In this way, doctors can compare different therapies.

In treatment studies for cancer of the liver, doctors are studying new anticancer drugs and drug combinations. They are also studying new ways to give chemotherapy, such as putting the drugs directly into the liver. Other research approaches include cryotherapy (surgery that uses extreme cold to destroy cancer cells) and combinations of several standard treatments.

Stage Explanation

Stages of Adult Primary Liver Cancer

Once adult primary liver cancer is found, more tests will be done to find out if the cancer cells have spread to other parts of the body (staging). The following stages are used for adult primary liver cancer:

- *Localized resectable.* Cancer is found in one place in the liver and can be totally removed in an operation.

- *Localized unresectable.* Cancer is found only in one part of the liver, but the cancer cannot be totally removed.

- *Advanced.* Cancer has spread through much of the liver or to other parts of the body.

- *Recurrent.* Recurrent disease means that the cancer has come back (recurred) after it has been treated. It may come back in the liver or in another part of the body.

Treatment Option Overview

How Adult Primary Liver Cancer Is Treated

There are treatments for all patients with adult primary liver cancer. Three kinds of treatment are used:

- surgery (taking out the cancer in an operation)
- radiation therapy (using high-dose x-rays to kill cancer cells)
- chemotherapy (using drugs to kill cancer cells)

Surgery may be used to take out the cancer or to replace the liver.

- Resection of the liver takes out the part of the liver where the cancer is found.

- A liver transplant is the removal of the entire liver and replacement with a healthy liver donated from someone else. Only a very few patients with liver cancer are eligible for this procedure.

- Cryosurgery is a type of surgery that kills cancer by freezing it.

Radiation therapy is the use of x-rays or other high-energy rays to kill cancer cells and shrink tumors. Radiation may come from a machine outside the body (external-beam radiation therapy) or from putting materials that contain radiation through thin plastic tubes (internal radiation therapy) in the area where the cancer cells are found. Drugs may be given with the radiation therapy to make the cancer cells more sensitive to radiation (radiosensitization).

Radiation may also be given by attaching radioactive substances to antibodies (radiolabeled antibodies) that search out certain cells

181

in the liver. Antibodies are made by the body to fight germs and other harmful things; each antibody fights specific cells.

Chemotherapy is the use of drugs to kill cancer cells. Chemotherapy for liver cancer is usually put into the body by inserting a needle into a vein or artery. This type of chemotherapy is called a systemic treatment because the drug enters the bloodstream, travels through the body, and can kill cancer cells outside the liver. In another type of chemotherapy called regional chemotherapy, a small pump containing drugs is placed in the body. The pump puts drugs directly into the blood vessels that go to the tumor.

If a doctor removes all the cancer that can be seen at the time of the operation, the patient may be given chemotherapy after surgery to kill any remaining cells. Chemotherapy that is given after surgery to remove the cancer is called adjuvant chemotherapy.

Hyperthermia (warming the body to kill cancer cells) and biological therapy (using the body's immune system to fight cancer) are being tested in clinical trials.

Hyperthermia therapy is the use of a special machine to heat the body for a certain period of time to kill cancer cells. Because cancer cells are often more sensitive to heat than normal cells, the cancer cells die and the tumor shrinks.

Biological therapy is the use of methods to get the body to fight cancer. Materials made by the body or made in a laboratory are used to boost, direct, or restore the body's natural defenses against disease. Biological therapy is sometimes called biological response modifier therapy or immunotherapy.

Treatment by Stage

Treatments for adult primary liver cancer depend on the stage of the disease the condition of the liver, and the patient's age and general health. Standard treatment may be considered, based on its effectiveness in patients in past studies, or participation into a clinical trial. Many patients are not cured with standard therapy, and some standard treatments may have more side effects than are desired. For these reasons, clinical trials are designed to find better ways to treat cancer patients and are based on the most up-to-date information. Clinical trials are ongoing in most parts of the country for most stages of adult liver cancer. For more information, call the Cancer Information Service at 1-800-4-CANCER (1-800-422-6237); TTY at 1-800-332-8615.

Localized Resectable Adult Primary Liver Cancer

Treatment is usually surgery (resection). Liver transplantation may be done in certain patients. Clinical trials are testing adjuvant systemic or regional chemotherapy following surgery.

Localized Unresectable Adult Primary Liver Cancer

Treatment may be one of the following:

1. Cryosurgery (in patients whose tumors can not be surgically removed).
2. Liver transplantation (in certain patients).
3. Regional chemotherapy, including local infusion of chemotherapy.
4. Systemic chemotherapy.
5. Surgery or cryosurgery followed by chemotherapy. Hyperthermia or radiation therapy with or without drugs to make the cancer cells more sensitive to radiation may be given in addition to chemotherapy.
6. Local injection of pure alcohol for small tumors.
7. Radiation therapy.

Advanced Adult Primary Liver Cancer

Treatment may be one of the following:

1. A clinical trial of biological therapy.
2. A clinical trial of chemotherapy.
3. A clinical trial of chemotherapy, radiation therapy, and drugs to make the cancer cells more sensitive to radiation (radiosensitizers).
4. A clinical trial of external radiation therapy plus chemotherapy followed by radiolabeled antibodies.

Recurrent Adult Primary Liver Cancer

Treatment of recurrent adult primary liver cancer depends on what treatment a patient has already received, the part of the body where the cancer has come back, whether the liver has cirrhosis, and other factors. Patients may wish to consider taking part in a clinical trial.

To Learn More

To learn more about adult primary liver cancer contact:

National Cancer Institute
Cancer Information Service
31 Center Drive, MSC 2580
Bethesda, MD 20892-2580
1-800-4-CANCER (1-800-422-6237)
TTY at 1-800-332-8615
http://www.nci.nih.gov.

CancerMail Service

To obtain a contents list, send e-mail to cancermail@icicc.nci.nih.gov with the word "help" in the body of the message.

CancerFax
301-402-5874, listen to recorded instructions.

The Cancer Information Service has booklets about cancer that are available to the public and can be sent on request.

- *In Answer to Your Questions About Liver Cancer*
- *What You Need To Know About Cancer*
- *Taking Time: Support for People with Cancer and the People Who Care About Them*
- *What Are Clinical Trials All About?*
- *Chemotherapy and You: A Guide to Self-Help During Treatment*
- *Radiation Therapy and You: A Guide to Self-Help During Treatment*
- *Eating Hints for Cancer Patients*
- *Advanced Cancer: Living Each Day*
- *When Cancer Recurs: Meeting the Challenge Again*

There are many other places where people can get material and information about cancer treatment and services. The social service office at a hospital can be checked for local and national agencies that help with getting information about finances, getting to and from treatment, getting care at home, and dealing with other problems.

Chapter 22

Childhood Liver Cancer

What Is Childhood Liver Cancer?

Childhood liver cancer, also called hepatoma, is a rare disease in which cancer (malignant) cells are found in the tissues of a child's liver. The liver is one of the largest organs in the body, filling the upper right side of the abdomen and protected by the rib cage. The liver has many functions. It plays an important role in making food into energy and also filters and stores blood.

Primary liver cancer is different from cancer that has spread from another place in the body to the liver (liver metastases).

There are two types of cancer that start in the liver (hepatoblastoma and hepatocellular cancer), based on how the cancer cells look under a microscope. Hepatoblastoma is more common in young children before age 3 and may be caused by an abnormal gene. Children of families whose members carry a gene related to a certain kind of colon cancer may be more likely to develop hepatoblastoma (genes carry the hereditary information that you get from your parents). Children infected with hepatitis B or C (viral infections of the liver) are more likely than other children to get hepatocellular cancer. Hepatocellular cancer is found in children from birth to age 4 or in children ages 12 to 15.

If a child has symptoms, the child's doctor may order special x-rays, such as a Computed Tomography (CT) scan or a liver scan. If a lump

National Cancer Institute (NCI), 2/99.

is seen on an x-ray, the child's doctor may remove a small amount of tissue from the liver using a needle inserted into the abdomen. This is called a needle biopsy and is usually done using an x-ray to guide the doctor. The child's doctor will have the tissue looked at under the microscope to see if there are any cancer cells.

A child's chance of recovery (prognosis) and choice of treatment depend on the stage of the child's cancer (whether it is just in the liver or has spread to other places), how the cancer cells look under a microscope (the histology), and the child's general state of health.

Stages of Childhood Liver Cancer

Once liver cancer is found, more tests will be done to find out if the cancer cells have spread to other parts of the body. This is called staging. The child's doctor needs to know the stage of disease in order to plan treatment. The following stages are used for childhood liver cancer:

Stage I

Stage I childhood liver cancer means the cancer can be removed with surgery.

Stage II

Stage II childhood liver cancer means that most of the cancer may be removed in an operation but very small (microscopic) amounts of cancer are left in the liver following surgery.

Stage III

Stage III childhood liver cancer means that some of the cancer may be removed in an operation, but some of the tumor cannot be removed and remains either in the abdomen or in the lymph nodes.

Stage IV

Stage IV childhood liver cancer means the cancer has spread to other parts of the body.

Recurrent

Recurrent disease means that the cancer has come back (recurred) after it has been treated. It may come back in the liver or in another part of the body.

Treatment Option Overview

How Childhood Liver Cancer Is Treated

There are treatments for all children with liver cancer. Three kinds of treatment are used:

- surgery (taking out the cancer in an operation)
- chemotherapy (using drugs to kill cancer cells).
- radiation therapy (using high-dose x-rays to kill cancer cells)

Surgery may be used to take out the cancer and part of the liver where the cancer is found. Sometimes the entire liver may be surgically removed and replaced by a liver transplant from a donor.

Chemotherapy uses drugs to kill cancer cells. Chemotherapy may be given to the child before surgery to help reduce the size of the liver cancer. The child may be given chemotherapy after surgery to kill any remaining cells. Chemotherapy given after surgery when the doctor has removed the cancer is called adjuvant chemotherapy. Chemotherapy for childhood liver cancer is usually put into the body through a needle in a vein or artery. This type of chemotherapy is called a systemic treatment because the drug enters the bloodstream, travels through the body, and can kill cancer cells outside the liver. In another type of chemotherapy, called direct infusion chemotherapy, drugs are injected directly into the blood vessels that go into the liver.

Sometimes a special treatment called chemo-embolization is used to treat childhood liver cancer. Chemotherapy drugs are injected into the main artery of the liver with substances that block or slow the flow of blood into the cancer. This lengthens the time the drugs have to kill the cancer cells and it also prevents the cancer cells from getting oxygen or other materials that they need to grow.

Radiation therapy uses x-rays or other high-energy rays to kill cancer cells and shrink tumors. Radiation may come from a machine outside the body (external radiation therapy) or from putting materials that produce radiation (radioisotopes) through thin plastic tubes in the area where the cancer cells are found (internal radiation therapy).

Treatment By Stage

Treatments for childhood liver cancer depend on the type (hepatoblastoma or hepatocellular carcinoma) and stage of the child's disease and their age and general health.

A child may receive treatment that is considered standard based on its effectiveness in a number of patients in past studies, or the parent may choose to have their child take part in a clinical trial. Not all patients are cured with standard therapy and some standard treatments may have more side effects than are desired. For these reasons, clinical trials are designed to test new treatments and to find better ways to treat cancer patients. Clinical trials are ongoing in many parts of the country for most stages of childhood liver cancer. For more information, call the Cancer Information Service at 1-800-4-CANCER (1-800-422-6237); TTY at 1-800-332-8615.

Stage I Childhood Liver Cancer

Stage I Hepatoblastoma

The child's treatment will probably be complete removal of the liver cancer by surgery followed by adjuvant chemotherapy.

Stage I Hepatocellular Carcinoma

Treatment will probably be complete removal of the liver cancer by surgery followed by adjuvant chemotherapy.

Stage II Childhood Liver Cancer

Stage II Hepatoblastoma

The child's treatment will probably be removal of the liver cancer by surgery followed by chemotherapy.

Stage II Hepatocellular Carcinoma

Treatment will probably be removal of the liver cancer by surgery followed by chemotherapy.

Stage III Childhood Liver Cancer

Stage III Hepatoblastoma

The child's treatment may be one or more of the following:

1. Chemotherapy to reduce the size of the tumor followed by surgery to remove as much of the cancer as possible.

2. Chemotherapy

3. Radiation therapy

4. Direct infusion of drugs into blood vessels going into the liver.

5. Liver transplant: Surgical removal of the liver followed by replacement with a donor's liver.

Stage III Hepatocellular Carcinoma

The child's treatment will probably be chemotherapy to reduce the size of the tumor followed by surgery to remove as much of the cancer as possible.

Stage IV Childhood Liver Cancer

Stage IV Hepatoblastoma

The child's treatment may be one or more of the following:

1. Chemotherapy to reduce the size of the tumor followed by surgery to remove as much of the cancer as possible followed by chemotherapy.

2. Surgical removal of cancer that has spread to the lungs.

3. Chemotherapy.

4. Radiation therapy followed by additional surgery.

5. Direct infusion of chemotherapy drugs into blood vessels going into the liver.

6. Chemotherapy drugs injected into the main liver artery with substances that block or slow the flow of blood (chemo-embolization chemotherapy).

7. Liver transplant: Surgical removal of the liver followed by replacement with a donor's liver.

8. Clinical trials are testing new therapies and may be considered for your child.

Stage IV Hepatocellular Carcinoma

The child's treatment will probably be chemotherapy to reduce the size of the tumor followed by surgery to remove as much of the cancer as possible.

Recurrent Childhood Liver Cancer

Recurrent Hepatoblastoma

Treatment depends on where the cancer recurred and how the cancer was treated before. Treatment may include additional surgery. Clinical trials are testing new therapies and may be considered.

Recurrent Hepatocellular Carcinoma

Clinical trials are testing new therapies and that may be considered.

What Is PDQ?

PDQ is a computer system that provides up-to-date information on cancer and its prevention, detection, treatment, and supportive care. PDQ is a service of the National Cancer Institute (NCI) for people with cancer and their families and for doctors, nurses, and other health care professionals.

To ensure that it remains current, the information in PDQ is reviewed and updated each month by experts in the fields of cancer treatment, prevention, screening, and supportive care. PDQ also provides information about research on new treatments (clinical trials), doctors who treat cancer, and hospitals with cancer programs. The treatment information in this summary is based on information in the PDQ summary for health professionals on this cancer.

How to Use PDQ

Cancer in children is rare. The majority of children with cancer are treated at cancer centers with special facilities to treat childhood cancers. There are organized groups of doctors and other health care professionals who work together by doing clinical trials to improve treatments for children with cancer.

PDQ can be used to learn more about current treatment of different kinds of cancer. You may find it helpful to discuss this information with your child's doctor, who knows your child and has the facts about your child's disease. PDQ can also provide the names of additional health care professionals and hospitals that specialize in treating children who have cancer.

Before your child begins treatment, you may want to consider entering your child in a clinical trial. PDQ can be used to learn more about the trials. A clinical trial is a research study that attempts to improve current treatments or find new treatments for people with cancer. Clinical trials are based on past studies and information discovered in the laboratory. Each trial answers specific scientific questions in order to find new and better ways to help people with cancer. During clinical trials, information is collected about new treatments, their risks, and how well they do or do not work. When a clinical trial shows that a new treatment is better than the treatment currently used as "standard" treatment, the new treatment may become the "standard" treatment. Children who are treated in clinical trials have the advantage of getting the best available therapy. In the United States, about two thirds of children with cancer are treated in a clinical trial at some point in their illness.

Listings of current clinical trials are available on PDQ. In the United States, there are two major groups (called cooperative groups) that organize clinical trials for childhood cancers: the Children's Cancer Group (CCG) and the Pediatric Oncology Group (POG). Doctors who belong to these groups or who take part in other clinical trials are listed in PDQ.

To learn more about cancer and how it is treated or to learn more about clinical trials for your child's kind of cancer, call the National Cancer Institute's Cancer Information Service. The number is 1-800-4-CANCER (1-800-422-6237); TTY at 1-800-332-8615. The call is free and a trained information specialist will be available to answer your cancer-related questions.

PDQ is updated whenever there is new information. Check with the Cancer Information Service to be sure that you have the most up-to-date information.

To Learn More

To learn more about childhood liver cancer,

National Cancer Institute
Cancer Information Service
31 Center Drive, MSC 2580
Bethesda, MD 20892-2580
1-800-4-CANCER (1-800-422-6237);
TTY at 1-800-332-8615.

The Cancer Information Service can also send you booklets. The following booklets may be helpful to you:

- *In Answer to Your Questions About Liver Cancer*

- *Young People with Cancer: A Handbook for Parents*

- *Talking with Your Child About Cancer*

- *Managing Your Child's Eating Problems During Cancer Treatment*

- *When Someone in Your Family Has Cancer*

The following general booklets on questions related to cancer may also be helpful:

- *Taking Time: Support for People with Cancer and the People Who Care About Them*

- *What Are Clinical Trials All About?*

- *Chemotherapy and You: A Guide to Self-Help During Treatment*

- *Radiation Therapy and You: A Guide to Self-Help During Treatment*

- *What You Need To Know About Cancer*

There are many other places where material about cancer treatment and information about services are available. Check the hospital social service office for local and national agencies that help with finances, getting to and from treatment, care at home, and dealing with other problems.

Part Six

Hepatitis

Chapter 23

The A, B, C, D, and E of Viral Hepatitis

The word "hepatitis" conjures up a vision of someone whose skin and/or conjunctiva is yellowed (jaundice) because of the deposition of bile pigments that a damaged liver is unable to remove from the circulating blood. Liver inflammation can be caused by factors such as alcohol abuse, some medications and trauma, as well as by certain viruses.

General dentists, oral surgeons, physicians, dental hygienists, dental assistants, nurses, and health profession students top the list of the people at high risk for whom vaccination protection is recommended. Since 1987, the American Dental Association has encouraged dentists and their staff members to take advantage of the hepatitis B vaccine and post-vaccination testing to protect themselves, their co-workers, and their patients from hepatitis B infection. In 1992, the ADA expanded this recommendation to include the vaccination of dental students, preclinical and clinical faculty, and staff against infectious diseases (for example, mumps, measles, rubella and hepatitis B).

The viral inflammation has some aspects that make the infected person potentially harmful to others. People may be chronically or acutely infected but not know that they have the disease because they have no symptoms. However, they still have the ability to spread the

This chapter contains text from "Hepatitis Statistics," and "Diagnosis and Treatment," © 1999, reprinted with permission of Hepatitis Foundation International, and "The A,B,C,D, and E of Viral Hepatitis," *Insights on Human Health*, National Institute of Dental Research.

disease. A person can become an asymptomatic chronic carrier of the disease after being infected with any one of the several hepatitis viruses (such as B, C, or D). The only protection against infection for the health care provider and the patient is vaccination.

The Five Types of Hepatitis

Viral hepatitis comprises at least five different viruses that differ in surface antigens, type of nucleic acid, mode of infection, length of viral incubation, and pathogenicity and the ability to produce a chronic disease that can progress to fulminating liver failure or hepatocellular carcinoma. All five forms of viral hepatitis can cause an acute illness, and all five have virulence and induce pathology primarily on the infected liver.

Hepatitis A Virus.

- Each year an estimated 152,000 HAV infections occur in the U.S. with 10 million cases worldwide.

- HAV causes an average of 30 missed days of work, resulting in approximately $2600 in lost wages. Medical care alone can cost $2800 for each hospitalized case.

- Children under the age of 5 often have no symptoms, whereas most adults will become ill.

- Approximately 100 people in the United States die each year from hepatitis A.

- The annual cost associated with hepatitis A is estimated at $200 million in the U.S. (1991 dollars).

Each hepatitis A virus, or HAV, is a small virus about .026 micrometers in diameter and is transmitted by the oral-fecal route. HAV can produce an acute illness with a viremia of four to eight weeks. Its debilitating symptoms are often flu-like: fever, fatigue, muscle and joint aches, as well as possible nausea, vomiting, and pain in the liver area.

Recovery may take as long as a year. The acute infection is clinically silent in approximately 90 percent of infected people. In about 10 percent of patients, acute HAV infection results in jaundice, but the risk of liver failure is very low, and there is no risk of chronicity. Recovery is associated with lifelong immunity. The virus is spread by eating contaminated food, drinking contaminated water or ice cubes, by close personal contact, or by sharing dirty needles. Each year in the United States 138,000 people become infected by HAV and 100 die of HAV.

Hepatitis B Virus.

- An estimated 140,000 Americans are infected each year with hepatitis B. Approximately 1–1.25 million people are chronically infected and are considered to be carriers of the virus.

- 300 million people in the world have chronic HBV.

- 70% of new cases occur among people age 15-39, of which 75% occur in teenagers.

- Each year 3,000–4,000 die from cirrhosis and 1,000 from primary liver cancer due to HBV infection in the U.S.

- 30-40% of people with HBV infection show no symptoms and can unknowingly pass HBV to others.

- About 30% of HBV cases are related to heterosexual activity, either unprotected sex with an infected person or multiple sexual partners.

- 22,000 pregnant women in the U.S. are chronically infected with HBV.

- Up to 90% of babies born to chronically infected mothers are infected at birth if they do not receive the HBIG (Hepatitis B Immune Globulin) and vaccine. Fifty to twenty-five percent of them will die of chronic liver disease, cirrhosis, or liver cancer before they reach middle age.

- 2-10% of adults and 25-50% of children under the age of 5 infected with HBV are unable to clear the virus from their bodies within six months and are considered to be chronically infected.

- HBV is 100 times more infectious than HIV (AIDS).

- Approximately 90% of adults infected with HBV will recover within six months and develop immunity.

- In 1994, 1,000 unvaccinated healthcare workers were infected with HBV.

- There is a 6-30% chance of HBV infection from a single needle stick contaminated with HBV if the HBIG and vaccine are not given.

- HBV can live on a dry surface for at least 7 days.

- The HBV vaccine provides immunity in over 95% of recipients.

- Since 1993, an increase in incidence was observed among sexually active heterosexuals, homosexual men, and injection drug users.

HBV, the cause of "serum hepatitis," is classified as a hepadnavirus. Electron micrographs of infected sera of people have shown three morphological forms of hepatitis B virus: complete, spherical, and filamentous. The complete virion (Dane particle) is about .042 mm. The spherical and filamentous forms of the virus represent viral coat material, or HBVsAg, produced in excess by the infected hepatocyte.

After infection of hepatocytes or mononuclear cells, viremia either is transient, lasts four to eight weeks, or is chronic. In 90 percent of infected people, acute infection is clinically silent or produces symptoms that mimic flu, including fever, headache, muscle ache, and fatigue. About 15 to 20 percent of patients develop short-term arthritis-like problems. In 10 percent of patients, acute infection can result in jaundice. In acute hepatitis with jaundice, the risk of fulminant liver failure is about 1:100. Ten percent of patients, irrespective of any acute reaction, can develop a chronic infection, either inactive or active. Patients with chronic active hepatitis caused by HBV have a high risk of developing cirrhosis. Antibodies against the HB surface antigen, HBsAg, can neutralize the virus, thus preventing infection. The antigen has been used as a vaccine since 1975 and became generally available in 1982.

Two other HBV antigens have been detected in humans: hepatitis B Core antigen, or HBcAg, which is not detectable free in the serum, and the hepatitis E antigen, HBeAg, associated with high infectivity. Antibody to the core antigen can be detected during acute illness, especially at the beginning of the illness, and antibody to the E antigen may point to a lower degree of infectivity and reduced likelihood of becoming a carrier.

HBV infection and its sequelae, however, still are one of the major causes of morbidity and death in man. Globally, more than 2 billion people are infected with HBV, and 350 million people are chronic carriers, at high risk of death from chronic active hepatitis, cirrhosis, and primary hepatocellular carcinoma. Between 1 million and 1.5

million people die each year of HBV infection, making it one of the major causes of morbidity and death worldwide. If the vaccine was used more widely, the disease could be prevented almost completely.

By the end of 1992, 41 countries worldwide crafted national policies to give HBV vaccine to all newborns. In some parts of the world, the major mode of transmission is from child to child or mother to child, and vaccinating newborns would break this cycle. The vaccine is 90 to 95 percent effective in preventing virus infection and the carrier state.

Although HBV vaccine is easily obtained in the United States each year, an estimated 300,000 people become infected. The virus is most commonly transmitted by shared needles, by high-risk sexual behavior, from a mother to her newborn, and in the health care setting. Saliva, blood, semen, tears, vaginal secretions, milk, and other bodily fluids are the major sources of infection. In approximately 30 to 40 percent of cases, the method of transmission is unknown.

Children are at the greatest risk. About 90 percent of babies who become infected at birth with HBV and up to half of the youngsters who are infected before the age of 5 years become chronic carriers. In an effort to eliminate chronic carriers, the U.S. Centers for Disease Control and Prevention, or CDC, recommends that all newborns be vaccinated. Other groups recommend that pregnant women be screened for HBsAg as part of their routine prenatal care. If they are infected, their babies should be given hepatitis B immune globulin as well as vaccine immediately after birth.

Dentists, oral hygienists, and oral surgeons who are routinely exposed to blood on the job are at the top of the list for contracting HBV. Safe and protective HBsAg vaccines against HBV exist. To be fully protective, three injections are required: the second injection one month after the first and the third injection six months later. The vaccine provides immunity for 10 to 20 years.

In 1987, the CDC estimated that 12,000 of the 300,000 hepatitis B virus infections occurred among health care workers, and approximately 250 of those people died as the result of infection. In 1991, 81 percent of the dentists who participated in the ADA's Health Screening Program, conducted each year at the ADA annual session, reported having received the HBV vaccine—a substantial increase from the 1987 level of 56 percent. Serologic data from the HSP for the years 1981 to 1989 indicated a decrease in the number of dentists naturally infected with HBV from 15 percent to 8 percent. Immunization and increasing use of universal precautions probably were responsible for the decrease.

Hepatitis C Virus.

- About 35,000 Americans contract hepatitis C each year.

- Currently, an estimated 3.9 million Americans, nearly 2% of the population, are chronically infected with the hepatitis C virus.

- Currently, transfusion-related hepatitis due to hepatitis C is a rare event.

- It is believed that 20% of patients with chronic hepatitis C will develop cirrhosis in 10-20 years. Liver failure and death may occur in 1/4 of those patients (5% overall) even though it may take many years.

- More than 85% of patients infected with HCV will remain chronically infected. Many can develop cirrhosis that may or may not have an impact on their life expectancy.

- 8,000-10,000 people die in the U.S. of hepatitis C related cirrhosis or cancer of the liver each year.

- Almost half of the 3,922 liver transplants in 1995 were performed on patients with hepatitis C.

- Transmission of HCV from infected mother to newborn may occur in 5-10% of deliveries.

Acute infection with hepatitis C virus, or HCV, is clinically silent in 95 percent of infected people. The remaining 5 percent develop jaundice. In 60 to 70 percent of patients exposed to HCV, a chronic infection develops that is associated with chronic hepatitis and fluctuating serum transaminase activities. Cirrhosis develops in 10 to 20 percent of these patients. The delay from initial infection to the development of cirrhosis usually is 10 to 30 years but sometimes is shorter (five to 10 years). With the advent of new tests to screen blood donors, a very small percentage of people with HCV currently became infected through blood transfusions. HCV appears to be spread mainly through unprotected sexual contact, shared needles, recipients of previously untested blood products, and health care workers, although the method of infection is unknown in many cases. HCV is the most common form of chronic viral hepatitis in the United States and appears to be a major factor in the 25,000 deaths each year that are caused by chronic liver disease.

Hepatitis D Virus (or Delta Hepatitis).

Infection with the hepatitis D virus, or HDV, is the severest form of viral hepatitis. It leads to cirrhosis in up to 70 percent of cases, often within a few years of the onset of disease. It accounts for less than 5 percent of the cases of chronic hepatitis. HDV occurs only in patients who have acute or chronic HBV hepatitis and are HBsAg-positive. HDV is coated by the HBV coat antigen HBsAg. An anti-HDV assay is available for diagnosing the infection, which should be suspected in patients who have chronic HBV infection but have clinical signs of acute hepatitis. Vaccine protection against HBV also serves against HDV.

Hepatitis E Virus.

Hepatitis E virus, or HEV, is an epidemic form of hepatitis that shares some characteristics with HAV, such as a lack of a chronic phase and enteric transmission primarily in underdeveloped countries with contaminated water supplies. Outbreaks have not been observed in the United States, but at least 20 epidemics have occurred in 17 other countries.

Diagnosis

Diagnosing any of the hepatitis viruses is generally done with tests that recognize either circulating viral antigens or circulating antibodies to viral antigens. Hepatitis E remains a diagnosis of exclusion, as clinically applicable serologic assays for it are not readily available.

> "Usually, acute viral hepatitis is self-limiting. Most patients experience complete recovery, with restoration of liver function and clearance of the virus."

Hepatitis A.

Tests for hepatitis A virus are available to screen for antibody to hepatitis A. The antibody is detectable at the onset of illness and persists for the patient's lifetime.

Hepatitis B.

A number of laboratory tests, including radioimmunoassay or enzyme-linked immunosorbent assay, can detect HBsAg. The antigen often appears before symptoms develop and disappears with recovery. If the antigen remains six months after recovery, the person may have chronic disease or be a carrier of the virus. Antibody to the antigen usually persists for many years and protects against further infection.

HBcAg cannot be detected in the blood, but antibody to the antigen can be detected at high levels during the beginning of the illness and decrease over time. In chronic carriers, high levels of antibody may persist for a lifetime.

HBe antigen and antibody to the antigen can be detected by commercial tests. Presence of the antigen indicates high infectivity.

Liver function tests often are diagnostic of hepatitis virus infection. High levels of the liver enzymes aspartate transaminase, or AST, and alanine transaminase, or ALT, are of particular importance.

Hepatitis C.

A new test is now available to detect antibody to hepatitis C. The antibody is present in 50 percent of people who have acute antibody and in almost all people who have hepatitis C.

Hepatitis D.

Until recently, this virus could be diagnosed only by liver biopsy. A blood test is now available to detect antibody to delta antigen (a protein found inside the hepatitis D virus).

Hepatitis E

Testing for anti-HEV is usually reserved for returning travelers from the developing world in whom hepatitis is present but other hepatitis viruses cannot be detected.

Treatment and Prevention

Hepatitis A

99% of those infected will recover without any serious aftereffects. There is no specific treatment for HAV other than treating symptoms, i.e., nausea, vomiting and diarrhea.

Individuals exposed to hepatitis A through household and close personal contact (anal/oral contact) or who plan to travel to developing countries where sanitary conditions are poor and the hepatitis A virus is prevalent, can receive temporary immunity (less than 3 months) by having 0.02- ml/kg immune globulin administered intramuscularly. For those exposed to HAV, immune globulin should be given as soon as possible after exposure and no later than 2 weeks. Vaccines are available to prevent HAV infection prior to exposure. These provide protection against the virus as early as 2 - 4 weeks after vaccination. Personal objects should not be shared and hands should be washed with soap and water following bowel movements and before food preparation. Immunization of children (2-18 years of age) consists of 2 or 3 doses of the vaccine. Adults need a booster dose 6-12 months following the initial dose of vaccine. Other individuals who should be vaccinated include: homosexual men; users of illicit injectable drugs; certain institutional workers (e.g., caretakers for the developmentally challenged); workers in day-care centers; and laboratory workers who handle live hepatitis virus. Patients with chronic liver disease should be vaccinated against hepatitis A.

Hepatitis B

The FDA approved treatment for HBV is interferon. Less than 50% of patients with chronic hepatitis B are candidates for interferon therapy. Initially, 40% of HBV patients treated will respond; however, a number will relapse when the treatment is stopped. In the long term, approximately 30-35% of eligible patients will benefit. The treatment, given by injection for several months, may have a number of side effects including flu-like symptoms, headache, nausea, loss of appetite, diarrhea, fatigue, and thinning of hair. Some patients experience depression. The type and severity of side effects differs for each individual. Interferon may interfere with the production of white blood cells and platelets by depressing the bone marrow. Blood tests are needed to monitor blood cells, platelets, and liver enzymes. Some HBV patients with advanced cirrhosis might be considered for liver transplant. Many new treatments are under investigation.

Safe and effective vaccines provide protection against hepatitis B for thirteen or more years. Three injections over a 6-12 month period are required to provide full protection. Children and adolescents (through age 18) and high risk individuals should be vaccinated. Unvaccinated individuals who have been exposed to HBV infected individuals through intimate contact or contact with infected blood or body fluids should receive an intramuscular injection of 0.06 ml/ kg hepatitis B immune globulin (HBIG) within 14 days of exposure and the hepatitis B vaccine. Newborns exposed to HBV at birth by an infected mother who is a carrier should receive 0.5 ml of HBIG plus the hepatitis B vaccine within 12 hours of birth and two additional doses of vaccine at one and six to twelve months of age. Individuals should practice safe sex and avoid contact with infected blood or other body fluids directly or on objects such as needles, razors, toothbrushes, etc. Sores and rashes should be covered with bandages and blood on any surface should be cleaned up with household bleach.

Hepatitis C

Currently, there are three types of interferon and a combination of interferon and ribavirin used to treat hepatitis C. Selection of patients for treatment may be determined by biochemical, virologic, and when necessary, liver biopsy findings, rather than presence or absence of symptoms. Interferon must be given by injection, and has a number of side effects including flu-like symptoms: headaches, fever, fatigue, loss of appetite, nausea, vomiting, depression, and thinning of hair. It may also interfere with the production of white blood cells and platelets by depressing the bone marrow. Periodic blood tests are required to monitor blood cells and platelets. Ribavirin can cause sudden, severe anemia and birth defects so women should avoid pregnancy while taking it and for 6 months following treatment. The severity and type of side effects differ for each individual. Treatment of children with HCV is under investigation.

While 50-60% of patients respond to treatment initially, lasting clearance of the virus occurs in about 10-40% of patients. Treatment may be prolonged and given a second time to those who relapse after initial treatment.

- Retreatment with bioengineered consensus interferon alone results in elimination of the virus in 58% of patients treated for one year. Side effects occur but the medication is usually well tolerated.

- Combined therapy (interferon and ribavirin) shows elimination of the virus in 47% after 6 months of therapy. Side effects from both drugs may be prominent.

Currently, almost one half of all liver transplants in the U.S. are performed for end-stage hepatitis C. However, reinfection of the transplanted liver by HCV occurs at a high rate. Fortunately, this infrequently requires a second transplant.

Anyone with hepatitis C should be vaccinated against hepatitis A and B and should not drink alcohol.

Try to maintain as normal a life as possible eating a well balanced diet, exercising, and keeping a positive attitude. Avoid depressing or overwhelming tasks, learn how to pace yourself, and rest when you feel tired. Plan physically exhausting tasks in the morning when your energy level is at its peak.

Hepatitis D

Interferon alfa-2b treatments may be beneficial to a small proportion of patients. Vaccination against HBV will prevent HDV.

Hepatitis E

Currently there is no treatment for HEV.

Conclusion

Recent breakthroughs in understanding hepatitis B make the future therapy of this disease promising. In the past few years, animal models have been developed for drug testing, and cell culture has been found that can allow replication of the virus. Other technological advances offer new areas for possible therapy for hepatitis, including monoclonal antibodies against HBsAg, HBV-antigen—specific T cells and antisense oligonucleotides. Many antiviral and immunomodulary agents are under evaluation, including interleukin-2, gamma interferon, acyclovir, ganciclovir, suramin, and combinations of drugs. Much work remains to be done.

Our best approach to the control and prevention of hepatitis is vaccination of susceptible populations, especially health care workers, with HBV vaccine and, under special circumstances, with HAV vaccine. We also must continue to observe good barrier protection techniques when dealing with patients.

For Additional Information

American Liver Foundation
75 Maiden Lane
Suite 603
New York, NY 10038
1-800-GO-LIVER (465-4837)

**Centers for Disease Control and Prevention/
National Center for Infectious Diseases**
Division of Viral and Rickettsial Diseases
Hepatitis Branch
Atlanta, Ga. 30333
1-888-443-7232 (The Hepatitis Hotline)

Hepatitis Foundation International
30 Sunrise Terrace
Cedar Grove, NJ 07009-1423, USA
(973) 239-1035 or (800) 891-0707
FAX: (973) 857-5044
E-Mail: mail@hepfi.org

National Digestive Diseases Information Clearinghouse
2 Information Way
Bethesda, Md. 20892-3570
1-301-654-3810

National Institute of Allergy and Infectious Diseases
Information Office
31 Center MSC 2520
Building 31, Room 7A50
Bethesda, Md. 20892
1-301-496-5717

Chapter 24

Hepatitis A

Hepatitis A Facts

Clinical Features

- Jaundice, fatigue, abdominal pain, loss of appetite, intermittent nausea, diarrhea.

Etiologic Agent

- Hepatitis A virus.

Incidence

- Estimated 125,000-200,000 total infections per year in the United States.

- 84,000-134,000 symptomatic infections per year.

- 100 deaths due to fulminant hepatitis per year.

Sequelae

- Prolonged or relapsing hepatitis (15%)

- No chronic infection

This chapter contains text from "Hepatitis A," Fact Sheet, Centers for Disease Control and Prevention (CDC), revised 6/8/98, and "Prevention of Hepatitis A Through Active or Passive Immunization," *Morbidity & Mortality Weekly Report*, December 27, 1996, Vol. 45/No.RR-15.

Prevalence

- 33% of Americans have evidence of past infection (immunity).

Costs

- Estimated $200 million (1991)dollars per year (medical and work loss).

Transmission

- Fecal-oral; food/waterborne outbreaks; bloodborne (rare)

Risk Groups

- Household/sexual contacts of infected persons;
- International travelers;
- Persons living in American Indian reservations, Alaska Native villages, and other regions with endemic hepatitis A;
- During outbreaks: day care center employees or attendees, homosexually active men, injecting drug users.

Surveillance

- National Notifiable Disease Surveillance System
- Viral Hepatitis Surveillance Program
- Sentinel Counties Studies

Trends

- Large nationwide outbreaks every decade (last in 1989)
- Cases increasing slightly during past several years

Prevention

- Hepatitis A vaccine is highly effective in preventing hepatitis A and provides the potential to have a substantial impact on the disease burden;
- Immune globulin administered pre- and post-exposure;
- Good hygiene and sanitation.

General Information

What Is Hepatitis A?

Hepatitis A is a liver disease caused by hepatitis A virus.

What Are the Signs and Symptoms of Hepatitis A?

Persons with hepatitis A virus infection may not have any signs or symptoms of the disease. Older persons are more likely to have symptoms than children. If symptoms are present, they usually occur abruptly and may include fever, tiredness, loss of appetite, nausea, abdominal discomfort, dark urine, and jaundice (yellowing of the skin and eyes). Symptoms usually last less than 2 months; a few persons are ill for as long as 6 months. The average incubation period for hepatitis A is 28 days (range: 15–50 days).

How Is Hepatitis A Diagnosed?

A blood test (IgM anti-HAV) is needed to diagnose hepatitis A. Talk to your doctor or someone from your local health department if you suspect that you have been exposed to hepatitis A or any type of viral hepatitis.

How Is Hepatitis A Virus Transmitted?

Hepatitis A virus is spread from person to person by putting something in the mouth that has been contaminated with the stool of a person with hepatitis A. This type of transmission is called "fecal-oral." For this reason, the virus is more easily spread in areas where there are poor sanitary conditions or where good personal hygiene is not observed.

Most infections result from contact with a household member or sex partner who has hepatitis A. Casual contact, as in the usual office, factory, or school setting, does not spread the virus.

What Products Are Available to Prevent Hepatitis A Virus Infection?

Two products are used to prevent hepatitis A virus infection: immune globulin and hepatitis A vaccine.

1. Immune globulin is a preparation of antibodies that can be given before exposure for short-term protection against hepatitis A and for persons who have already been exposed to

hepatitis A virus. Immune globulin must be given within 2 weeks after exposure to hepatitis A virus for maximum protection.

2. Hepatitis A vaccine has been licensed in the United States for use in persons 2 years of age and older. The vaccine is recommended (before exposure to hepatitis A virus) for persons who are more likely to get hepatitis A virus infection or are more likely to get seriously ill if they do get hepatitis A. The vaccines currently licensed in the United States are HAVRIX(®) (manufactured by SmithKline Beecham Biologicals) and VAQTA(®) (manufactured by Merck & Co., Inc).

Hepatitis A Vaccine and Immune Globulin

What Are the Dosages and Schedules for Hepatitis A Vaccines?

Table 24.1. Recommended Dosages of HAVRIX(®)[1]

Vaccinee's age (years)	Dose (EL.U.)[2]	Volume (mL)	No. doses	Schedule (mos)[3]
2-18	720	0.5	2	0,6-12
>18	1,440	1.0	2	0,6-12

[1]*Hepatitis A vaccine, inactivated, SmithKline Beecham Biologicals.*
[2]*ELISA units.*
[3]*0 months represents timing of the initial dose; subsequent numbers represent months after the initial dose.*

Table 24.2. Recommended Dosages of VAQTA(®)[1]

Vaccinee's age(years)	Dose (U)[2]	Volume (mL)	No. doses	Schedule (mos)[3]
2-17	25	0.5	2	0,6-18
>17	50	1.0	2	0,6

[1]*Hepatitis A vaccine, inactivated, Merck & Co., Inc.*
[2]*Units.*
[3]*0 months represents timing of the initial dose; subsequent numbers represent months after the initial dose.*

How Are Hepatitis A Vaccines Made?

There is no live virus in hepatitis A vaccines. The virus is inactivated during production of the vaccines similar to Salk-type inactivated polio vaccine.

Is Hepatitis A Vaccine Safe?

Yes, hepatitis A vaccine has an excellent safety profile. No serious adverse events have been attributed definitively to hepatitis A vaccine. Soreness at the injection site is the most frequently reported side effect.

Any adverse event suspected to be associated with hepatitis A vaccination should be reported to the Vaccine Adverse Events Reporting System (VAERS). VAERS forms can be obtained by calling 1-800-822-7967.

Is Immune Globulin Safe?

Yes. No instance of transmission of HIV (the virus that causes AIDS) or other viruses has been observed with the use of immune globulin administered by the intramuscular route. Immune globulin can be administered during pregnancy and breast-feeding.

Is Immune Globulin in Short Supply?

Yes. This shortage is expected to continue necessitating a prioritization of indications for the use of immune globulin.

Can Other Vaccines Be Given at the Same Time that Hepatitis A Vaccine Is Given?

Yes. Hepatitis B, diphtheria, polio virus (oral and inactivated), tetanus, oral typhoid, cholera, Japanese encephalitis, rabies, yellow fever vaccine, or immune globulin can be given at the same time that hepatitis A vaccine is given, but at a different injection site.

How Long Does Immunity Last after Hepatitis A Vaccination?

Although data on long-term protection are limited, estimates based on modeling techniques suggest that protection will last for at least 20 years.

When Are Persons Protected after Receiving Hepatitis A Vaccine?

Protection against hepatitis A begins four weeks after the first dose of hepatitis A vaccine. Check with your doctor for when the next dose is due.

Can Hepatitis A Vaccine Be Given after Exposure to Hepatitis A Virus?

No, hepatitis A vaccine is not licensed for use after exposure to hepatitis A virus. In this situation, immune globulin should be used.

Should Pre-Vaccination Testing Be Done?

Pre-vaccination testing is done only in specific instances to control cost (e.g., persons who were likely to have had hepatitis A in the past). This includes persons who were born in countries with high levels of hepatitis A virus infection, elderly persons, and persons who have clotting factor disorders and may have received factor concentrates in the past.

Should Post-Vaccination Testing Be Done?

No.

Can a Patient Receive the First Dose of Hepatitis A Vaccine from One Manufacturer and the Second (Last) Dose from Another Manufacturer?

Yes. Although studies have not been done to look at this issue, there is no reason to believe that this would be a problem.

What Should Be Done if the Second Dose of Hepatitis A Vaccine Is Delayed?

The second dose should be administered as soon as possible. There is no need to repeat the first dose.

Can Hepatitis A Vaccine Be Given during Pregnancy or Lactation?

We don't know for sure, but because vaccine is produced from inactivated hepatitis A virus, the theoretical risk to the developing fetus is expected to be low. The risk associated with vaccination, however, should be weighed against the risk for hepatitis A in women who may be at high risk for exposure to hepatitis A virus.

Can Hepatitis A Vaccine Be Given to Immunocompromised Persons? (e.g., Persons on Hemodialysis or Persons with AIDS)

Yes.

Persons Who Should Receive Hepatitis A Vaccine

Hepatitis A vaccination provides protection before one is exposed to hepatitis A virus. Hepatitis A vaccination is recommended for the following groups who are at increased risk for infection and for any person wishing to obtain immunity.

Persons Traveling To or Working in Countries that Have High or Intermediate Rates of Hepatitis A.

All susceptible persons traveling to or working in countries that have high or intermediate rates of hepatitis A should be vaccinated or receive immune globulin before traveling. Persons from developed countries who travel to developing countries are at high risk for hepatitis A. Such persons include tourists, military personnel, missionaries, and others who work or study abroad in countries that have high or intermediate levels of hepatitis A. The risk for hepatitis A exists even for travelers to urban areas, those who stay in luxury hotels, and those who report that they have good hygiene and that they are careful about what they drink and eat.

Children in Communities that Have High Rates of Hepatitis A and Periodic Hepatitis A Outbreaks.

Children living in communities that have high rates of hepatitis A (e.g., American Indian, Alaska Native) should be routinely vaccinated beginning at 2 years of age. High rates of hepatitis A are generally found in these populations, both in urban and rural settings. In addition, to effectively prevent epidemics of hepatitis A in these communities, vaccination of previously unvaccinated older children is recommended within 5 years of initiation of routine childhood vaccination programs. Although rates differ among areas, available data indicate that a reasonable cutoff age in many areas is 10-15 years of age because older persons have often already had hepatitis A. Vaccination of children before they enter school should receive highest priority, followed by vaccination of older children who have not been vaccinated.

Men Who Have Sex with Men

Sexually active men (both adolescents and adults) who have sex with men should be vaccinated.

Hepatitis A outbreaks among men who have sex with men have been reported frequently. Recent outbreaks have occurred in urban areas in the United States, Canada, and Australia.

Illegal-Drug Users

Vaccination is recommended for injecting and noninjecting illegal-drug users if local health authorities have noted current or past outbreaks among such persons.

During the past decade, outbreaks have been reported among injecting-drug users in the United States and in Europe.

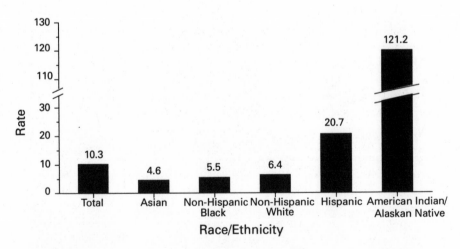

Figure 24.1. *Rates Per 100,000 Population of Reported Hepatitis A Cases, by Race/Ethnicity—United States.*

Persons Who Have Occupational Risk for Infection

Persons who work with hepatitis A virus-infected primates or with hepatitis A virus in a research laboratory setting should be vaccinated. No other groups have been shown to be at increased risk for hepatitis A virus infection because of occupational exposure.

Outbreaks of hepatitis A have been reported among persons working with non-human primates that are susceptible to hepatitis A virus infection, including several Old World and New World species. Primates that were infected were those that had been born in the wild, not those that had been born and raised in captivity.

Persons Who Have Chronic Liver Disease

Persons with chronic liver disease who have never had hepatitis A should be vaccinated, as there is a higher rate of fulminant (rapid onset of liver failure, often leading to death) hepatitis A among persons with chronic liver disease. Persons who are either waiting for or have received liver transplants also should be vaccinated.

Persons Who Have Clotting-Factor Disorders

Persons who have never had hepatitis A and who are administered clotting-factor concentrates, especially solvent detergent-treated preparations, should be given hepatitis A vaccine.

All persons with hemophilia (Factor VIII, Factor IX) who receive replacement therapy should be vaccinated because there appears to be an increased risk of transmission from clotting-factor concentrates that are not heat inactivated.

Groups for Whom Hepatitis A Vaccine Is Not Routinely Recommended

Food Service Workers

Foodborne hepatitis A outbreaks are relatively uncommon in the United States; however, when they occur, intensive public health efforts are required for their control.

Although persons who work as food handlers have a critical role in common-source foodborne outbreaks, they are not at increased risk for hepatitis A because of their occupation. Consideration may be given to vaccination of employees who work in areas where community-wide outbreaks are occurring and where state and local

215

health authorities or private employers determine that such vaccination is cost-effective.

Sewerage Workers

In the United States, no work-related outbreaks of hepatitis A have been reported among workers exposed to sewage.

Health-care Workers

Health-care workers are not at increased risk for hepatitis A. If a patient with hepatitis A is admitted to the hospital, routine infection control precautions will prevent transmission to hospital staff.

Children Under 2 Years of Age

Because of the limited experience with hepatitis A vaccination among children under 2 years of age, the vaccine is not currently licensed for this age-group.

Day-care Attendees

The frequency of outbreaks of hepatitis A is not high enough in this setting to warrant routine hepatitis A vaccination. In some communities, however, day-care centers play a role in sustaining community-wide outbreaks. In this situation, consideration should be given to adding hepatitis A vaccine to the prevention plan for children and staff in the involved center(s).

Travel and the Prevention of Hepatitis A

Who Should Receive Protection Against Hepatitis A before Travel?

All susceptible persons traveling to or working in countries that have high or intermediate rates of hepatitis A should be vaccinated or receive immune globulin before traveling. Persons from developed countries who travel to developing countries are at high risk for hepatitis A. Such persons include tourists, military personnel, missionaries, and others who work or study abroad in countries that have high or intermediate levels of of hepatitis A. The risk for hepatitis A exists even for travelers to urban areas, those who stay in luxury hotels, and those who report that they have good hygiene and that they are careful about what they drink and eat.

How Soon before Travel Should the First Dose of Hepatitis A Vaccine Be Given?

Protection against hepatitis A virus infection begins four weeks before travel. Check with your doctor about when the next dose is due.

What Should Be Done if a Person Cannot Receive Hepatitis A Vaccine?

Travelers who are allergic to a vaccine component or who elect not to receive vaccine should receive a single dose of immune globulin (0.02 mL/kg), which provides effective protection against hepatitis A for up to 3 months. Travelers whose travel period exceeds 2 months should be administered immune globulin at 0.06 mL/kg; administration must be repeated if the travel period exceeds 5 months. Note!! Immune globulin is in very short supply and the supply is often not adequate for use in this setting.

If Travel Starts Sooner than 4 Weeks Prior to the First Vaccine Dose, What Should Be Done?

Because protection may not be complete until 4 weeks after vaccination, persons traveling to a high-risk area less than 4 weeks after

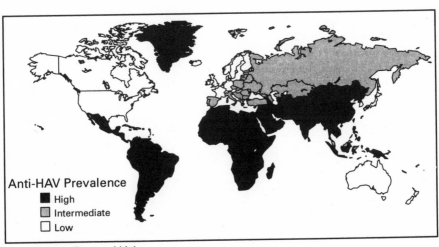

Anti-HAV Prevalence
■ High
▨ Intermediate
□ Low

*Low, intermediate, and high.
†This map generalizes available data, and patterns may vary within countries.

Figure 24.2. Patterns of Hepatitis A Virus Infection Worldwide

the initial dose of hepatitis A vaccine should also be given immune globulin (0.02 mL/kg), but at a different injection site.

Note: Immune globulin is in very short supply and the supply is often not adequate for use in this setting. Therefore, the first dose of hepatitis A vaccine should be administered as soon as travel to a high-risk area is planned.

What Should Be Done for Travelers Who Are Less than 2 Years of Age to Protect Them from Hepatitis A Virus Infection?

Immune globulin is recommended for travelers less than 2 years of age because the vaccine is currently not licensed for use in this age group.

Note: Immune globulin is in very short supply and the supply is often not adequate for use in this setting.

The use of commercial sources and trade names is for identification and does not imply endorsement by the Public Health Service or the U.S. Department of Health and Human Services.

Chapter 25

Hepatitis B

Chapter Contents

Section 25.1

What You Need to Know about Hepatitis B

"What Do I Need to Know about Hepatitis B," National Institute of Diabetes and Digestive and Kidney Diseases (NIDDK), NIH Publication No. 97-4228, October 1997, updated February 20, 1998.

What Is Hepatitis B?

Hepatitis B is a liver disease. Hepatitis (HEP-ah-TY-tis) makes your liver swell and stops it from working right.

You need a healthy liver. The liver does many things to keep you alive. The liver fights infections and stops bleeding. It removes drugs and other poisons from your blood. The liver also stores energy for when you need it.

What Causes Hepatitis B?

Hepatitis B is caused by a virus. A virus is a germ that causes sickness. (For example, the flu is caused by a virus.) People can pass viruses to each other. The virus that causes hepatitis B is called the hepatitis B virus.

How Could I Get Hepatitis B?

Hepatitis B spreads by contact with an infected person's blood, semen, or other body fluid. You could get hepatitis B by

- having sex with an infected person without using a condom
- sharing drug needles
- getting a tattoo or body piercing with dirty tools that were used on someone else
- getting pricked with a needle that has infected blood on it (health care workers can get hepatitis B this way)
- sharing a toothbrush or razor with an infected person

- an infected woman can give hepatitis B to her baby at birth or through her breast milk

You cannot get hepatitis B by

- shaking hands with an infected person
- hugging an infected person
- sitting next to an infected person.

What Are the Symptoms?

Hepatitis B can make you feel like you have the flu. You might

- feel tired
- feel sick to your stomach
- have a fever

- not want to eat
- have stomach pain
- have diarrhea

Some people have

- dark yellow urine
- light-colored stools

- yellowish eyes and skin

Some people don't have any symptoms. If you have symptoms, or think you might have hepatitis B, go to a doctor.

What Are the Tests for Hepatitis B?

To check for hepatitis B, the doctor will test your blood. These tests show if you have hepatitis B and how serious it is.

The doctor may also do a liver biopsy. Biopsy (BYE-op-see) is a simple test. The doctor removes a tiny piece of your liver through a needle. The doctor checks the piece of liver for signs of hepatitis B and liver damage.

How Is Hepatitis B Treated?

Treatment for hepatitis B may involve:

- A drug called interferon (in-ter-FEAR-on). It is given through shots. Most people are treated for 4 months.

- Surgery. Over time, hepatitis B may cause your liver to stop working. If that happens, you will need a new liver. The surgery is called a liver transplant. It involves taking out the old, damaged liver and putting in a new, healthy one from a donor.

How Can I Protect Myself?

You can get the hepatitis B vaccine. A vaccine is a drug that you take when you are healthy that keeps you from getting sick. Vaccines teach your body to attack certain viruses, like the hepatitis B virus.

The hepatitis B vaccine is given through three shots. All babies should get the vaccine. Infants get the first shot within 12 hours after birth. They get the second shot at age 1 to 2 months and the third shot between ages 6 to 18 months.

Older children and adults can get the vaccine, too. They get three shots over 6 months. Children who have not had the vaccine should get it. You need all of the shots to be protected. If you miss a shot, call your doctor or clinic right away to set up a new appointment.

You can also protect yourself and others from hepatitis B if you

- use a condom when you have sex,
- don't share drug needles with anyone,
- wear gloves if you have to touch anyone's blood,
- don't use an infected person's toothbrush, razor, or anything else that could have blood on it,
- also, if you get a tattoo or body piercing, make sure it is done with clean tools.

For More Information

American Liver Foundation
75 Maiden Lane, Suite 603
New York, NY 10038
Tel: (800) 465-4837 (GO-LIVER)

Hepatitis Foundation International
30 Sunrise Terrace
Cedar Grove, NJ 07009-1423
Tel: (800) 891-0707

National Institute of Digestive Diseases Information Clearinghouse (NDDIC)
2 Information Way
Bethesda, MD 20892-3570

Section 25.2

Understanding Your Hepatitis B Blood Tests

Reprinted with permission of the Hepatitis B Foundation © 1998.

Disclaimer: This information should not be used as personal medical advice. Since every situation is unique, each person needs to discuss specific questions, concerns, and treatment options with their own health care provider.

Understanding your hepatitis B blood test results can be confusing, so it is important to discuss them carefully with your health care provider. It is helpful if you request a written copy of your blood tests so that you can be sure you know your results.

Before explaining the tests, here are two basic medical terms:

- Antigen—this is a substance that sets off an alarm in your body to protect itself (e.g. hepatitis B virus)

- Antibody—this is produced by the body to protect itself from an antigen. Antibodies bind to and often inactivate antigens.

Common Blood Tests for Hepatitis B Infection

HBsAg (hepatitis B surface antigen)—This is the outer surface of the hepatitis B virus that triggers an antibody response. HBsAg "positive" or "reactive" means that the person is infected with HBV and can potentially pass it on to others who are in close daily contact.

Anti-HBs (antibody to hepatitis B surface antigen)—The presence of antibodies indicates that a person has been exposed to HBV, but successfully cleared the virus from their body and is no longer contagious to others. The antibody protects the body from any future exposure to HBV infection-a person has been "naturally immunized". Antibodies are also produced from the HBV vaccine series.

223

Anti-HBc (antibody to hepatitis B core)—This test is used to identify a past or present HBV infection. It is produced during and after acute HBV infection. The core antigen is part of the hepatitis B virus and the antibody to the core antigen is usually present in chronic carriers. However, if it is present with a "positive" anti-HBs (protective antibodies), then it is associated with recovery from an infection and this person is not a carrier. The interpretation of this test depends on the first two test results.

Additional Blood Tests for Hepatitis B Carriers

E-Antigen—This is a viral protein that is secreted by HBV infected cells. Its presence indicates high levels of virus in the blood which increases a carrier's infectiousness to others who are in close contact. If this test is negative, but a person is known to be HBsAg positive, then it indicates low levels of virus in the blood, which decreases one's infectiousness. This test is often used to monitor the effectiveness of some HBV therapies, whose goal is to convert a carrier to "e-antigen negative".

E-Antibody—Carriers who stop producing e-antigen sometimes produce e-antibodies. The clinical significance of this result is uncertain.

Liver Function Tests (or Liver Enzymes)—Includes blood tests that assess the general state of the liver and biliary system. When elevated above normal values, the ALT (alanine aminotransferase) and AST (aspartate aminotransferase) tests indicate damage to liver cells. The ALT and AST are enzymes that are located in liver cells and leak out into the bloodstream when liver cells are injured.

AFP (Alpha-FetoProtein)—This is a normal protein produced in the developing fetus. Pregnant women will have elevated AFP's. Other adults, however, should not have much AFP in their blood. In a chronic carrier, high levels of AFP could indicate the possibility of liver cancer since this kind of tumor produces AFP.

Ferritin—Iron is stored in the liver in the form of Ferritin. Increased levels of Ferritin means there is a high iron storage. This could result from an increased iron intake in the diet (vitamin supplements, food cooked in iron pots, etc.). An elevation can also occur from a destruction of liver cells causing leakage of Ferritin. More research is needed to understand the relationship between elevated Ferritin and liver tumors.

High-Risk Groups for Hepatitis B

The following groups are at risk for hepatitis B. Most people in these groups should be tested and/or vaccinated depending on individual risk factors.

- Immigrants/refugees from areas of high HBV prevalence (Asia, parts of Africa, Southern Italy, Eastern Europe, and Amazon Basin)
- Children born in the US to immigrants/refugees who come from areas of high HBV prevalence
- Adoptees and their families from countries where HBV is endemic (see above)
- Alaskan natives/Pacific Islanders
- Clients/staff of institutions for the developmentally disabled
- Injecting drug users
- Sexually active homosexual and bisexual men
- Sexually active adults and teenagers with more than one sexual partner in six months
- People who have sexually transmitted diseases
- Close household contacts and sexual partners of HBV carriers
- Hemodialysis patients
- Inmates of long-term correctional facilities
- Recipients of certain blood products
- Health, Dental, and Emergency Care personnel who have contact with blood
- Infants born to HBV+ women (national recommendation is that all pregnant women should be screened for hepatitis B)

HBV Vaccination

There are currently two vaccines available, both synthesized using scientific DNA technology. There is no possibility of contracting any disease from the vaccine itself! It takes three injections over a six-month schedule to provide full protection against HBV. The vaccine has been in use worldwide for over 15 years with only a few mild side effects reported. Since 1991, the Centers for Disease Control and Prevention (CDC) have recommended that all infants receive the HBV vaccine. There are an increasing number of states that now require HBV vaccination for school entrance. Check with your school for their requirements.

For More Information

Hepatitis B Foundation
700 East Butler Avenue
Doylestown, PA 18901-2697
(215) 489-4900
E-mail: info@hepb.org

Section 25.3

Hepatitis B and the Vaccine that Protects You

This information was produced by the Centers for Disease Control and Prevention (CDC); Hepatitis Branch, National Center for Infectious Diseases; and the National Immunization Program; August 12, 1998, revised February 5, 1999.

What Is Hepatitis B?

Hepatitis B is a serious disease caused by the hepatitis B virus (HBV) which is present in the blood and body fluids of an infected individual. The virus can be transmitted from mother to baby at birth as well as through unprotected sexual intercourse, and unsterilized needles. HBV infection can cause acute illness that leads to loss of appetite; tiredness; pain in muscles, joints, or stomach; diarrhea or vomiting; and yellow skin or eyes (jaundice). HBV can also cause chronic infection, especially in infants and children, that leads to liver damage (cirrhosis), liver cancer, and death. Each year in the United States, an estimated 200,000 people have new HBV infections, of whom more than 11,000 people are hospitalized and 20,000 remain chronically infected. Overall, an estimated 1.25 million people in the United States have chronic HBV infection, and 4,000 to 5,000 people die each year from hepatitis B related chronic liver disease or liver cancer (Centers for Disease Control and Prevention (CDC), 1990; Margolis, 1991; West, 1992).

How Is Hepatitis B Vaccine Used to Prevent Hepatitis B and Its Related Complications?

Hepatitis B vaccine prevents both HBV infection and those diseases related to HBV infection. It has been available since 1982. Hepatitis B vaccines currently available in the United States are made using recombinant DNA technology, and contain only a portion of the outer protein of HBV or hepatitis B surface antigen [HBsAg] (Emini, 1986; Stephenne, 1990). The vaccine does not contain any live components. The vaccine is given as a series of three intramuscular doses. More than 95% of children and adolescents, and more than 90% of young, healthy adults develop adequate antibody to the recommended series of three doses (Szmuness, 1980; Zajac, 1986; Andre, 1989). Persons who respond to hepatitis B vaccine are protected against acute hepatitis B as well as the chronic consequences of HBV infection, including cirrhosis and liver cancer (CDC, 1991 a; Hadler, 1992).

For Whom Is Hepatitis B Vaccine Recommended?

The Advisory Committee on Immunization Practices (ACIP) recommends hepatitis B vaccine for everyone 18 years of age and younger, and for adults over 18 years of age who are at risk for HBV infection (CDC, 1991 a,b; 1996). Hepatitis B vaccine has been recommended as a routine infant vaccination since 1991, and as a routine adolescent vaccination since 1995 (CDC, 1991,CDC 1996). Adults who are at increased risk of HBV infection and who should receive the vaccine include: sexually active heterosexual adults with more than one sex partner in the prior 6 months or a history of a sexually transmitted disease; homosexual and bisexual men; illicit injection drug users, persons at occupational risk of infection; hemodialysis patients; household and sex contacts of persons with chronic HBV infection; and clients and staff of institutions for the developmentally disabled; (CDC, 1991 b).

Why Not Vaccinate Children in those Families Where There Is the Highest Risk of HBV Infection, Rather than Vaccinating All Infants/ Children?

Routine immunization of infants and adolescents is recommended for several reasons. One is that there is a large disease burden attributable to HBV infections that occur among children. Approximately 30,000 infants and children were infected each year before routine infant hepatitis B immunization began and CDC estimates that one-third of the chronic HBV infections in the United States come from infected infants and young children. The majority of these infections occur among children of mothers who are not infected with HBV and thus would not be prevented by perinatal hepatitis B prevention programs. Other than for infants born to HBV infected pregnant women, there is no way to identify and selectively vaccinate those children at risk of infection (Margolis, 1991).

Another reason we vaccinate infants and older children is that it will provide them protection against exposure to HBV infection when they are older adolescents and adults. While most HBV infections occur among older adolescents and young adults, vaccination of persons in high-risk groups has generally not been a successful public health strategy. In addition, about 30% of persons do not know where they acquired their acute HBV infection (Alter, 1990).

Is Hepatitis B Vaccine Safe?

Hepatitis B vaccines have been shown to be very safe when given to infants, children or adults (CDC, 1991 a; Greenberg, 1993). More than 20 million persons have received hepatitis B vaccine in the United States and more than 500 million persons have received the vaccine worldwide. The most common side effects from hepatitis B vaccination are pain at the injection site and mild to moderate fever (Szmuness, 1980; Francis, 1982; Zajac, 1986; Stevens, 1985; Andre, 1989; Greenberg, 1993). Studies show that these side effects are reported no more frequently among those vaccinated than among persons not receiving vaccine (Szmuness, 1980; Francis, 1982). Among children receiving both hepatitis B vaccine and diphtheria-tetanus-pertussis (DTP) vaccine, these mild side effects have been observed no more frequently than among children receiving DTP vaccine alone (CDC, 1991 a; Greenberg, 1993).

Is There an Association Between Hepatitis B Vaccine and Serious Side Effects?

Serious side effects reported after receiving hepatitis B vaccine are very uncommon (Andre, 1989; CDC, 1991 a; Greenberg, 1993). There is no confirmed scientific evidence that hepatitis B vaccine causes chronic illness, including multiple sclerosis, chronic fatigue syndrome, rheumatoid arthritis, or autoimmune disorders. There is no risk of HBV infection from the vaccine.

Large-scale hepatitis B immunization programs in Taiwan, Alaska, and New Zealand have observed no association between vaccination and the occurrence of serious adverse events. Furthermore, surveillance of adverse events in the United States after hepatitis B vaccination have shown no association between hepatitis B vaccine and the occurrence of serious adverse events including Guillain-Barre' syndrome, transverse myelitis, optic neuritis, and seizures (Shaw, 1988; CDC, 1991 a; Chen, 1991; Niu, 1996; Niu 1998 CDC, unpublished data).

A low rate of anaphylaxis (hives, difficulty breathing, shock) has been observed in vaccine recipients based on reports to the Vaccine Adverse Event Reporting System (VAERS), with an estimated incidence of 1 in 600,000 vaccine doses distributed. One case has been reported in 100,763 children (10-11 years old) vaccinated with recombinant vaccine in British Columbia and no cases were observed in 166,757 children vaccinated in New Zealand. Although none of the persons who developed anaphylaxis died, anaphylactic reactions can be life-threatening, and therefore further vaccination with hepatitis B vaccine is contraindicated in persons with a history of anaphylaxis after a previous dose of vaccine. There have been rare reports of hair loss after hepatitis B vaccination, with the majority of individuals regrowing their hair (Wise, 1997). Studies are in progress to better quantify the possible slight risk of hair loss.

Any presumed risk of adverse events associated with hepatitis B vaccination must be balanced with the expected 4,000 to 5,000 HBV-related liver disease deaths that would occur without immunization, assuming a 5% lifetime risk of HBV infection.

Does Hepatitis B Vaccination Cause Demyelinating Diseases Such as Multiple Sclerosis (MS)?

The scientific evidence to date does not support hepatitis B vaccination causing multiple sclerosis (MS) or other demyelinating diseases.

Multiple sclerosis is a disease of the central nervous system characterized by the destruction of the myelin sheath surrounding neurons, resulting in the formation of "plaques". MS is a progressive and usually fluctuating disease with exacerbations (patients feeling worse) and remissions (patients feeling better) over many decades. Eventually, in most patients, remissions do not reach baseline levels and permanent disability and sometimes death occurs. The cause of MS is unknown. The most widely held hypothesis is that MS occurs in patients with a genetic susceptibility and that some environmental factors "trigger" exacerbations. MS is 3 times more common in women than men, with diagnosis usually made as young adults.

The concern that hepatitis B vaccination may cause MS or exacerbate it derives from case reports and media attention in France and, more recently, televised news reports in the United States. However, it is possible that these MS case reports are purely coincidental to hepatitis B vaccination. Carefully controlled studies (currently underway) are needed to determine the nature of these reports.

Other than these case reports, what then is the current scientific evidence that hepatitis B vaccination causes MS or other demyelinating diseases? First, extensive pre-licensure clinical trials did not document such an effect. Second, hundreds of millions of persons worldwide have been immunized without developing MS (or any other autoimmune disease). This finding provides important negative evidence as well as an appropriate framework for assessing this possible association-namely, that if vaccination causes MS, it does so extremely rarely.

Third, prospective studies of MS patients have shown that exacerbations appeared to be more frequent after nonspecific viral illnesses (Sibley, 1985). This is presumably due to generalized stimulation of the immune system that occurs with such infections (Owen, 1980). Given the intent of immunizations is to stimulate the immune system, it is not surprising therefore that exacerbations of MS have been reported after various vaccinations (Poser, 1994). Given the large number of vaccinations administered worldwide, it is also not surprising that surveillance systems in the U.S., France, and elsewhere (Quast, 1991), have received some reports of MS temporally (coincidentally) associated with vaccinations. As with all such case reports, however, they only constitute signals of possible causal associations. Further controlled studies are necessary to establish causation.

A recent (and largest to date) multi-center randomized double-blind placebo controlled trial of influenza immunization in 104 MS patients failed to show any difference in attack rate or disease progression over 6 months between vaccines and placebo recipients (Miller, 1997). This study suggests that even if the vaccine can exacerbate MS, it must do so only among a small minority of MS patients.

Fourth, whether vaccinations actually cause an overall excess of MS in the population (vs. being just one of multiple possible triggers for MS in genetically susceptible individuals, without causing an excess of MS) can only be evaluated in a population-based study. If vaccination only rarely exacerbates MS in MS patients, if at all (Miller, 1997), it is hard to imagine physiologically that vaccinations would cause an excess of MS.

Although scientific evidence to date does not support hepatitis B vaccination causing multiple sclerosis (MS) or other demyelinating diseases a study is currently being organized in the Vaccine Safety Datalink project at CDC because of public concern about this issue in France and elsewhere and because there is little available research on this specific topic (Chen, 1997). Computerized medical records on approximately 5 million or 2% of the U.S. population are available in this study. It will probably be at least one year, however, before any results are available

In the meantime, the concern regarding a suggested association between vaccination and MS or any other chronic illness must be weighed against the very strong evidence that vaccines have in protecting against disease and death.

How Is Vaccine Safety Monitored after It Is Licensed for Use?

The Vaccine Adverse Event Reporting System (VAERS) ensures the safety of vaccines distributed in the United States. VAERS reports are usually submitted by health care professionals or vaccine manufacturers, however any one can submit a report to VAERS. VAERS is administered, monitored and analyzed jointly by the Centers for Disease Control and Prevention and the Food and Drug Administration. Persons who wish to report a possible health effect related to a vaccine should notify their health care provider and can also call the VAERS program at 1-800-822-7967.

Where Can I Find More Information about Hepatitis B and Hepatitis B Vaccine?

Further information regarding hepatitis B and hepatitis B vaccine can be obtained by contacting the Hepatitis Hotline of the Hepatitis Branch, CDC at 1-888-4HEP-CDC (or 1-888-443-7232) and by contacting your local or state health department. For information about vaccines contact the National Immunization Program, CDC Information Hotline at 1-800-232-2522; or visit the CDC National Immunization Program website at http:/www.cdc.gov/nip/, or the CDC Hepatitis Branch website at http://www.cdc.gov/ncidod/diseases/hepatitis/

References

Alter MJ, Hadler SC, Margolis HS, et al. The changing epidemiology of hepatitis B in the United States. Need for alternative vaccination strategies. *JAMA* 1990;263:1218-22.

Andre FE. Summary of safety and efficacy data on a yeast derived hepatitis B vaccine. *Am J Med*. 1989;87(Suppl 3A): 14s-20s.

Centers for Disease Control and Prevention. Protection against viral hepatitis: Recommendations of the Advisory Committee on Immunization Practices (ACIP). *MMWR*. 1990;39:5-22.

Centers for Disease Control and Prevention. Hepatitis B virus: A comprehensive strategy for eliminating transmission in the United States through Universal Childhood Vaccination. *MMWR*. 1991;40 (RR-13):1-17.

Centers for Disease Control and Prevention. Immunization of Adolescents: Recommendations of Advisory Committee on Immunization Practices, American Academy of Pediatrics, American Family Physicians and American Medical Association.. *MMWR*. 1996; 45 (RR-13):1-14.

Centers for Disease Control and Prevention. Update on Adult Immunization: Recommendations of the Immunization Practices Advisory Committee (ACIP). *MMWR*. 1991;40 (RR-12);30-33.

Chen D-S. Control of hepatitis B in Asia: mass immunization program in Taiwan. In: Hollinger FB, Lemon SM, Margolis HS, eds. Viral hepatitis and liver disease. Baltimore: Williams and Wilkins, 1991:716-719.

Chen RT, Glasser J, Rhodes P, et al. The Vaccine Safety Datalink Project: A New Tool for Improving Vaccine Safety Monitoring in the United States. *Pediatrics* 1997;99:765-73.

Emini EA, Eliis RW, Miller WJ, et al: Production and immunologic analysis of recombinant hepatitis B vaccine. J infect. 1986;13 (Suppl A):3-9.

Francis DP, Hadler SC, Thompson SE, et al. Prevention of hepatitis B vaccine: report from the Centers for Disease Control multicenter efficacy trial among homosexual men. *Ann Intern Med.* 1982;97:362-6.

Greenberg DP. Pediatric experience with recombinant hepatitis B vaccines and relevant safety and immunization studies. *Pediatr Infect Dis J.* 1993;12:438-445.

Hadler SC, Margolis HS. Hepatitis B Immunization: vaccine types, efficacy, and indications for immunization. In: Remington JS, Swartz MN, eds. Current Clinical Topics in Infectious Diseases. Boston Mass: *Blackwell Scientific Publications;* 1992:282-308.

Margolis HS, Alter MJ, Hadler SC. Hepatitis B: evolving epidemiology and implications for control. Semin Liver Dis. 1991;11:84-92.

Miller AE, Morgante LA, Buchwald LY et al. A multi center, randomized double-blind placebo controlled trial of influenza immunization in multiple sclerosis. *Neurology* 1997:48:312-314.

Niu MT, Davis DM, Ellenberg S. Recombinant hepatitis B vaccination of neonates and infants: emerging safety data from the Vaccine Adverse Event Reporting System. *Pediatr Inf Dis J* 1996;15:771-6.

Niu MT, Rhodes P, Salive M, Lively T, et. al. Comparative safety data of two recombinant hepatitis B vaccines in children: data from the Vaccine Adverse Event Reporting System (VAERS) and Vaccine Safety Datalink (VSD). *J Clin Eidemiol* 1998;51:503-10.

Owen RL, Dau PC, Johnson KP, Spitler LE. Immunologic mechanisms in multiple sclerosis: exacerbation by type A hepatitis and skin test antigen. *JAMA* 1980;244:2307-2309.

Poser CM. Notes on the pathogenesis of multiple sclerosis. *Clinical Neuroscience* 1994;2:258-265.

Quast U, Herder C, Zwisler O. Vaccination of patients with encephaloymelitis disseminata. *Vaccine* 1991;9:228-230.

Shaw FE, Graham DJ, Guess HA, et al. Postmarketing surveillance for neurologic adverse events reported after hepatitis B vaccination. *Am J Epidemiol*. 1988;127:337-352.

Sibley WA et al. Clinical viral infections and multiple sclerosis. *Lancet* 1985;1:1313-1315.

Stephenne J. Development and production aspects of a recombinant yeast-derived hepatitis B vaccine. *Vaccine*. 1990;8:S69-73.

Stevens CE, Toy PT, Tong MJ, et al. Perinatal hepatitis B virus transmission in the Unites States: prevention by passive-active immunization. *JAMA*. 1985; 253:1740-1745.

Strom BL, ed. *Pharmacoepidemiology*. Sussex: John Wiley & Sons, 1994.

Szmuness W, Stevens CE, Harley EJ, et al. Hepatitis B vaccine: demonstration of efficacy in a controlled clinical trial in a high risk population in the United States. *N Engl J Med*. 1980;303:833-841.

West DJ, Margolis HS. Prevention of hepatitis B virus infection in the United States: a pediatric perspective. *Pediatr Infect Dis J*. 1992;11:866-874.

Wise RP, Kiminyo KP, Salive ME. Hair loss after routine immunizations. *JAMA*. 1997;278:1176-1178.

Zajac BA, West DJ, McAleer WJ, Scolnick EM. Overview of clinical studies with hepatitis B vaccine made by recombinant DNA. *J Infect*. 1986;13(Suppl A):39-45.

For Additional Reference

World Health Organization. Scare of multiple sclerosis from hep B vaccine "quite unfounded". *Vaccine and Immunization News*: The newsletter of the global programme for vaccines and immunization, World Health Organization. 1997; No. 4: p. 8.

World Health Organization. No evidence that hepatitis B vaccine causes multiple sclerosis. *Weekly Epidemiological Record*, World Health Organization. 1997; No. 21: pp. 149-152.

Section 25.4

If You Are a Hepatitis B Carrier

Reprinted with permission © 1998 "Advice to Carriers,"
Hepatitis B Foundation.

A chronic carrier of Hepatitis B Virus (HBV) is someone who has the hepatitis B virus in their blood and can pass the disease on to others.

Some people who have been infected with the Hepatitis B Virus (HBV) continue to produce the virus for long periods of time, even though they may not have obvious symptoms. These people are usually called "healthy carriers" because although they feel healthy, they carry the virus in their bloodstream.

Although HBV is associated with liver disease, people who are diagnosed as carriers should feel reassured that their lives can be long and healthy.

Advice for All Carriers of HBV Who Are Otherwise in Good Health

1. **Contact a physician skilled in liver diseases.**

   This should be a Gastroenterologist, Hepatologist, or Internist with a special interest in liver disease. If you are interested in finding a liver specialist in your area, information is available from the Hepatitis B Foundation at http://www2.hepb.org/ hepb where a Directory of Liver Specialists is maintained or call (215) 489-4900.

2. **Get regular check-ups.**

   These should include exams specifically designed to detect liver disease including liver cancer and cirrhosis.

   For those over 15 years of age: Schedule regular visits with the doctor This may be yearly, every six months, or more

235

frequently depending on what you and your doctor decide is best. The doctor will perform a physical exam, will order blood tests for HBV markers (liver function enzymes and alpha feto protein) and may arrange for ultra-sound imaging of your liver.

For those under 15 years of age: Schedule visits with your child's doctor. Your visits may be once per year or more frequently depending on your child's situation. Your doctor will perform a physical exam and order blood tests for HBV markers, liver function enzymes and alpha fetoprotein.

These tests are necessary to detect liver disease at the earliest stages and to monitor any progression of liver disease. In the unlikely event that such advancing disease does occur, you may choose from the currently available therapies. Be sure to discuss treatment options with your doctor before starting any program.

3. **If you are pregnant**

   HBV is passed from mothers who are carriers to their newborn children at the time of delivery. If you are a pregnant carrier, be certain that you doctors are aware of your HBV status and arrange to protect your newborn against HBV with hepatitis B immune globulin and the vaccine within hours of delivery. This procedure prevents the newborn from becoming infected with HBV from the mother 95% of the time.

4. **Be sure your close contacts and household members are vaccinated against HBV.**

   If you are a carrier, your blood and body fluids may contain infectious HBV and may infect other people. Therefore, your household partners, sexual partners, and other people with whom you have close contact should be vaccinated against HBV.

5. **Be careful not to spread your blood to others**.

   Cover all cuts with a bandage. Properly discard of tampons and feminine napkins soiled by menstrual blood. Do not donate blood or organs. Avoid unprotected sex with anyone who has not been vaccinated. Follow good personal hygiene practices, and do not share any items that could spread your blood to others including your toothbrush, nail clippers, pierced ear-rings, shaving razors, or needles.

HBV Disinfection: Wear latex or rubber gloves when clean-ing any blood spills, vomit, diarrhea, and other bodily secre-tions to avoid contact with potentially infectious materials. Clean all spills with a diluted chlorine bleach solution (mix one part household bleach with nine parts water). Household alcohol such as rubbing alcohol will also disinfect HBV. Dis-card cleaning materials and the bodily fluids into a plastic bag and tie securely. Dispose of properly in the garbage can. Wash your hands thoroughly with soap and warm water. If clothes become soiled with potentially infectious materials, wash them in a diluted solution of bleach.

6. **Diet**

   No specific diet has been shown to help in treating hepatitis B. However, eating green and yellow vegetables, particularly cabbage, broccoli, and cauliflower are good for the liver. They tend to protect it against chemicals and toxins in the environ-ment. Following the American Cancer Society's diet, which in-cludes foods low in fat, low in cholesterol, and high in fiber, is beneficial for your entire body as well as your liver.

7. **Do not drink alcohol**. It is very poisonous to your liver.

8. **Avoid other liver toxins**

   Mold on old rice, popcorn, and peanuts is toxic to your liver.

   If you have chronic liver disease, avoid raw seafood because of the risk of vibrio infection.

   Do not inhale large amounts of fumes from paint, paint thin-ner, glue, or household cleaning products. Some of these prod-ucts contain phenols, which are chemicals that can be toxic to your liver.

9. **Consult your doctor before taking any prescribed or over-the-counter medications** to avoid adverse drug inter-actions which could damage your liver.

10. **Promote Cure Research** by supporting organizations dedi-cated to the cause of helping those already infected with HBV.

For Additional Information

Hepatitis B Foundation
700 East Butler Avenue
Doylestown, PA 18901-2697
(215) 489-4900
E-mail: info@hepb.org

Section 25.5

Adoption and Hepatitis B

There are many issues you need to be aware of when adopting a child. One of these is hepatitis B. It is essential, if you plan to adopt a child, that you are informed about hepatitis B and how it may affect the life of the child and your family.

Many people wish to adopt children from countries other than the United States. Potential adoptive families need to be aware that the hepatitis B virus (HBV) is highly prevalent in regions such as Asia, parts of Africa, South America, and Eastern Europe. Children from these regions are often infected with the virus from their birth mothers who have HBV and unknowingly pass the disease on to their children during delivery.

Children of intravenous drug users are also at risk for being carriers of HBV, as their mothers can pass the disease on to them at birth.

Your agency should be able to tell you if a child has been tested for HBV. However, results of the test should not adversely influence your decision to adopt. If you are concerned about the results of the test, you can contact the Hepatitis B Foundation to speak with a parent who has adopted a child with HBV, or you can join a support group in your area.

Finding out that the child you wish to adopt is a carrier of HBV can be upsetting, but should not be a cause for alarm. You can be reassured that your child will most likely enjoy a long and healthy life. Most carriers of the disease experience no symptoms for decades.

The key to successful adoption of a child with HBV is to be prepared with accurate information about the disease and to protect yourself with the HBV vaccine prior to the child's arrival.

You will need to be prepared for certain issues that may arise when you find out the child you wish to adopt is a carrier of HBV. The following suggestions are compiled by the Hepatitis B Foundation and its support group for parents. These are not conclusive recommendations, but rather, guidelines which may help you decide how best to approach your personal situation. Each family is unique, and each community is different, so adjust your decisions accordingly.

Parents of Carriers

Finding out that your child is a carrier of HBV can be a very stressful experience. The good news is that your child will most likely enjoy a long and healthy life, as most carriers of the disease experience no symptoms for decades.

As a parent of an HBV carrier, you will face certain issues as your child grows. These are not conclusive recommendations, but rather, guidelines which may help you decide how best to approach your personal situation. Each family is unique, and each community is different, so adjust your decisions accordingly.

Protecting Your Family

If your child is a carrier of HBV you need to protect your family from the virus. All parents, siblings, extended family members, childcare providers and others coming into close contact with the carrier should be vaccinated.

Telling Others

Know the Facts

If people are unfamiliar with HBV, there is a possibility they will become alarmed when told your child is a carrier. The key to minimizing this is to know the facts. It is essential to know that HBV is not transmitted casually, but only through blood, sex and needles. Precautions should be taken in the handling of everyone's blood and secretions—not just your child's. Inform people that not only is there a readily available vaccine against HBV, but that the American Academy of Pediatrics now recommends that all children under 16 years of age be vaccinated.

Who Should You Tell? Use Your Judgment.

You must use personal discretion and sound judgment in deciding who to tell about your child's HBV status. Laws vary from state to state, but often there are no specific laws that address disclosure of HBV status. You also do not necessarily have a "duty" to inform others of your child's HBV status. However, you must be careful that you are not endangering others.

Know the Risk

You need to consider whether your child is at high or low risk for exposing others to his or her blood (e.g. consider age, frequency of accidents, nosebleeds, biting, etc.), the possible adverse impact such a disclosure could have on your child's life, and the degree of risk a caretaker has for exposure (frequent vs. occasional contact).

Note: The "Americans with Disabilities Act" (1992) is a federal law that may protect against discrimination related to chronic HBV.

What Should You Say?

Know your facts, use simple explanations, and remain calm. Emphasize that your child is healthy and poses no risk if all blood spills are handled carefully, and that the blood of all children should be handled carefully.

The Centers for Disease Control (CDC) recommends that everyone use "universal precautions" when dealing with both children and adults. This means that in case of an accident, everyone's blood and bodily fluids should be treated as if is infected. Wear gloves when coming into contact with all potentially infectious materials and always follow strict disinfection procedures.

Disinfection:

Wear rubber or latex gloves when cleaning up spills. Keep a spray bottle filled with a diluted solution of bleach (one part bleach to nine parts water). If blood, vomit, or other bodily fluids are spilled, spray the area with the bleach, allow to stand for one minute and wipe clean.

If blood is spilled on clothing, the clothing should be washed in a diluted solution of bleach. Household alcohol, such as rubbing alcohol, will also kill the virus. Discard the towels or cleaning materials in a plastic bag and tie the bag securely. Wash your hands thoroughly with soap and water after cleaning spills.

Disinfection procedures should be followed when accidents happen with anyone's blood and secretions, not just the carrier's blood and secretions.

When telling others, consider saying something like this:

"Treat my child as you should treat every child—with care. You know the risk my child poses, but you don't know the risk that other children might present."

If possible, give literature to reinforce your facts. The Hepatitis B Foundation can provide literature to you to distribute to other parents and teachers.

For Additional Information

Hepatitis B Foundation
700 East Butler Avenue
Doylestown, PA 18901-2697
(215) 489-4900
E-mail: info@hepb.org

Chapter 26

Hepatitis C

Chapter Contents

Section 26.1

What You Need to Know about Hepatitis C

Excerpted from "What Do I Need To Know about Hepatitis C," *FDA Consumer*, March-April 1999.

Hepatitis C Is a Liver Disease.

Hepatitis (HEP-ah-TY-tis) makes your liver swell and stops it from working right.

You need a healthy liver. The liver does many things to keep you alive. The liver fights infections and stops bleeding. It removes drugs and other poisons from your blood. The liver also stores energy for when you need it.

Hepatitis C Is Caused by a Virus.

A virus is a germ that causes sickness. (For example, the flu is caused by a virus.) People can pass viruses to each other. The virus that causes hepatitis C is called the hepatitis C virus.

Hepatitis C Spreads by Contact with an Infected Person's Blood.

You Could Get Hepatitis C by

- Sharing drug needles

- Getting pricked with a needle that has infected blood on it (hospital workers can get hepatitis C this way)

- Getting a tattoo or body piercing with dirty tools that were used on someone else

- Having sex with an infected person. However, this does not happen very often

You Can NOT Get Hepatitis C by

- Shaking hands with an infected person
- Hugging an infected person
- Kissing an infected person
- Sitting next to an infected person

If You Had a Blood Transfusion or Organ Transplant Before 1992, You Might Have Hepatitis C.

Before 1992, doctors could not check blood for hepatitis C, and some people received infected blood. If you had a blood transfusion or organ transplant before 1992, ask a doctor to test you for hepatitis C.

What Are the Symptoms?

Many people with hepatitis C don't have symptoms. However, some people with hepatitis C feel like they have the flu. So, you might

- Feel tired
- Feel sick to your stomach
- Have a fever
- Not want to eat
- Have stomach pain
- Have diarrhea

Some people have

- Dark yellow urine
- Light-colored stools
- Yellowish eyes and skin

If you have symptoms, or think you might have hepatitis C, go to a doctor.

What Are the Tests for Hepatitis C?

To check for hepatitis C, the doctor will test your blood. These tests show if you have hepatitis C and how serious it is.

The doctor may also do a liver biopsy. Biopsy (BYE-op-see) is a simple test. The doctor removes a tiny piece of your liver through a needle. The doctor checks the piece of liver for signs of hepatitis C and liver damage.

How Is Hepatitis C Treated?

Hepatitis C is treated with a drug called interferon. Interferon (inter-FEAR-on) is given through shots. If the drug does not work after

3 months, treatment will be stopped. If the drug does work, you will be treated with it for a year. Interferon doesn't work for everyone, so doctors are developing and testing other drugs.

You may need surgery if you have hepatitis C for many years. Over time, hepatitis C can cause your liver to stop working. If that happens, you will need a new liver. The surgery is called a liver transplant. It involves taking out the old, damaged liver and putting in a new, healthy one from a donor.

How Can I Protect Myself?

You can protect yourself and others from hepatitis C:

- Don't share drug needles with anyone

- Wear gloves if you have to touch anyone's blood

- Don't use an infected person's toothbrush, razor, or anything else that could have blood on it

- If you get a tattoo or body piercing, make sure it is done with clean tools

- If you or your partner has hepatitis C, ask a doctor if you should use a condom during sex.

- If you have hepatitis C, don't give your blood or plasma. The person who receives it could become infected with the virus.

For More Information

American Liver Foundation
75 Maiden Lane, Suite 603
New York, NY 10038
Tel: (800) 465-4837 (GO-LIVER)

Hepatitis Foundation International
30 Sunrise Terrace
Cedar Grove, NJ 07009-1423
Tel: (800) 891-0707

National Digestive Diseases Information Clearinghouse (NDDIC)
2 Information Way
Bethesda, MD 20892-3570
E-mail: nddic@info.niddk.nih.gov

Section 26.2

New Treatment Helps Some, But Cure Remains Elusive

"Hepatitis C," *FDA Consumer*, March-April 1999.

Elaine Moreland knew she wasn't imagining the symptoms. Fatigue, migraines, nausea, memory loss, anxiety, and dizziness all were wreaking havoc in her life. Yet doctor after doctor could find nothing wrong with her. Some said she was depressed. Others blamed hypochondria.

Finally, in 1992, after suffering for several years, she went to another doctor in tears. "I told him that I was not leaving his office until he found something," she says. Through extensive testing, he did. Moreland, then 32, had hepatitis C.

The nation's most common blood-borne infection, hepatitis C is estimated to affect some 4 million Americans in its chronic form. Eventually, as many as 70 percent of them will develop liver disease, according to the national Centers for Disease Control and Prevention.

In congressional testimony last year, former Surgeon General C. Everett Koop, M.D., called hepatitis C "a disease these millions will carry for a decade or more—possibly spreading to others—while it develops into a serious threat to their health."

Hepatitis C is one of five currently identified viruses—hepatitis A, B, C, D, and E—all of which can attack and damage the liver. Widely viewed as one of the most serious of the five, the hepatitis C virus (HCV) is spread primarily through contact with infected blood and can cause cirrhosis (irreversible and potentially fatal liver scarring), liver cancer, or liver failure. Hepatitis C is the major reason for liver transplants in the United States, accounting for 1,000 of the procedures annually. The disease is responsible for between 8,000 and 10,000 deaths yearly.

Some estimates say the number of HCV-infected people may be four times the number of those infected with the AIDS virus. "One of the main differences is that hepatitis C doesn't kill as quickly as AIDS," says Jay Hoofnagle, M.D., director of digestive diseases and nutrition at the National Institute of Diabetes and Digestive and Kidney Diseases.

Presently, there is no vaccine or other means of preventing hepatitis C infection. HCV exists in many different forms, called genotypes, confounding researchers in their quest to develop a vaccine effective for all variations. Also, HCV mutates frequently within infected patients, so even if an effective vaccine is developed, it could be rendered useless by a new strain of mutant virus.

Once HCV is contracted, treatment or the body's defenses can cure a small portion of patients. In most others, however, HCV's frequent mutations allow it to evade the immune system, defeating attempts to develop a cure. Some treatments are available, but they don't work for all patients. The most recent is one that combines a genetically engineered biological drug (interferon) with the drug ribavirin.

Who Is at Risk?

High-risk activities for acquiring hepatitis C include:

- injecting illegal drugs—this risk exists even if the drug abuse only lasted for a short time or occurred many years ago

- receiving organs from donors whose blood contained HCV

- getting pricked with a needle that has infected blood on it— mainly a risk for health-care workers

- frequently being exposed to blood products such as those used to treat hemophilia or chronic kidney failure

- "snorting" cocaine using shared equipment

- getting a tattoo or body piercing with unsterile instruments that were used on someone infected with HCV

- using an infected person's toothbrush, razor, or anything else that may have blood on it

- engaging in high-risk sexual behavior, such as having multiple partners or failing to use condoms.

In the recent past, people receiving blood transfusions were a main risk group for HCV infections. That is because before 1990, there was no reliable screening test of the blood supply for the virus, so many were unwittingly infected. At the time, the risk of HCV infection was about 1 in 200 units of blood, says CDC. In May 1990, the Food and Drug Administration licensed an enzyme immunoassay (EIA) test for HCV, which indicates the presence of HCV antibodies in blood samples. But this test had a high rate of false positives (see "Identifying Recipients of Contaminated Blood" in this section). Two years later, the agency approved a more sensitive and reliable EIA test, which has helped lower the odds of contracting hepatitis C from donated blood to 1 in 100,000 units. In February, FDA approved an improved test for confirming positive results from screening tests.

Acquiring HCV through sex between monogamous partners has not been conclusively demonstrated and appears to be rare. Studies have shown that less than 5 percent of spouses of patients with chronic hepatitis C become infected. But some of these studies include data from countries where hepatitis C is common in the general population. Likewise, transmission of HCV from infected mother to infant also is rare and results in infection of the infant in only about 5 percent of cases. There is no evidence that breast-feeding spreads HCV.

In about 10 percent of acute hepatitis C cases and 30 percent of chronic cases, the source of the infection cannot be identified. These "sporadic" infections, says the National Institute of Diabetes and Digestive and Kidney Diseases, are likely caused by infection through contamination of cuts, wounds or medical injections with the blood or body fluids of infected persons. Also, some infected patients may not provide truthful information about potential exposure, especially regarding past drug abuse. Further, some health experts say there may be an as-yet unknown pathway for the virus. Most experts agree, however, that HCV cannot be acquired through casual contact with an infected person such as shaking hands, hugging, or even kissing. It also is not spread by sneezing, coughing, or sharing eating utensils or drinking glasses.

Treating the Disease

Some patients learn they have hepatitis C through a routine physical or when they donate blood and a blood test shows elevated liver enzymes. Others have symptoms (see "Hepatitis C: Types and Symptoms" in this section). Further testing for HCV antibodies using the EIA test and a supplemental test such as the "Western blot" or HCV-RNA detection can positively identify the infection. A liver biopsy shows disease manifested by damage already done to the liver.

Once diagnosed, CDC recommends the following:

- Stop using alcohol

- See a doctor regularly

- Don't start any new medicines or use over-the-counter, herbal, or other drugs without consulting with a doctor

- Get vaccinated against hepatitis A, a food and water borne virus, if liver damage is present.

One of the only approved treatments for chronic hepatitis C, especially for patients with consistently elevated liver enzymes or mild-to-moderate liver damage, is the biological drug interferon alpha, marketed as Intron A by Schering Corp. and Roferon-A by Roche Laboratories Inc. Amgen Inc. also has an approved drug derived from interferon alpha called Infergen. Hepatitis C patients must inject interferon themselves, usually three times a week. In about 25 percent of patients, the drug has a pronounced effect, reducing HCV to very low levels in the blood. However, if the drug is ineffective after three months, doctors probably will discontinue it.

Doctors also may prescribe Rebetron, a Schering product that combines interferon with the antiviral drug ribavirin. Approved in June 1998 for patients who have relapsed after interferon therapy and expanded in December 1998 to include patients never treated with interferon, this combination therapy appears to suppress blood levels of HCV more effectively than a first or repeat course of interferon alone. In clinical trials, about 45 percent of relapsed patients treated with the combination sustained reduced HCV levels for six months after discontinuing therapy, compared with 5 percent of relapsed patients who were retreated with interferon alone. These results were reinforced by a study published last Nov. 19 in the New England Journal of Medicine showing the combination to be significantly more effective in suppressing HCV levels.

"We've learned from research in other viral diseases that combination therapies rather than [a single drug] may offer the best potential for effective treatment," says John Hutchison, M.D., medical director of liver transplantation at Scripps Clinic and Research Foundation.

Bill Ruttman, 44, a Lansdale, Pa., hepatitis C patient, has taken the combination treatment since October 1998. As a result, his HCV levels have dropped to undetectable levels, and his once-elevated liver enzyme levels have "normalized," which he says is good news because for now, he feels the disease has been slowed down. "I'm extremely happy in that regard," he says.

Ruttman's successful therapy has come at a price, however, because of Rebetron's side effects. He suffers from extreme fatigue and has to nap often during the day, and he sleeps restlessly at night. He also has bouts of depression and is currently unable to work. His side effects are typical of those experienced by patients taking interferon alone as well as the combination therapy.

Because side effects can be serious, patients should be closely monitored by their doctors. Ribavirin can cause anemia, and interferon is associated with both psychosis and suicidal behavior, though the latter occurs in 1 to 2 percent of patients. Both interferon and ribavirin present significant potential risks for pregnant women, including possible fetal death or malformations. Female patients and female partners of male patients must not become pregnant while receiving this therapy and for six months after completing therapy.

Some patients who take interferon or the combination complain of flu-like side effects such as fever, chills, and body aches. Many side effects, such as muscle aches and low-grade fever, can be managed. Some side effects may be reduced by giving the drug at night or lowering the dosage. Side effects are often more severe during the first few weeks of treatment, especially after the first injection.

Patient Elaine Moreland says her interferon therapy caused "just about every one of the [side effects] listed in the drug handout sheets—severe muscle cramps, hair loss, nervousness, heart palpitations, fatigue, sweating, headaches, and blurry vision." Ultimately, she says, treatment was stopped because it wasn't working. Because of the potential side effects, she is holding off on further therapy in the hope that improved treatments may soon be available. "I'm waiting to see what comes down the pike unless signs start to point to serious progression of my disease."

Currently, chronic hepatitis C patients who do not respond to therapy have few options. In many, cirrhosis or other damage will eventually cause the liver to stop functioning. In these cases, a liver transplant is the only recourse. However, even new livers often become infected with the virus. But because HCV usually progresses slowly, says Jay Hoofnagle, many transplant recipients can live normal lives for many years despite the infection.

On the Horizon

A major focus of hepatitis C research is development of a cell culture through which scientists can study HCV outside the human body. By understanding how the virus replicates and how it injures cells, researchers may be able to develop ways to control the virus as well as drugs to block it.

Several drugs currently under study show some promise as future treatments for the disease. They include thymosin, amantadine, and other forms of interferon.

"What we really need, of course, is a vaccine against this disease," Surgeon General David Satcher, M.D., told a congressional committee last year. "However, we cannot underestimate the complexity of this task, particularly because of the rapid rate at which the virus mutates." Researchers at the National Institute of Allergy and Infectious Diseases say a vaccine is likely 10 years away.

One research hurdle was cleared in 1997 when NIAID scientists and FDA researcher Stephen Feinstone, M.D., independently cloned an infectious hepatitis C virus. NIAID director Anthony Fauci, M.D., says the work "will enable scientists to better understand the factors and mechanisms that determine whether the virus is cleared from the body or produces a chronic infection."

Another obstacle to research progress is the need for more funding. Though hepatitis C has taken a back seat in recent years to appropriations for many other more visible public health problems such as AIDS, the situation is improving. Direct funding for hepatitis C research at the National Institutes of Health was $25.3 million in 1997, but has increased to over $34 million in 1999. Private efforts have bolstered funding as well. For example, country music entertainer Naomi Judd, herself a hepatitis C patient who was forced to retire in 1991, started the Naomi Judd Research Fund to help find a cure for the disease. Through the fund, she has helped the American Liver Foundation raise over a million dollars.

Meanwhile, federal and private groups are escalating efforts to educate primary care physicians and the public about the disease. And through the Internet and local support groups, hepatitis C sufferers are finding what patient Bill Ruttman calls "a community."

As for those just diagnosed with the disease, patient Elaine Moreland has this advice: "Try to find a good doctor who is knowledgeable about HCV. Become active in your own medical treatment. Read all you can about the disease. Above all, try to keep a positive attitude and know you're not alone in the fight."

Identifying Recipients of Contaminated Blood

Before 1992, tests to detect antibodies to the hepatitis C virus in the nation's blood supply were unreliable or nonexistent. As a result, many patients who received blood then may have contracted the virus unknowingly. To identify them so they can receive treatment, the Department of Health and Human Services is sponsoring a "lookback" program that is tracking down and informing about 300,000 people who received suspected HCV-contaminated blood before 1992. HHS agencies, including FDA and the Health Care Financing Administration, will ensure that recipients of blood that initially tested negative for antibodies to HCV, but was collected from donors who later tested positive for the antibodies, are informed by letter that they may have received blood containing HCV. As part of the lookback program, the national Centers for Disease Control and Prevention is leading educational programs for health-care professionals and the public to bring greater awareness of the disease.

Hepatitis C: Types and Symptoms

Infection with hepatitis C may cause symptoms right away, not for years, or sometimes not at all. With the acute form of the disease, symptoms such as fatigue, nausea, and dark urine typically show up within six months. About one-fourth of patients with acute hepatitis C recover completely with treatment. But according to the National Institute of Diabetes and Digestive and Kidney Diseases, the other estimated 75 percent of these patients will progress eventually to the long-term, or chronic, form of the disease, with detectable HCV in their blood.

Chronic hepatitis C, however, varies widely in its severity and outcome. It can lie dormant for 10 years or more before symptoms appear. Some patients will have no symptoms of liver damage, and their liver enzymes will stay at normal levels (elevated enzymes are one indication of liver disease). A liver biopsy, in which the doctor removes a tiny piece of liver with a needle, may show some degree of chronic hepatitis, but it may be mild.

Other patients, however, will have severe hepatitis C, with detectable HCV in their blood, liver enzymes elevated as much as 20 times more than normal, and a prognosis of ultimately developing cirrhosis and end-stage liver disease. Another group of patients falls somewhere in the middle, with few or no symptoms, mild- to-moderate elevation of liver enzymes, but with an uncertain prognosis.

According to the National Institute of Diabetes and Digestive and Kidney Diseases, at least 20 percent of chronic hepatitis C patients develop cirrhosis, but this process can take 10 to 20 years from the onset of infection. As many as 5 percent of chronic patients, after 20 to 40 years, develop liver cancer. Other studies show that those with cirrhosis develop liver cancer within 17 years.

Patients with no symptoms sometimes learn they have the disease when a routine physical or blood donation shows elevated levels of liver enzymes, which can indicate hepatitis C, as well as other liver disorders.

Other patients, however, have symptoms that prompt them to seek medical attention, including:

- yellowish eyes or skin (jaundice)
- fatigue, or an extreme feeling of being tired all the time
- pain or tenderness in the right upper quadrant of the body
- persistent nausea or pains in the stomach
- lingering fever
- loss of appetite
- diarrhea
- dark yellow urine or light-colored stools
- If you have any of these symptoms, see a doctor right away.

For More Information

Contact any of the following organizations for more on hepatitis C, its treatment, support groups, and Internet mailing lists.

American Liver Foundation
75 Maiden Lane, Suite 603
New York, NY 10038
1-800-GO LIVER (1-800-465-4837)
URL: http://www.liverfoundation.org

Hepatitis C Foundation
1502 Russett Drive
Warminster, PA 18974
(215) 672-2606
URL: http://www.hepcfoundation.org

Hepatitis Foundation International
30 Sunrise Terrace
Cedar Grove, NJ 07009-1423
1-800-891-0707
URL: http://www.hepfi.org

National Digestive Diseases Information Clearinghouse
2 Information Way
Bethesda, MD 20892-3570
301-654-3810
URL: http://www.niddk.nih.gov

In addition, two helpful publications are available on-line from the national Centers for Disease Control and Prevention or by calling CDC at (404) 332-4555:

- Hepatitis C Fact Sheet—www.cdc.gov/ncidod/diseases/hepatitis/ c/fact.htm

- Hepatitis C Questions and Answers—www.cdc.gov/ncidod/diseases/hepatitis/c/faq.htm

—John Henkel

John Henkel is a staff writer for *FDA Consumer*.

Section 26.3

Chronic Hepatitis C: Current Disease Management

National Institute of Diabetes and Digestive and Kidney Diseases (NIDDK), NIH Publication No. 97-4230, August 1997, updated September 20, 1998.

Introduction

The hepatitis C virus (HCV) is one of the most important causes of chronic liver disease in the United States. It accounts for about 20 percent of acute viral hepatitis, 60 to 70 percent of chronic hepatitis, and 30 percent of cirrhosis, end-stage liver disease, and liver cancer.

Almost 4 million Americans, or 1.8 percent of the U.S. population, are infected with HCV. Hepatitis C causes an estimated 8,000 to 10,000 deaths annually in the United States.

A distinct and major characteristic of hepatitis C is its propensity to cause chronic liver disease. At least 75 percent of patients with acute hepatitis C ultimately develop chronic infection, and most of these patients have accompanying chronic liver disease.

Chronic hepatitis C varies greatly in its course and outcome. At one end of the spectrum are patients who have no signs or symptoms of liver disease and completely normal levels of serum liver enzymes. Liver biopsy usually shows some degree of chronic hepatitis, but the degree of injury is usually mild and the overall prognosis may be good. On the other end of the spectrum are patients with severe hepatitis C who have symptoms, HCV RNA in serum, and elevated serum liver enzymes, and who ultimately develop cirrhosis and end-stage liver disease. In the middle of the spectrum are many patients who have few or no symptoms, mild to moderate elevations in liver enzymes, and a prognosis that is uncertain. The best estimates are that at least 20 percent of patients with chronic hepatitis C develop cirrhosis, a process that generally takes 10 to 20 years. After 20 to 40 years, a smaller percentage of patients with chronic disease develop liver cancer.

Chronic hepatitis C can cause cirrhosis, liver failure, and liver cancer. Approximately 20 percent of patients develop cirrhosis within 10 to 20 years of the onset of infection. Liver failure resulting from chronic hepatitis C is one of the most common reasons for liver transplants in the United States. Hepatitis C might be the most common cause of primary liver cancer in the developed world. In Italy, Spain, and Japan at least half of liver cancers could be related to HCV. Men, alcoholics, cirrhosis patients, people over age 40, and those infected for 20 to 40 years are more likely to develop HCV-related liver cancer.

Risk Factors and Transmission

HCV is spread primarily by contact with blood and blood products. Blood transfusions and the use of shared, unsterilized, or incompletely sterilized needles and syringes have been the most important causes of the spread of HCV in the United States. With the introduction of routine blood screening for antibody to HCV in 1990 and improvements in these tests in 1992, transfusion-related hepatitis C has virtually disappeared. At present, injection drug use is the most common risk factor for contracting the disease. However, many patients acquire hepatitis C without any known episode of exposure to blood or to drug use.

The major high-risk groups for hepatitis C are the following:

- People who had blood transfusions before 1992 and the availability of highly accurate anti-HCV screening

- Patients who have frequent exposure to blood products, such as patients with chronic renal failure, hemophilia, or malignancies requiring chemotherapy

- Health care workers who suffer needle-stick accidents

- Injection drug users, including those who used drugs for a brief period only, long in the past

- Persons with high-risk sexual behavior, multiple partners, and sexually transmitted diseases

- Persons who use cocaine, particularly with intranasal administration, using shared equipment

Sexual Transmission

Sexual transmission of hepatitis C between monogamous partners appears to be uncommon. Whether hepatitis C is spread by sexual contact is not conclusively proven and studies have been contradictory. Less than 5 percent of spouses of patients with chronic hepatitis C become infected. The risk of infection appears to correlate with the length of marriage and viral titers in the affected spouse; however, the studies reporting spouse transmission were confounded by other risk factors, such as other shared known sources of exposure, and came from areas of the world where hepatitis C is common in the general population.

Maternal-Infant Transmission

Maternal-infant transmission is also uncommon. In most studies, only 5 percent of infants born to infected women become infected. The disease in the newborn is usually mild and subclinical. The risk of maternal-infant spread correlates best with the viral titer in the mother. Breast-feeding has not been linked to HCV's spread.

Sporadic Transmission

Sporadic transmission, when the source of infection cannot be identified, occurs in about 10 percent of cases of acute hepatitis C and in 30 percent of cases of chronic hepatitis C. These cases are also referred to as sporadic or community-acquired infections. The sources are probably inapparent parenteral exposures, such as cuts, wounds, or medical injections. Some may be due to sexual transmissions.

The Hepatitis C Virus

HCV is a small (50 nm in diameter), enveloped, single-stranded RNA virus of the family Flaviviridae. The genome of the virus mutates rapidly, and the resultant changes in the envelope protein may explain how it escapes clearance by the immune system. There are at least 6 major genotypes and more than 30 subtypes of HCV. The different genotypes have different geographic distributions. Genotypes 1a and 1b are the most common in the United States. Genotypes 2 and 3 are present in only 10 to 20 percent of patients. Overall there is little difference in the severity of disease or outcome of patients infected with different genotypes. However, patients with genotypes 2 and 3 are more likely to respond to alpha interferon treatment.

Clinical Symptoms and Signs

Symptoms

Many people with chronic hepatitis C are asymptomatic of liver disease. If symptoms are present, they are usually mild, non-specific, and intermittent. They may include:

- Fatigue
- Mild right upper quadrant pain or tenderness
- Nausea
- Poor appetite
- Muscle and joint pains

Signs

Similarly, the physical exam is likely to be normal or show only mild hepatomegaly or tenderness. Some patients have vascular spiders or palmar erythema.

Clinical Features of Cirrhosis

Once a patient develops cirrhosis or if the patient has severe disease, symptoms and signs are more prominent. In addition to fatigue, the patient may complain of muscle weakness, poor appetite, nausea, weight loss, itching, dark urine, fluid retention, and abdominal swelling. Physical findings of cirrhosis may include:

- Enlarged liver
- Enlarged spleen
- Jaundice
- Muscle wasting
- Excoriations.

Extra-Hepatic Manifestations

One to two percent of people with hepatitis C develop extra-hepatic manifestations. The most common of these is cryoglobulinemia, which is marked by

- Skin rashes, such as purpura, vasculitis, or urticaria
- Joint and muscle aches
- Kidney disease
- Neuropathy
- The presence of cryoglobulins, rheumatoid factor, and low complement levels in serum

Other extra-hepatic manifestations of chronic hepatitis C are

- Glomerulonephritis (which may be linked to cryoglobulinemia)
- Porphyria cutanea tarda (which occurs in patients with many forms of liver disease).

Diseases that are less well documented to be related to hepatitis C are

- Seronegative arthritis
- Keratoconjunctivitis sicca (Sjögren's syndrome)
- Non-Hodgkin's type, B-cell lymphomas

Serologic Tests

Enzyme Immunoassay

Anti-HCV is detected by enzyme immunoassay (EIA). The third-generation test (EIA-3) used today is more sensitive and specific than previous tests. However, as with all enzyme immunoassays, false positive results are a problem with the EIA-3. False positive reactions are particularly common among patients with rheumatoid factor or high levels of immunoglobulins, and when stored serum samples are tested. Therefore, in most situations a positive EIA test should be confirmed by using another method such as recombinant immunoblot assay (RIBA) or polymerase chain reaction (PCR) amplification for HCV RNA.

Other problems with EIA tests are that immunocompromised patients may not produce enough antibodies for detection with EIA and patients with acute hepatitis may test negative for anti-HCV when they first present to the physician. Antibody is present in almost all patients by 1 month after onset of acute illness; thus patients with acute hepatitis who initially test negative may need followup testing.

Recombinant Immunoblot Assay

Immunoblot assays are used to confirm anti-HCV reactivity. These tests are also called "Western blots"; serum is incubated on nitrocellulose strips on which four recombinant viral proteins are blotted. Color changes indicate that antibodies are adhering to the proteins. An immunoblot is considered positive if more than one protein reacts and considered indeterminate if only one positive band is detected. Early in the course of acute hepatitis C, patients often have an indeterminate immunoblot, developing antibody reactivity to the other proteins with time. This test is routinely done in blood banks when an anti-HCV positive sample is found by EIA. Immunoblot assays are highly specific and valuable in verifying anti-HCV reactivity. Indeterminate tests require further follow-up testing, including attempts to confirm the specificity by testing for HCV RNA.

PCR Amplification

PCR amplification can detect low levels of HCV RNA in serum. Testing for HCV RNA is a reliable way of demonstrating that hepatitis C infection is present and is the most specific test for infection. Testing for HCV RNA by PCR is particularly useful when aminotransferases are normal or only slightly elevated, when anti-HCV is not present, or when several causes of liver disease are possible. This method also helps in diagnosing hepatitis C in people who are immunosuppressed, have recently had an organ transplant, or have chronic renal failure. At present, however, there are no FDA-approved PCR assays for general use, although commercial test systems are available. Many commercial laboratories offer their own PCR assays, which are not subject to strict independent quality controls. Thus, the reliability and specificity of the PCR technique is not standardized. In addition, the PCR technique is expensive and prone to technical or laboratory error. When ordering HCV RNA testing by PCR, it is important that the physician use an excellent laboratory that is willing to document standardization of the test.

Biochemical Indicators of HCV Infection

- In chronic hepatitis C, increases in the alanine and aspartate aminotransferases range from 0 to 20 times the upper limit of normal.

- Alanine aminotransferase (ALT) levels are usually higher than aspartate aminotransferase (AST) levels, but that finding may be reversed in patients who have cirrhosis.

- Alkaline phosphatase and gamma glutamyl transpeptidase are usually normal. If elevated, they may indicate cirrhosis.

- Rheumatoid factor and low platelet and white blood cell counts are frequent in patients with cirrhosis, providing clues to the presence of advanced disease.

- The enzymes lactate dehydrogenase and creatine kinase are usually normal.

- Albumin levels and prothrombin time do not increase until late stage disease.

- Iron and ferritin levels may be slightly elevated.

Quantification of HCV RNA in Serum

Several methods are available for measuring the titer or level of virus in serum, which is an indirect assessment of viral load. These methods include a quantitative PCR and a branched DNA (bDNA) test. Both assays are reasonably accurate, but there may be spontaneous variation in levels by 3- to 5-fold over time. These assays have been helpful in elucidating the nature of hepatitis C, but they are not generally clinically helpful. Thus, in HCV infection, viral load does not correlate with severity of illness or poor prognosis (as it seems to in HIV infection). When attempting to assess whether hepatitis C is present, these tests should not be ordered; instead, the more sensitive and reliable qualitative PCR for HCV RNA is needed.

Genotyping and Serotyping of HCV

There are six known genotypes and more than 30 subtypes of hepatitis C. The genotype of infection is helpful in defining the epidemiology of hepatitis C. The only clinical usefulness of knowing the genotype or serotype (genotype-specific antibodies) relates to interferon therapy. Patients with genotypes 2 and 3 are two to three times more likely to respond to alpha interferon therapy. However, the genotype of infection should not determine whether alpha interferon therapy is offered, as it is an imperfect predictor of response.

Normal Serum ALT Levels

Some patients with chronic hepatitis C have normal serum alanine aminotransferase (ALT) levels, even when tested on multiple occasions. In this and other situations in which the diagnosis of chronic hepatitis C may be questioned, the presence of anti-HCV alone should be confirmed by a supplemental test such as an immunoblot assay. Testing for HCV RNA may be helpful to confirm the presence of viremia.

Liver Biopsy

Liver biopsy is not necessary for diagnosis, but it is helpful for grading the severity of disease and staging the degree of fibrosis and permanent architectural damage. Hematoxylin and eosin stains and Masson's trichrome stain are used to grade the amount of necrosis and inflammation and to stage the degree of fibrosis. Specific immunohistochemical stains for HCV have not been developed for routine use. Liver biopsy is also helpful in ruling out other causes of liver disease, such as alcoholic liver injury or iron overload.

HCV causes the following changes in liver tissue:

- Necrosis and inflammation around the portal areas, so-called "piecemeal necrosis"

- Necrosis of hepatocytes and focal inflammation in the liver parenchyma

- Inflammatory cells in the portal areas ("portal inflammation")

- Fibrosis, with early stages being confined to the portal tracts, intermediate stages being expansion of the portal tracts and bridging between portal areas or to the central area, and late stages being frank cirrhosis characterized by architectural disruption of the liver with fibrosis and regeneration.

Grading and staging of hepatitis by assigning scores for severity are helpful in managing patients with chronic hepatitis. The degree of inflammation and necrosis can be assessed as none, minimal, mild, moderate, or severe. The degree of fibrosis can be assessed similarly. Scoring systems are particularly helpful in clinical studies on chronic hepatitis.

Immunostaining

Immunostaining using polyclonal or monoclonal antibodies to detect HCV antigens in the liver has been reported to be useful. However, these tests are not commercially available, and even in the hands of research investigators, immunostaining detects HCV antigens in liver tissue in only 60 to 70 percent of patients with chronic hepatitis C—largely in those with high levels of HCV in serum. This test also requires special handling of liver tissue and thus is not appropriate for routine clinical use.

Diagnosis

Hepatitis C is most readily diagnosed when serum aminotransferases are elevated and anti-HCV is present in serum.

Acute Hepatitis C

Acute hepatitis C is diagnosed on the basis of symptoms of acute disease such as jaundice, fatigue, and nausea, along with marked increases in serum ALT (greater than 10-fold elevation), and presence of anti-HCV or de novo development of anti-HCV.

Diagnosis of acute disease can be problematic as anti-HCV is not always present when the patient presents to the physician with symptoms. In 30 to 40 percent of patients, anti-HCV is not detected until

2 to 8 weeks after onset of symptoms. Acute hepatitis C can also be diagnosed by testing for HCV RNA, but a more practical approach is to repeat the anti-HCV testing a month after onset of illness. HCV RNA testing should be reserved for patients with acute hepatitis in whom the diagnosis still cannot be made by conventional tests for hepatitis A, B, and C.

Chronic Hepatitis C

Chronic hepatitis C is diagnosed when anti-HCV is present and serum aminotransferase levels remain elevated for more than 6 months. Testing for HCV RNA (by PCR) can help confirm the diagnosis and documents that viremia is present; more than 95 percent of patients with chronic infection will have the viral genome detectable in serum by PCR.

Diagnosis of hepatitis C is problematic in patients who cannot produce anti-HCV because they are immunosuppressed or immunoincompetent. Thus, HCV RNA testing may be required for patients with a solid organ transplant or who are taking corticosteroids or have agammaglobulinemia. Diagnosis is also difficult in patients with anti-HCV who have another form of liver disease that might be responsible for the liver injury, such as alcoholism, iron overload, or autoimmunity. In these situations, the anti-HCV may represent a false positive reaction, previous HCV infection, or mild hepatitis C occurring on top of another liver condition.

Differential Diagnosis

The major conditions that can be confused clinically with chronic hepatitis C include

- Autoimmune hepatitis
- Nonalcoholic steatohepatitis (fatty liver)
- Sclerosing cholangitis
- Wilson's disease
- Alpha-1-antitrypsin deficiency-related liver disease
- Medication-induced liver disease.

Treatment

Alpha interferon is currently the only approved treatment for hepatitis C. It improves serum aminotransferase levels in 50 percent of patients during treatment, and a majority of these patients also become negative for HCV RNA by PCR. However, many of these patients relapse once interferon is discontinued. In patients who relapse, the reappearance of HCV RNA and rise of serum ALT levels usually occurs within 1 to 3 months after treatment; only rarely does it occur later. A sustained, long-term response (defined as no relapse at least 6 months after stopping interferon) occurs in 10 to 15 percent of patients who are treated for 6 months and 20 to 25 percent of those treated for 1 year.

Characteristics that predict a good response to interferon are absence of cirrhosis, a short duration of infection, low levels of HCV RNA in serum, and viral genotypes 2 and 3. None of these features are perfect predictors, but they can help in evaluating the chances of success.

Who Should Be Treated?

Patients with anti-HCV, HCV RNA, elevated aminotransferase levels, and evidence of chronic hepatitis on liver biopsy should be offered therapy with alpha interferon. A recent NIH Consensus Development Conference recommended that all patients with fibrosis on liver biopsy or at least moderate degrees of inflammation and necrosis should be treated, and that patients with milder histological disease be managed on an individual basis. Patient selection should not be based on symptoms, mode of acquisition, genotype of HCV, or serum HCV RNA levels.

Patients found to have cirrhosis through liver biopsy can be offered therapy if they do not have signs of decompensation, such as ascites, persistent jaundice, wasting, variceal hemorrhage, or hepatic encephalopathy. However, interferon therapy is less likely to be successful in patients with cirrhosis than those without, and therapy has not been proven to improve survival or ultimate outcome.

Children and patients older than 60 years also should be managed on an individual basis, as the benefit in these patients has not been well documented. In these indefinite situations, the indications for therapy should be reassessed at regular intervals. In view of the rapid developments in hepatitis C today, better therapies may soon be available, at which point expanded indications for therapy would be appropriate.

In patients with clinically significant extra-hepatic manifestations, such as cryoglobulinemia and glomerulonephritis, long-term maintenance therapy with alpha interferon aimed at suppression of the disease may be needed rather than a 12-month course aimed at eradication of HCV RNA. In these patients, continuous therapy can be given despite persistence of HCV RNA in serum if clinical symptoms and signs resolve on therapy.

Who Should Not Be Treated?

Therapy is inadvisable outside of prospective controlled trials in patients who have

- Clinically decompensated cirrhosis due to hepatitis C

- Normal aminotransferase levels

- Severe depression or other neuropsychiatric syndromes

- Autoimmune disease that is not well controlled (rheumatoid arthritis, psoriasis)

- Active substance or alcohol abuse

- Immunosuppression, particularly those who have had a solid-organ transplant.

Patients with bone marrow compromise or cytopenias, such as low platelet counts (<75,000 cells/mm3) or neutropenia (<1,000 cells/mm3), should be treated with caution and frequent monitoring of cell counts.

Finally, the effects of interferon on the fetus are not well known. Female patients should agree to avoid becoming pregnant during therapy, and male patients should practice adequate forms of birth control until therapy is completed.

Current Optimal Treatment Regimens

In the United States, the approved regimen for alpha interferon is 3 million units (mu) by subcutaneous injection three times a week for 6 to 12 months. A recent NIH Consensus Development Conference recommended that therapy be given for 12 months. Treatment should be stopped early if aminotransferase levels do not improve and HCV RNA does not become undetectable within 12 weeks. Late responses are extremely rare, and continuing therapy provides no further benefit. Furthermore, therapy should be stopped if side effects are too troublesome. In some patients, lowering the dose to 2 mu may be necessary because of side effects; however, breakthrough with reappearance of HCV RNA and rises in ALT levels often occurs when the dose is reduced.

Options for Patients Who Do Not Respond to Treatment

Few options exist for patients who either do not respond to therapy or who respond and later relapse. Patients who relapse after a 6-month course of interferon may respond to a second, longer course of therapy (lasting 12 to 18 months), particularly if they became and remained HCV RNA negative during therapy. New treatments are needed for those who do not respond to interferon at all. The most promising is ribavirin, an oral nucleoside analog, which is now being evaluated in combination with alpha interferon in large clinical trials. This combination may improve the long-term response rate above that achieved with interferon alone. Thus, the results of these trials may change recommendations regarding therapy.

Brief Recommendations for Evaluating and Monitoring Interferon Therapy

Before Beginning Interferon Treatment

- Do a liver biopsy to confirm the diagnosis, assess the grade and stage of disease, and rule out other diagnoses. In situations where a liver biopsy is contraindicated, such as clotting disorders, interferon can be given without a pretreatment liver biopsy.

- Measure serum HCV RNA by PCR to document that viremia is present.

- Measure blood counts and aminotransferases to establish the baseline for these values.

- Measure levels of serum thyroid-stimulating hormone (TSH) to rule out subclinical thyroid disease, which is common in patients with liver disease.

- Counsel the patient about the relative risks and benefits of treatment. Side effects should be thoroughly discussed.

During Treatment

- Measure blood counts (including platelets) and aminotransferases at 2- to 8-week intervals.

- Measure aminotransferase levels and HCV RNA by PCR at 3 months. If ALT is still elevated and HCV RNA is present, stop interferon treatment. If either ALT is normal or HCV RNA is undetectable or both (they usually improve together), continue therapy for 9 more months.

- Assess side effects, particularly psychological problems, regularly.

- Measure TSH levels every 6 months during therapy.

- At the end of therapy, test aminotransferases and HCV RNA to assess whether there is an end-of-treatment response.

After Treatment

- Measure aminotransferases every 8 weeks for 6 months.
- If aminotransferases are still normal 6 months after stopping treatment, measure serum HCV RNA by PCR to assess whether a "sustained" virological and biochemical response has occurred. If aminotransferases are normal and HCV RNA is negative at 6 months, the chance for a long-term "cure" is excellent; relapses have rarely been reported after this point.

Side Effects of Treatment

Common side effects of alpha interferon (occurring in more than 10 percent of patients) include

- Fatigue
- Muscle aches
- Nausea and vomiting
- Skin irritation at the injection site
- Low grade fever
- Weight loss
- Headache
- Irritability
- Depression
- Mild bone marrow suppression
- Hair loss (reversible)

Most of these side effects are mild to moderate in severity and can be managed. They are worse during the first few weeks of treatment, especially with the first injection. Thereafter, side effects diminish. Acetaminophen may alleviate the muscle aches and low-grade fever, and side effects may be less troublesome if interferon is taken in the evening. Fatigue and depression are occasionally so troublesome that the dose of interferon should be decreased or therapy stopped early. Depression and personality changes can occur on interferon therapy and be quite subtle and not readily admitted by the patient. These side effects need careful monitoring.

Uncommon side effects (occurring in less than 2 percent of patients) include

- Autoimmune disease (especially thyroid disease)
- Severe bacterial infections
- Marked thrombocytopenia
- Marked neutrophilia
- Seizures
- Depression with suicidal ideation or attempts
- Retinopathy (microhemorrhages and cotton wool spots)
- Hearing loss

Rare side effects include acute congestive heart failure, renal failure, visual loss, pulmonary fibrosis, and sepsis. Deaths have been reported from suicide and sepsis.

A unique side effect is paradoxical worsening of disease. This is assumed to be caused by induction of autoimmune hepatitis, but its pathogenesis is really unknown. Because of this possibility, aminotransferases should be monitored. If ALT levels rise to greater than twice the baseline values, interferon should be stopped and the patient monitored. Some patients with this complication have required corticosteroid therapy to control the hepatic injury.

The Future of Hepatitis C: Research

Basic Research

A major focus of hepatitis C research is developing a tissue culture system that will enable researchers to study HCV outside the human body. Animal models and molecular approaches to the study of HCV are also important. Understanding how the virus replicates and how it injures cells would be helpful in developing a means of controlling the virus and to screen for new drugs that would block the virus.

Diagnostic Tests

Reliable and inexpensive assays for measuring HCV RNA and antigens in the blood and liver are needed. Although current tests for anti-HCV are quite sensitive, a small percentage of patients with hepatitis C test negative for anti-HCV (false negative reaction), and a percentage of patients who test positive are not infected (false positive reaction). Also, there are patients who have resolved the infection but still test positive for anti-HCV. Convenient tests to measure HCV in serum and to detect HCV antigens in liver tissue would be helpful.

New Treatments

New therapies are needed for hepatitis C. Agents being evaluated include

- Other forms of alpha interferon
- Beta interferon
- Thymosin
- Amantadine
- Nucleoside analogs, including ribavirin
- Combinations of alpha interferon and ribavirin

Most information suggests that all forms of alpha and beta interferon give similar results, although the optimal dose for each preparation may be different. Nucleoside analogs are the major forms of antiviral medications used to treat AIDS and herpes virus infections. Most nucleoside analogs such as AZT and acyclovir act mostly on DNA viruses. Among nucleoside analogs currently being used, ribavirin has been shown to be potentially helpful in hepatitis C. Alone, ribavirin has limited efficacy. It lowers aminotransferases in 30 to 50 percent of patients, but it does not reduce the amount of virus, and virtually all patients relapse when treatment is ended. A more promising approach to therapy is the combination of alpha interferon and ribavirin, which in small studies appears to lead to a higher long-term response rate than alpha interferon alone.

Researchers are actively trying to develop new antiviral agents for hepatitis C. Most interesting will be specific inhibitors of HCV-derived enzymes such as protease and polymerase inhibitors. Molecular approaches to treating hepatitis C are also being investigated, such as using antisense oligonucleotides, which are small complementary segments of DNA that bind to viral RNA and inhibit viral replication. All of these approaches remain experimental and have not been applied to humans. The serious nature and the frequency of hepatitis C in the population make the search for new therapies of prime importance.

Prevention

At present, the only means of preventing new cases of hepatitis C are to screen the blood supply, encourage health professionals to take blood and body fluid precautions, and inform people about high-risk behaviors. Programs to promote needle exchange offer some hope in decreasing hepatitis C spread among injection drug users. Vaccines and immune globulin products do not exist for hepatitis C, and development in the near future seems unlikely because these products would require antibodies to all the genotypes and variants of hepatitis C. Nevertheless, advances in immunology and innovative approaches to immunization make it likely that some form of vaccine will eventually be developed for hepatitis C.

Selected Review Articles and References

Alter, M. J. (1996). Epidemiology of hepatitis C. *European Journal of Gastroenterology & Hepatology, 8*, 319-323.

American Medical Association. (1995). *Prevention, diagnosis, and management of viral hepatitis: A guide for primary care physicians* [Fact sheet]. Chicago, IL.

Centers for Disease Control and Prevention. (Accessed 1996, Nov. 25). *Hepatitis A to E.* http://www.cdc.gov/ncidod/diseases/hepatitis/slideset/httoc.htm.

Centers for Disease Control and Prevention, National Center for Infectious Diseases. (1993). *Hepatitis C prevention* [Brochure]. Washington, DC: U.S. Government Printing Office.

Hoofnagle, J. H., & Di Bisceglie, A. M. (1997). The treatment of chronic viral hepatitis. *New England Journal of Medicine, 336*(5), 347-356.

Lemon, S. M., & Thomas, D. L. (1997). Vaccines to prevent viral hepatitis. *New England Journal of Medicine, 336*(5), 196-204.

McDonnell, W. M., & Lok, A. S. (1996). Testing for hepatitis C virus RNA in serum: When and how? *Viral Hepatitis Reviews, 2*(2), 81-83.

Proceedings of the National Institutes of Health Consensus Development Conference (1997). Management of hepatitis C. *Hepatology, 26* (Supplement 1).

Strader, D. B., & Seeff, L. B. (1996). The natural history of chronic hepatitis C infection. *European Journal of Gastroenterology & Hepatology,* 8(4), 324-328.

Patient Education

Disease management should begin with patient education about the disease and general recommendations on how to prevent transmission and avoid further injury. Patients need to know the cause of the disease, possible complications, and how the condition may affect their life. A few important recommendations should be given to all patients with chronic hepatitis C:

- Do not donate blood, semen, or tissues.

- Do not share razors, toothbrushes, or other items that might be contaminated with blood.

- If you have more than one sexual partner, follow safe sexual practices or use condoms.

- If you are in a monogamous, long-term relationship, sexual transmission is unlikely. Currently, no changes in sexual practices are recommended, although you may choose to modify your behavior or use condoms or other barriers. Your sexual partner should be tested for anti-HCV.

- You do not need to avoid normal social and work interactions, such as being with family members, preparing food, eating together, shaking hands, and kissing and hugging others, including children.

- It is safe for women with chronic hepatitis C to become pregnant. Breast-feeding is also considered safe. Children born to women with hepatitis C should be tested for evidence of infection, aminotransferases, and anti-HCV at 1 year of age.

- You should avoid alcohol use; abstinence from alcohol is recommended. Having more than one alcoholic drink per day is unwise.

- You should be vaccinated against hepatitis A and hepatitis B; you may need to be tested for antibodies to these diseases before vaccination.

- You should visit your physician every 6 to 12 months to check for symptoms and signs of liver disease and to test for serum aminotransferases, bilirubin, and albumin.

- You should be careful about taking medications that might be harmful to the liver and remind your physician of your hepatitis when you get a prescription for another condition.

Patient Education Resources

The National Digestive Diseases Information Clearinghouse (NDDIC) has patient education materials on hepatitis C. To obtain free copies, contact the clearinghouse at

National Digestive Diseases Information Clearinghouse (NDDIC)
2 Information Way
Bethesda, MD 20892-3570
E-mail: nddic@info.niddk.nih.gov

Patient education materials are also available from

American Liver Foundation
75 Maiden Lane, Suite 603
New York, NY 10038
Tel: (800) 465-4837

Hepatitis Foundation International
30 Sunrise Terrace
Cedar Grove, NJ 07009-1423
Tel: (800) 891-0707

Section 26.4

First Home Test for Hepatitis C Virus

FDA Talk Paper April 29, 1999.

The FDA has approved the first over-the-counter blood collection kit for testing for antibodies to hepatitis C virus (HCV), the nation's most common blood-borne infection and a major cause of liver damage.

With the kit, which does not require a prescription, the user collects a sample of blood at home and mails it to a designated laboratory for analysis. The results are available anonymously by phone through a unique identification number.

HCV is spread primarily through contact with infected blood. It is responsible for 8,000 to 10,000 deaths in the United States annually. Many people have the disease long before it is detected.

The kit—the Hepatitis C Check, made by Home Access Health Company of Hoffman Estates, Ill.—contains instructions for use, the personal identification number, a lancet for obtaining a drop of blood, filter paper, and a mailer. The user collects a blood sample on the filter paper and sends it to the laboratory. The lab tests the sample with a FDA-licensed test for antibodies to HCV and confirms any positive sample with a different FDA-licensed test for antibodies to HCV.

The results are available four to 10 business days from receipt of the blood sample and can be obtained anonymously by phone from an automated system or from a healthcare counselor.

The test shows whether a person has ever contracted the hepatitis C virus, unless he was exposed in the previous six months, which may be too early for the test to detect. However, it does not show whether the infection is active now. This must be determined by a physician with additional testing and evaluation of the individual.

As part of the test system, Home Access Health provides a telemedicine service, which offers education and counseling about HCV and, if desired, referral to a physician.

Approval of the collection kit was based on clinical studies to determine safety and effectiveness conducted by the manufacturer.

Home Access Health tested the product in approximately 1,200 people. Study participants used the collection kit and also had their blood obtained twice—by a finger stick and from their vein—by a healthcare professional.

The study showed that, when the home user collected an adequate sample of blood, the test results were similar to test results for blood that was drawn by a healthcare professional.

Hepatitis affects some 4 million Americans in its chronic form. HCV is one of five currently identified hepatitis viruses—A, B, C, D, and E—all of which can attack and damage the liver. HCV, one of the most serious of the five, can cause cirrhosis (irreversible and potentially fatal liver scarring), liver cancer, or liver failure. Hepatitis C is the major reason for liver transplants in the United States.

Individuals at high-risk for acquiring hepatitis C include those who:

- received blood transfusions or organ transplants prior to 1992 before the blood supply could be reliably screened for the virus;

- inject illegal drugs;

- get pricked with an infected needle;

- or engage in high-risk sexual behavior with an HCV-infected person.

Last year, the U.S. Public Health Service announced a look-back program designed to identify chronic carriers of HCV so they can receive treatment and counseling. The plan includes a direct notification effort to reach people who received a blood transfusion from a donor, mostly before 1992, who later tested positive for HCV, and an education effort directed at all people at risk for hepatitis C.

Further Information

Home Access Hepatitis C Check Service
(888) 888-HEPC
www.homeaccess.com

Chapter 27

Autoimmune Hepatitis

What Is Hepatitis?

When cells in the body are injured by such things as chemicals or infection, the area that is wounded becomes inflamed. Hepatitis is inflammation of the liver, which in turn causes damage to individual liver cells. It is most often caused by viral infection. However, it can also be caused by alcohol, certain drugs, chemicals or poisons, or other diseases.

Hepatitis may be either acute or chronic. In acute hepatitis, the inflammation develops quickly and lasts only a short period of time. The patient usually recovers completely, but it can take up to several months. Occasionally, a person fails to recover fully, and the hepatitis becomes chronic. In other words, it continues at a smoldering pace. Chronic hepatitis can develop over a number of years without the patient ever having acute hepatitis or even feeling sick. As the liver repairs itself, fibrous tissue develops, much like a scar forms after a cut or injury to the skin heals. Advanced scarring of the liver is called cirrhosis. Over time, cirrhosis irreversibly damages the liver, eventually ending in liver failure.

What Is Autoimmune Hepatitis?

The immune system consists of different types of white blood cells that help to fight infections. Some of these cells produce antibodies.

Reprinted with permission © 1998, "Hepatitis," Chek Med Systems, Inc.

Antibodies act as warriors. They defend the body by destroying bacteria, viruses, and other foreign materials. There are different kinds of antibodies, each fighting against a specific foreign substance. Thus, the immune system protects the body against outside invasion by germs. But sometimes, the immune system mistakenly recognizes the body's own organs as foreign. It can develop antibodies against these organs. This can cause various illnesses, such as rheumatoid arthritis and lupus. These illnesses are called autoimmune disorders because the body is literally fighting against itself.

When the immune system attacks the liver in this way, it is called autoimmune hepatitis. Autoimmune hepatitis is not caused by a virus or bacteria, so it is not a contagious disease. Exactly what triggers the immune system against the liver is unknown. The inflammation is usually chronic, and without treatment it can cause serious injury to the liver.

Symptoms and Diagnosis

Autoimmune hepatitis occurs mainly in adolescent or young adult women (about 70% of the time). However, there have also been cases of older women and men developing the disease. Early symptoms are the same as those for most types of hepatitis: fatigue, abdominal discomfort, and aching joints. These early symptoms are sometimes mild and mistaken for other illnesses, such as the flu. So, it is wise for people with these symptoms to consult a physician. When autoimmune hepatitis progresses to severe cirrhosis, there may be jaundice (yellow coloring to the skin and eyes), marked swelling of the abdomen from fluid inside the abdomen, intestinal bleeding, or mental confusion.

The physician often suspects autoimmune hepatitis from the patient's medical history. For example, patients with other autoimmune diseases—thyroiditis, ulcerative colitis, diabetes mellitus, vitiligo (a patchy loss of pigment in the skin), Sjogren's syndrome (a condition causing dry eyes and mouth)—are more likely to have autoimmune hepatitis. A definite diagnosis of autoimmune hepatitis is obtained with blood testing. Two antibodies that may develop in the blood are the ANA (antinuclear antibody) and the SMA (smooth muscle antibody). Also, a certain type of blood protein called gamma globulin is frequently elevated. A liver biopsy is always needed to determine how much inflammation and scarring has developed. This exam is performed under local anesthesia. A slender needle is inserted through the right lower chest to extract a small piece of liver tissue.

The tissue is then examined under a microscope. This information allows the physician to tailor the treatment to each individual patient.

Treatment

The treatment of autoimmune hepatitis is aimed at curbing the autoimmune response, and therefore the damage to liver cells. It is most effective when begun at an early stage of the disease. In most cases, the initial treatment is with a cortisone drug, usually prednisone (trade names: Deltasone, Orasone). Sometimes a second drug, such as Imuran, may be added. The medication is taken daily, usually for at least a year. The physician may attempt to taper and stop treatment if the patient is doing well. However, a relapse often occurs, and the medication then must be restarted and taken indefinitely. There may be side effects with prednisone, such as swelling of the face, retention of fluid, and weight gain. Long-term treatment with these drugs may also cause loss of bone. This can lead to osteoporosis, or even severe damage to joints such as the shoulder and knee. Therefore, the physician uses the lowest dosage possible to decrease symptoms, improve liver tests, and slow liver damage.

Unfortunately, a few patients do not respond well to treatment, especially if the disease is diagnosed late and cirrhosis is well advanced. When the patient no longer responds to treatment with medication and liver damage is severe, a liver transplant is considered.

Liver Transplantation

Liver transplantation is now an accepted form of treatment for chronic, severe liver disease. Advances in surgical techniques and the use of new drugs to suppress rejection have dramatically improved the success rate of transplantation. The outcome for patients with autoimmune hepatitis is excellent. Survival rates for this condition at transplant centers are well over 90 percent, with a good quality of life after recovery.

Summary

Autoimmune hepatitis is inflammation of the liver. The inflammation is a result of the immune system developing antibodies against the liver. It is not a contagious disease, but it is a serious chronic disease that can lead to irreversible cirrhosis, and eventually to liver failure. However, the outlook for patients with autoimmune hepatitis is generally very favorable. With early diagnosis, drug treatment to prevent serious liver damage is effective in most patients. For those few patients who do not respond to other treatment, successful liver transplantation is now a standard form of therapy when liver damage is severe.

Chapter 28

Neonatal Hepatitis

What Is Neonatal Hepatitis?

Neonatal hepatitis is inflammation of the liver that occurs only in early infancy, usually between one and two months after birth. About 20% of the infants with neonatal hepatitis were infected by a virus that caused the inflammation before birth by their mother or shortly after birth. These include cytomegalovirus, rubella (measles), and hepatitis A, B, or C viruses. In the remaining 80% of the cases no specific virus can be identified as the cause, but many experts suspect that a virus is to blame.

What Are the Symptoms and How Is It Diagnosed?

The infant with neonatal hepatitis usually has jaundice (yellow eyes and skin), that appear at one to two months of age, is not gaining weight and growing normally, and has an enlarged liver and spleen. The infant cannot absorb vitamins for proper growth.

The jaundice is caused by the child's bile ducts becoming inflamed and enlarged, blocking the flow of bile into the small intestine for digestion of fats and absorption of vitamins. This results in the yellow pigment of bile seeping into the blood stream, causing the yellowing of the skin and eyes. In the 80% of the cases where there is no virus identified as the cause, a liver biopsy is performed, where a small piece

Reprinted with permission © 1997, American Liver Foundation, 1-800-GO-LIVER.

of the liver is taken out of the child with a needle and examined with a microscope.

The biopsy will often show that four or five liver cells are combined into a large cell that still functions, but not as well as a normal liver cell. This type of neonatal hepatitis is sometimes called "giant cell hepatitis."

The symptoms of neonatal hepatitis are similar to another infant liver disease, biliary atresia, in which the bile ducts are destroyed for reasons that are not understood. The infant with biliary atresia is also jaundiced and has an enlarged liver, but is growing well and does not have an enlarged spleen. These symptoms, along with a liver biopsy and blood tests, are needed to distinguish biliary atresia from neonatal hepatitis.

What Are the Complications?

Patients with neonatal hepatitis caused by rubella or cytomegalovirus are at risk of developing an infection of the brain that could lead to mental retardation or cerebral palsy. Many of these infants will also have permanent liver disease from the destruction of liver cells and the resulting scarring (cirrhosis).

Infants with giant cell hepatitis usually recover (80% of cases) with little or no scarring to their liver. Their growth pattern resumes as bile flows normally into the small intestine for digestion and to absorb vitamins.

About 20% of the infants with neonatal giant cell hepatitis develop chronic liver disease and cirrhosis. Their liver becomes very hard, due to the scarring, and the jaundice does not disappear by six months of age. Infants who reach this point in the disease eventually will require a liver transplant.

Because of the blockage of the bile ducts and the damage caused to liver cells, infants with chronic neonatal hepatitis will not be able to digest fats and will not be able to absorb vitamins A, D, E, and K. The lack of vitamin D leads to poor bone and cartilage development (rickets). Vitamin A is also needed for normal growth and good vision. Vitamin K deficiency is associated with easy bruising and a tendency to bleed, whereas the lack of vitamin E results in poor coordination.

Chronic neonatal hepatitis will lead to the inability of the liver to eliminate toxins in the bile. This causes itching, skin eruptions, and irritability.

How Is Neonatal Hepatitis Treated?

There is no specific treatment for neonatal hepatitis. Vitamin supplements are usually prescribed and many infants are given phenobarbital, a drug used to control seizures, but which also stimulates the liver to excrete additional bile. Formulas containing more easily digested fats are also given to the infant.

Neonatal hepatitis caused by the hepatitis A virus also usually resolves itself within six months, but cases that are the result of infection with the hepatitis B or hepatitis C viruses most likely will result in chronic liver disease. Infants who develop cirrhosis ultimately will need a liver transplant.

Can Neonatal Hepatitis Be Spread to Others?

Infants with neonatal hepatitis caused by the cytomegalovirus, rubella, or the hepatitis A, B, and C viruses may transmit the infection to others who come in close contact with the infant.

These infected infants should not come into contact with pregnant women because of the possibility that the woman will transmit the virus to her unborn child.

Chapter 29

Hepatitis A and B Vaccinations

Hepatitis B Vaccination

Eradication of hepatitis B is possible through a comprehensive vaccination program. The Centers for Disease Control and Prevention, the American Academy of Pediatrics, and the American Academy of Family Physicians recommend that all newborns, infants, children 11-12 years of age, and especially sexually active teenagers, be vaccinated against Hepatitis B Virus infection (HBV). The Vaccines for Children Program provides hepatitis B vaccine to young people under the age of 19 years who are on Medicaid, have no insurance, or whose insurance does not cover immunizations. Parents and guardians are encouraged to have their children vaccinated at an early age to prevent the serious complications that can occur when youngsters under the age of five are infected. The incidence of HBV infection, a sexually transmitted disease 100 times more infectious than AIDS, is the highest between the ages of 15 and 39.

Safe and effective vaccines are available and require three injections to obtain immunity. Hepatitis B vaccine is given as an intramuscular injection and can be given at the same time as other vaccinations. It can be given in a number of schedules, all of which provide excellent protection. For infants, vaccination can begin at

This chapter includes text from "Hair Loss after Receiving Vaccinations: Questions and Answers," Centers for Disease Control and Prevention (CDC), November 1997, and "Hepatitis A and B Vaccination," © 1997 Hepatitis Foundation International, reprinted with permission.

birth. A second dose at 1-2 months of age and the third dose at 6-18 months of age may be given. The Hepatitis B vaccine is marketed in combination with Haemophilus Influenza Type b (Hib). Check with your physician. For older children, adolescents, or adults, vaccination should be completed within 6 months.

All women should be screened with the hepatitis B surface antigen test during pregnancy to determine if they are a carrier (chronically infected) of HBV. If not treated, 85%-95% of infants born to HBV infected mothers may become carriers. This can be prevented by giving these infants an injection of Hepatitis B Immune Globulin (HBIG) and their first dose of HB vaccine within 12 hours after delivery. This treatment will prevent 90% of chronic HBV infections. The vaccine is safe to be given during pregnancy. Children, adults, and teenagers who are household or sexual contacts of HBV carriers are at risk of HBV infection. These persons should be vaccinated as soon as possible.

Hepatitis A Vaccination

Vaccines to protect against infection with the hepatitis A virus (HAV) have been shown to be safe and effective in preventing hepatitis A when given prior to exposure.

Hepatitis A is spread from person to person by anal/oral contact, by putting something in the mouth that has been contaminated with infected feces (stool), and fecal contamination of food and water. The highest rates of infection occur in children—often with no symptoms. Children commonly pass HAV to adults who can become quite ill. Good hand washing with soap and water after using the toilet or changing diapers will prevent transmission. Diaper changing tables in day care centers, if not cleaned properly or changed after each use, can be a source of contamination and transmission of the virus. Food handlers occasionally become infected and have been associated with large outbreaks.

It is anticipated that hepatitis A vaccine will eventually be given routinely to infants to prevent hepatitis A in the United States; however, it is not currently licensed for children less than 2 years of age.

Persons who are at high risk of hepatitis A, including those traveling or working in developing countries, homosexual men, and users of illicit drugs, should be vaccinated. Children in populations that experience repeated epidemics of hepatitis A should be routinely vaccinated including Alaska Native, American Indian, Pacific Islander, and certain closed religious communities. Hepatitis A vaccination is also being used to control epidemics of hepatitis A in other communities.

Clinical trials show the vaccine, which is made from inactivated hepatitis A virus to stimulate the body's immune system to combat hepatitis A virus, to be highly effective in preventing hepatitis A.

The recommended dosages and schedules vary according to the person's age and which vaccine is used. Children 2 years of age and older, as well as adults need more than one shot of vaccine for long-term protection. Patients with significant liver disease and persons with clotting factor disorders should consider being vaccinated for hepatitis A and B. Check with your doctor or nurse to determine how many shots are needed and when to return for the next dose.

Questions and Answers

What Is in the Hepatitis B Vaccine?

Two types of hepatitis B vaccines are currently licensed in the United States. The two are 1) the recombinant hepatitis B vaccine and 2) the plasma-derived vaccine, which is no longer being produced in the United States.

The commonly used vaccine is recombinant hepatitis B vaccine, which is produced by using common baker's yeast. The vaccines contain no more than 95% Hepatitis B surface antigen protein, and no more than 5% of yeast-derived protein. The vaccine also includes very tiny amounts of other additives such as aluminum hydroxide and thimerosal which help to stabilize and preserve the vaccine.

What Other Side Effects Are Associated with the Hepatitis B Vaccine?

Most persons who receive hepatitis B vaccine have no side effects at all. Of persons who do experience side effects the most common include pain at the injection site (3%-29% of persons vaccinated), and mild fever (1%-6% of persons vaccinated).

As with any medication or vaccine, there is a very small risk that serious problems, even death could occur from someone having a serious allergic reaction.

Is It Still a Good Idea to Get a Hepatitis B Shot?

Yes. Immunizations are the best protection against vaccine preventable diseases, such as hepatitis B.

Getting the disease is much more likely to cause serious illness than getting the vaccine. Each year an estimated 4,000 persons die of hepatitis B-related cirrhosis, and more than 800 die of hepatitis B-related liver cancer.

What Should I Do if I Believe that I Have Had a Reaction or Have Side Effects from Hepatitis B Vaccine or Any Vaccine?

You should contact your health care provider if you suspect you have had a reaction or side effects from a vaccine. You or your health care provider should also report this information to the Vaccine Adverse Effects Reporting System at 1-800-822-7967.

For Additional Information

Hepatitis Foundation International
30 Sunrise Terrace
Cedar Grove, NJ 07009-1423, U.S.A.
Phone: 800-891-0707
FAX: 973-857-5044
E-Mail: mail@hepfi.org

Chapter 30

Occupational Hepatitis

Occupational Safety and Health Administration (OSHA) Health Hazard Definitions

Although safety hazards related to the physical characteristics of a chemical can be objectively defined in terms of testing requirements (e.g., flammability), health hazard definitions are less precise and more subjective. Health hazards may cause measurable changes in the body—such as decreased pulmonary function. These changes are generally indicated by the occurrence of signs and symptoms in the exposed employees—such as shortness of breath, a non-measurable, subjective feeling. Employees exposed to such hazards must be apprised of both the changes in body function and the signs and symptoms that may occur to signal that change.

The determination of occupational health hazards is complicated by the fact that many of the effects or signs and symptoms occur commonly in non-occupationally exposed populations, so that effects of exposure are difficult to separate from normally occurring illnesses. Occasionally, a substance causes an effect that is rarely seen in the population at large, such as angiosarcomas caused by vinyl chloride exposure, thus making it easier to ascertain that the occupational exposure was the primary causative factor. More often, however, the

---

This chapter contains text from "Epidemiologic Notes and Reports Outbreak of Occupational Hepatitis—Connecticut," MMWR Weekly February 27, 1987, and Occupational Safety and Health Administration (OSHA) Standard 1910.1200 App A–Complete.

effects are common, such as lung cancer. The situation is further complicated by the fact that most chemicals have not been adequately tested to determine their health hazard potential, and data do not exist to substantiate these effects.

There have been many attempts to categorize effects and to define them in various ways. Generally, the terms "acute" and "chronic" are used to delineate between effects on the basis of severity or duration. "Acute" effects usually occur rapidly as a result of short-term exposures, and are of short duration. "Chronic" effects generally occur as a result of long-term exposure, and are of long duration.

The acute effects referred to most frequently are those defined by the American National Standards Institute (ANSI) standard for Precautionary Labeling of Hazardous Industrial Chemicals (Z129.1-1982)—irritation, corrosivity, sensitization, and lethal dose. Although these are important health effects, they do not adequately cover the considerable range of acute effects that may occur as a result of occupational exposure, such as, narcosis.

Similarly, the term chronic effect is often used to cover only carcinogenicity, teratogenicity, and mutagenicity. These effects are obviously a concern in the workplace, but again, do not adequately cover the area of chronic effects, excluding, for example, blood dyscrasias (such as anemia), chronic bronchitis, and liver atrophy.

The goal of defining precisely, in measurable terms, every possible health effect that may occur in the workplace as a result of chemical exposures cannot realistically be accomplished. This does not negate the need for employees to be informed of such effects and protected from them.

The following are effects which may occur that affect the liver.

- **Hepatotoxins:** Chemicals that produce liver damage

- **Signs and Symptoms:** Jaundice; liver enlargement

- **Chemicals:** Carbon tetrachloride; nitrosamines

Occupational Hepatitis

On September 28, 1986, a previously healthy, 40-year-old male factory worker who had experienced several days of abdominal pain and nausea was seen at the emergency room at Yale-New Haven Hospital, New Haven, Connecticut. Liver function tests revealed an elevated aspartate aminotransferase (AST) level of 949 U/L (normal = 35 U/L). Alkaline phosphatase and bilirubin assays were all normal.

290

Hepatitis A IgM antibody and hepatitis B surface antigen and antibody were negative, as was an abdominal ultrasound.

Further history revealed that the patient had become ill after working for 2 weeks at a plant where fabrics are coated with a polyurethane polymer. He had no history of significant alcohol use or blood transfusions. When the patient was removed from the workplace, his symptoms resolved. Subsequent liver function tests have revealed partial resolution of his hepatitis. However, 2 months later, his alanine aminotransferase (ALT) level was still elevated at 207 U/L (normal = 32 U/L), and his AST level was 49 U/L. Within 1 month, three other co-workers were seen with similar symptoms and liver enzyme abnormalities.

Inspection of the patients' workplace showed that large quantities of dimethylformamide (DMF), a solvent which is widely used in manufacturing acrylic fibers and polyurethanes, was being used in poorly ventilated areas. DMF and smaller quantities of other solvents including toluene; methyl ethyl ketone; and 1,1,1 trichloroethane were mixed with polyurethane polymer, coated onto the fabric, and then evaporated from the polyurethane-coated fabric as it dried. The company has 66 employees, most of who work directly in the production of polyurethane-coated materials. The employees are generally young (mean age = 35 years) and healthy.

Forty-five of the employees agreed to have liver screening tests, including AST, ALT, bilirubin, g-glutamyl transpeptidase (GGT), alkaline phosphatase, and lactate dehydrogenase. Thirty of the 45 employees screened had elevated levels of AST, ALT, or GGT. Eleven had elevations that were more than twice the normal level for one or more of these liver enzymes. In all but one employee, the ALT level was greater than the AST level. In addition, workers directly involved with producing the polyurethane-coated material had higher liver enzyme elevations than did nonproduction workers.

Based on these findings, the professional staff at the Yale Occupational Medicine Program urged immediate termination of the production process until protective engineering controls had been adequately installed. These instructions have been followed. This cohort of workers will be followed to help ascertain whether DMF causes chronic liver damage.

Occupationally Induced Liver Disease

Although the hepatotoxic effects of industrial chemicals such as carbon tetrachloride, chlordecone (kepone), and monovinyl chloride are widely known, occupationally induced liver disease is regarded by some as a historic problem. However, there is continuing evidence that chemically induced hepatic disease is an important occupational health problem for selected U.S. workers. This outbreak of subacute hepatic disease, occurring during routine workplace exposure to DMF, without evidence of a chemical spill or accidental release, further emphasizes the importance of this problem.

Because of its excellent solvent properties and lack of volatility, DMF is widely used in manufacturing polymerized films, fibers, and coatings, particularly in acrylic and spandex fabrics. It is readily absorbed through the skin and lungs, metabolized by the liver, and excreted in urine.

There are precedents that reinforce the possibility that serious human hepatotoxins may not have yet been recognized. For some of the most severe occupational hepatotoxins, such as trinitrotoluene, dimethylnitrosamine, polychlorinated biphnyls, and tetrachloroethane, the epidemiologic identification of human liver disease preceded an adequate exploration of animal hepatotoxicity. On the other hand, human liver disease for the organochloride insecticide, kepone, reached national attention through reports in the lay press in the mid-1970's, although parallel animal toxicities had been demonstrated a decade earlier.

Adverse human effects from DMF and other dimethylamides merit a much closer look. Perhaps this review should also include the classes of halogenated hydrocarbons and nitroaromatics from which the most damaging identified hepatotoxins have emerged.

Part Seven

Genetically Based
Liver Disease

Chapter 31

Alagille Syndrome

Alagille syndrome is an inherited disorder that mimics other forms of prolonged liver disease seen in infants and young children. However, a group of unusual features in other organ systems distinguishes Alagille syndrome from other liver and bile duct diseases in infants.

Children with Alagille Syndrome usually have a liver disease characterized by a progressive loss of the bile ducts within the liver over the first year of life and narrowing of bile ducts outside the liver. This leads to a buildup of bile in the liver, causing damage to liver cells. Scarring may occur and lead to cirrhosis in about 30 to 50 percent of affected children.

Symptoms of the illness are jaundice, pale, loose stools, and poor growth within the first three months of life. Later there is persistent jaundice, itching, fatty deposits in the skin, and stunted growth and development during early childhood. Frequently the disease stabilizes between ages 4 and 10 with an improvement in symptoms.

Other features which help establish the diagnosis include abnormalities in the cardiovascular system, the spinal column, the eye and the kidneys. Narrowing of the blood vessel connecting the heart to the lungs (pulmonary artery) leads to extra heart sounds but rarely problems in heart function. The shape of the bones of the spinal column may look like the wings of a butterfly on x-ray but almost never cause any problems with function of the nerves in the spinal cord.

More than 90 percent of children with Alagille Syndrome have an unusual abnormality of the eyes. An extra, circular line on the surface of the eye requires specialized eye examination to detect and does not lead to any disturbances in vision. In addition, some children have various abnormalities in their kidneys that may lead to minor changes in kidney function.

Many physicians believe that there is a specific facial appearance shared by most of the children with Alagille Syndrome that makes them easily recognizable. The features include a prominent, broad forehead, deep-set eyes, a straight nose, and a small pointed chin.

Alagille Syndrome is generally inherited only from one parent and there is a 50 percent chance that each child will develop the syndrome. Each affected adult or child may have all or only a few of the features of the syndrome. Frequently a parent or brother or sister of the affected child will share the facial appearance, heart murmur, or butterfly vertebrae, but will have a completely normal liver and bile ducts.

Treatment of Alagille Syndrome is based on trying to increase the flow of bile from the liver, maintain normal growth and development, and prevent or correct any of the specific nutritional deficiencies that often develop. Because bile flow from the liver to the intestine is slow in Alagille Syndrome, medications designed to increase the flow of bile are frequently prescribed, including Phenobarbital, Questran, or Colistipol. This may decrease the damage in the liver and improve the digestion of fat in foods that are eaten.

Also, itching caused by the buildup of bile in the blood and skin may be relieved. Other drugs are also used to relieve itching (Benadryl, Atarax). Elevations in blood cholesterol also respond to the medications used to increase bile flow. Elevated blood cholesterol levels can lead to small yellow deposits of cholesterol on the skin of knees, elbows, palms, eyelids, and other surfaces that are frequently rubbed. Lowering blood cholesterol usually causes the cholesterol skin deposits to improve. Although these are unsightly, they are almost never associated with any dangerous symptoms.

Although reduced flow of bile into the intestine leads to poor digestion of dietary fat, a specific type of fat can still be well digested and therefore infant formulas containing high levels of medium-chain triglycerides (MCT) are usually substituted for conventional formulas. Trade names are Pregestamil or Portagen. Some infants can grow adequately on breast milk if additional MCT oil is given. Foods containing fat may lead to looser, greasy stools later in childhood. However, the benefits from the calories and vitamins in the fat that is absorbed usually leads to the recommendation that the child not be put on a low-fat diet. There are no other dietary restrictions. Occasionally, MCT oil is also prescribed as a nutritional supplement.

Problems with fat digestion and absorption may lead to deficiency of fat-soluble vitamins—A, D, E, and K. Vitamin A deficiency causes night blindness and red eyes. Vitamin D deficiency causes softening and fractures of the bones and teeth (rickets). Vitamin E deficiency causes a disabling disease of the nervous system and muscles, and vitamin K deficiency causes bleeding problems. Deficiencies of these vitamins can be diagnosed by blood tests and usually can be corrected by large oral doses. If the child's system cannot absorb vitamins given by mouth, vitamin injections into the muscle are necessary.

Sometimes surgery is necessary during infancy to help establish the diagnosis of Alagille Syndrome by direct examination of the bile duct system. However, surgical reconstruction of the bile duct system is not recommended because bile can still flow from the liver and there is presently no procedure that can correct for the loss of the bile ducts within the liver. Occasionally liver cirrhosis advances to a stage where the liver fails to perform its functions. Liver transplantation is then considered.

The overall life expectancy for children with Alagille Syndrome is unknown, but depends on several factors: the severity of scarring in the liver, whether heart or lung problems develop because of the narrowing in the pulmonary artery, and the presence of infections or other problems related to poor nutrition. Many adults with Alagille Syndrome are leading normal lives.

Although Alagille Syndrome was first described in the English medical literature in 1975, it is now becoming recognized more frequently among children with chronic forms of liver disease. Diagnosis can be established by microscopic examination of liver biopsy specimens, a stethoscope examination of the child's heart and chest, a special eye examination (slit-lamp exam), an x-ray of the spinal column, and an ultrasound (sonogram) examination of the abdomen.

Treatment is primarily medical and not surgical. Patients generally have a much better outcome than children with some of the other liver diseases that may present at the same age.

For More Information

American Liver Foundation
75 Maiden Lane, Suite 603
New York, NY 10038
1-800-GO LIVER (465-4837); Fax: 212-483-8179
E-mail: webmail@liverfoundation.org
URL: http://www.liverfoundation.org

Chapter 32

Alpha-1-Antitrypsin Deficiency

Alpha-1-antitrypsin deficiency is a hereditary disease that may lead to hepatitis and cirrhosis. It is the most common genetic cause of liver disease in children. Adults are also affected and may have lung involvement with emphysema as well as liver disease. The protein alpha-1-antitrypsin is a substance made in the liver. It plays an important role preventing the breakdown of enzymes in various organs of the body.

A child must inherit the tendency from both parents to develop the disease, alpha-1-antitrypsin deficiency. The incidence of the disease in the United States is approximately 1:2000 live births. Fortunately, for reasons that are not understood, only 10-20% of the babies born with the deficiency will have liver disease. Decreased levels of the serum protein, alpha-1-antitrypsin, lead to liver damage with scarring and abnormal liver function.

The disease most often appears in the newborn period with jaundice, swelling of the abdomen, and poor feeding. It may also appear in late childhood or adulthood and be detected because of fatigue, poor appetite, swelling of the abdomen and legs, or abnormal liver tests.

The diagnosis is made by blood tests when the serum level of alpha-1-antitrypsin is low and standard liver function tests are abnormal. Other tests such as urine collection, ultrasound examination, or tests using specialized X-ray techniques may be necessary. A biopsy

---

of the liver (sampling liver tissue with a needle or by operation) is usually performed to look for liver injury. Relatives who are carriers but do not have the disease can also be diagnosed by blood tests.

Currently, there is no cure for this disease. However, certain abnormalities can be treated or controlled. Treatment is designed to maintain normal nutrition, to provide the liver and the body with essential nutrients, and to identify complications early in order to treat them better. Multiple vitamins and vitamins E, D, and K are often given. When jaundice is severe or itching appears, phenobarbital or cholestyramine may be used. If the disease progresses, excess body fluid may occur and can be treated with diuretics.

Patients who develop cirrhosis (scarring of the liver) have changes in blood flow through the liver which produce other complications: nosebleeds, bruising, excess body fluid, enlarged veins in the inside of the stomach and esophagus (varices). Occasionally, increases in pressure in these veins make them leak, and internal bleeding may result. Increased sleepiness after eating protein (due to increased blood ammonia levels) and increased risk of infection may be late complications.

The long-term outcome of the disease is variable. Approximately 25% of affected patients develop cirrhosis and its complications, but 75% of individuals will not have any significant liver disease after the newborn period. Some patients with cirrhosis lead relatively normal lives for relatively long periods of time. The reason for this difference is not known. Liver transplantation can be done when liver failure develops and interferes with normal functioning at school, work, or in the home.

Chapter 33

Galactosemia

Galactosemia is a rare hereditary disease leading not only to cirrhosis in infants, but more seriously, to early devastating illness if not diagnosed quickly.

This disease is caused by elevated levels of galactose (a sugar in milk) in the blood resulting from a deficiency of the liver enzyme required for its metabolism (breakdown). To have the disease, a child must inherit the tendency from both parents. The incidence of the disease is approximately 1:20,000 live births. For each pregnancy, in such a family, there is a 1 in 4 chance a baby will be born with the deficiency. Because of the potential disastrous side effects of late diagnosis, many states have mandatory neonatal screening programs for galactosemia. The disease usually appears in the first days of life following the ingestion of breast milk or formula. Vomiting, liver enlargement, and jaundice are often the earliest signs of the disease, but bacterial infections (often severe), irritability, failure to gain weight, and diarrhea may also occur. If unrecognized in the newborn period, the disease may produce liver, brain, eye, and kidney damage.

Blood tests can make the diagnosis. The disease is detected by measuring the level of enzyme in red blood cells, white blood cells, or liver. Affected patients have no enzyme activity; carriers (parents) have intermediate enzyme activity (about 1/2 the normal level). A

Reprinted with permission, © 1997 American Liver Foundation, 1-800-GO-LIVER.

galactose tolerance test should never be done, as it may be harmful. Affected infants who ingest galactose will excrete it in large quantities in their urine where it can also be detected. If the infant is vomiting, and not taking milk, the test can be negative. If the disease is suspected, the diagnosis should be confirmed by blood testing.

Treatment is based on elimination of galactose from the diet. This may be done in the early neonatal period by stopping breast feeding and by the administration of diets which contain no lactose or galactose, (Nutramigen, Pregestimil). This diet should be compulsively followed, and continued for years, and possibly for life. The red blood cell levels of galactose or its metabolites (Galactose-l-phosphate) may be used as a monitor to gauge the adherence to the diet and restriction of galactose. It is also recommended that mothers of affected infants be placed on a galactose-free diet during the subsequent pregnancy. This may somewhat modify symptoms present at birth. With early therapy, any liver damage which occurred in the first few days of life will nearly completely heal. Galactosemia should be considered in any jaundiced infant because of beneficial effects of early dietary restriction.

Additional Information

American Liver Foundation

75 Maiden Lane, Suite 603
New York, NY 10038
1-800-GO LIVER (465-4837)
Fax: 201-256-3214
E-mail: info@liverfoundation.org
URL: http://www.liverfoundation.org

Chapter 34

Gaucher Disease

Diagnosis and Treatment

There are three forms of Gaucher disease: Types I, II, and III. Type I is the most common form of the disease. The signs and symptoms of this form of the disease vary greatly from one person to another. The most common symptom is an enlarged spleen, which is generally painless. Other symptoms may include an enlarged liver, frequent nosebleeds, bruising, bone pain, and a lack of energy. Some people may experience only a few of these symptoms, while others may have many. One person may have bone problems, while another may have only an enlarged spleen. Symptoms can be present in any combination. In addition, children with Type I Gaucher disease may be shorter than their peers and have delayed puberty.

Type II is much less common than type I. Symptoms usually appear in an infant several months after birth. The disease affects the infant's nervous system, resulting in an inability to support the head and difficulty breathing. Infants with this type of disease usually die by the time they are 2 years old.

Type III is also less common than type I. It is characterized by a combination of symptoms from both Type I and Type II. This form of the disease affects the person's central nervous system. As a result,

This chapter includes the following articles reprinted with permission from the University of Pittsburgh: © 1997 "Gaucher Disease: Diagnosis and Treatment," and © 1997 "Gaucher Disease: A Clinical Trial of Gene Therapy."

people with Type III may experience irregular eye movement, seizures, and mental retardation.

Who Is At Risk for Gaucher Disease?

Gaucher disease may occur among every nationality and ethnic group, but it is most common among Jews of Eastern European descent (Ashkenazi Jews). Type I Gaucher disease, in fact, is the most common genetic disease among Jews. An estimated one in 10 Ashkenazi Jews is a carrier of Gaucher disease. Types II and III, however, are not more prevalent among the Jewish population.

How Do People Get Gaucher Disease?

Gaucher disease is hereditary, meaning that it is passed from parents to children. Many parents are carriers of the disease. Carriers are people who do not have the disease or any of its symptoms, but who can pass it on to their children. When both parents are carriers, their children may be affected with the disease, may be carriers, or may neither have the disease nor be carriers. In this way, the disease can seem to skip generations.

Because carriers have no disease symptoms, most parents are unaware whether they are carriers. It can be very difficult for parents to learn that they are carriers, and to accept that their children may be carriers or may have the disease. These are normal reactions. Parents may also have questions about the risks to their children or future children. Genetic counseling is available to explain how Gaucher disease is inherited, to describe the tests that can identify carriers, and to help families deal with the many emotions they face.

How Is Gaucher Disease Diagnosed?

A blood test is used to determine whether a person experiencing symptoms has Gaucher disease. A blood test is also used to identify people who may be carriers of Gaucher disease but do not have any symptoms.

Is There an Effective Treatment for Gaucher Disease?

A few years ago, enzyme replacement therapy became available as the first effective treatment for Gaucher disease. The treatment consists of a modified form of the glucocerebrosidase enzyme given intravenously. It takes approximately two hours for a person to receive the treatment, and the treatment is usually given every two weeks. Enzyme replacement therapy can stop and often reverse the symptoms of Gaucher disease. Disadvantages of the enzyme treatment are its high cost and the fact that it is a lifelong process.

Is There a Cure for Gaucher Disease?

Currently there is no cure for Gaucher disease. But researchers at the Pittsburgh Genetics Institute are investigating ways to correct the genetic defect using gene therapy techniques. Clinical trials may be available in the near future.

A Clinical Trial of Gene Therapy

Gaucher disease is an inherited disease caused by mutations (DNA changes) in the gene that codes for an enzyme called glucocerebrosidase (GC). The enzyme GC is responsible for breaking down a fatty substance called glucosylceramide. In Gaucher disease, the mutated GC gene produces too little functional GC, so glucosylceramide is not broken down properly and it accumulates in the liver, spleen, and bone marrow and, on rare occasions, in the brain. This is what causes the typical symptoms of Gaucher disease, including enlarged organs, bone deterioration with multiple fractures, and in some patients progressive nervous system degeneration.

The gene therapy clinical trial is a study to evaluate gene therapy as a treatment for Gaucher disease. We hope that information obtained during the trial will benefit future patients with Gaucher disease. We do not know if patients participating in the trial will benefit directly from it. Depending on the outcome, trial participants currently receiving enzyme replacement therapy eventually may be able to decrease and/or discontinue treatment.

What Treatments Are Available for Gaucher Disease?

Bone marrow transplantation. Bone marrow transplantation has been used successfully in the past to treat a few people with Gaucher disease. However the treatment requires a marrow donor and has a 10 percent to 25 percent risk of fatal complications, which make it an unacceptable approach for most patients with Gaucher disease.

Gaucher symptoms are caused by accumulation of glucosyl-ceramide in one particular cell type—the macrophage. Macrophages come from the bone marrow. The fact that bone marrow transplantation can successfully treat Gaucher disease is significant. This tells us that replacement of defective cells with "normal" cells halts the course of the disease and causes existing symptoms to decrease or disappear.

Enzyme replacement therapy. Enzyme replacement therapy with modified GC has been available as a treatment for Gaucher disease since the early 1990s. The GC used for therapy is extracted from human placentas or generated in the laboratory and the chemically modified to target it to macrophages. Patients receive the modified enzyme by intravenous infusion. Treatments are usually given every two weeks, and it takes about two hours for a person to receive the treatment.

Approximately 800 people worldwide are receiving enzyme replacement therapy. The disease has stopped getting worse in the majority of these patients, and most have also experienced a reversal of disease symptoms. The main drawback to enzyme replacement therapy is that it involves lifelong infusions. It is also very expensive.

What Is Somatic Cell Gene Therapy?

If successful, somatic cell gene therapy may provide a cure for Gaucher disease, not just a treatment. The gene therapy clinical trial involves:

- injecting the patient with a substance called G-CSF to stimulate release of stem cells from the bone marrow into the blood

- collecting the stem cells from the patients blood

- inserting a healthy copy of the GC gene into the autologous (patient's own) stem cells

- returning the "corrected" stem cells to the patient, where they take up residence in the bone marrow and produce cells such as macrophages.

"Somatic" indicates that the corrected cells are not reproductive cells. This means the transferred gene will not be passed on to the patient's children.

Why Is Gene Therapy Expected to Work in People with Gaucher Disease?

Successful gene therapy for Gaucher disease requires that the therapeutic GC gene be transferred effectively into stem cells that, when returned to the body, will produce "corrected" macrophages. In other words, the transferred gene must work correctly and produce sufficient amounts of functional GC.

Researchers at the University of Pittsburgh Medical Center believe they have found a way to effectively transfer the therapeutic gene into patients. Some stem cells are members of a family called CD34 cells. In the laboratory, when a normal copy of the GC gene is inserted into CD34 cells, the cells produce two to four times the normal level of GC. This is a good sign because it indicates that the transferred GC gene is functioning in cells that produce new macrophages.

How Is Somatic Cell Gene Transfer Accomplished?

The most efficient way to transfer and express genes in human cells is through the use of viruses that act as gene carriers. The viruses are modified so that they can still infect human cells but can no longer multiply and cause disease. Modified viruses used for this purpose are called vectors.

The vector used in this clinical trial is a retroviral vector. When retroviruses infect cells, they incorporate their genetic materials into the DNA of the cell. Using this natural ability of retroviruses, therapeutic genes can be introduced into cells.

What Does the Study Involve and How Is It Different From Existing Treatments?

- Administration of G-CSF by subcutaneous (beneath the skin) injection.

- Collection of bone marrow-producing cells by leukopheresis beginning on the fifth day after the initial G-CSF injection.

- Separation of CD34 cells from other white blood cells.

- Exposure of CD34 cells to the retroviral vector that carries the GC gene.

- Testing of transduced (corrected) CD34 cells for their ability to produce enzyme and for contaminants.

- Return of corrected cells by intravenous infusion.

Response to the treatment is measured by changes in the size of the spleen and liver, and by bone x-rays, bone marrow biopsies, and monthly blood tests.

Is There a Special Program for People with Gaucher Disease?

The Pittsburgh Genetics Institute has a Gaucher Disease Diagnosis and Treatment Program at the University of Pittsburgh Medical Center.

The director of the program is John A. Barranger, MD, PhD. Dr. Barranger was instrumental in the development of enzyme replacement therapy for people with Gaucher disease. He joined the Pittsburgh Genetics Institute in 1990 to continue his 17-year search for a cure for Gaucher disease.

The Gaucher Disease Diagnosis and Treatment Program offers diagnosis, treatment, and genetic counseling for people with Gaucher disease and their families.

For More Information or to Schedule an Appointment

Call Erin Rourk, MS, CGC
Program Coordinator
(800) 334-7980

Chapter 35

Hereditary Hemochromatosis

Preview

Hereditary hemochromatosis, once thought to be rare is the most common genetic disorder in the United States. Nonetheless, the condition often goes undetected and untreated until its severe effects have become apparent. What clues can lead to the diagnosis, and how can they be spotted in patients, before significant morbidity has occurred? In this chapter, Drs. McDonnell and Witte discuss the diagnosis and management of this under recognized problem as well as the various issues involved in screening.

An Illustrative Case of Hemochromatosis

A 47 year old, white, male presented with complaints of fatigue and nonspecific musculoskeletal aches and pains. History taking and physical examination offered no clues to the cause of his symptoms. Laboratory testing showed a normal complete blood count and normal glucose and Thyrotropin levels, but his alanine aminotransferase (ALT) was 50% above the normal.

The elevated ALT level had also been detected during a routine evaluation several months earlier and warranted further evaluation.[1] The patient had no high-risk social behaviors and was a regular blood

"Hereditary Hemochromatosis: Preventing Chronic Effects of this Under-diagnosed Disorder," Office of Genetics & Disease Prevention, Centers of Disease Control and Prevention (CDC), 1997.

309

donor. Laboratory testing showed a serum iron level of 147 μg/dL (micrograms per deciliter), total iron binding capacity 225 μg/dL, and transferrin saturation of 65%. A second transferrin saturation test, performed after fasting and exclusion of dietary iron and vitamin C supplements for at least 24 hours, revealed a saturation of 76%. Additional testing showed the following values: serum iron 168 μg/dL, total iron binding capacity, 220 μg/dL; and serum 550 μg/L (normal, 20 to 400 μg/L). Sedimentation rate was normal. The results were strongly suggestive of hemochromatosis.[2]

The patient was referred to a specialist in iron overload disease, who recommended a liver biopsy because of the patient's age, abnormal liver enzyme levels, and elevated serum ferritin concentration. Histologic examination revealed Perls' stain grade 2 iron, primarily in hepatic parenchymal cells, and minimal inflammation. The hepatic iron index (hepatic iron concentration [mol/g dry weight] divided by patient's age [years] was 2.1. An index of 1.9 or higher is used to differentiate hemochromatosis from other liver diseases.

The patient received weekly phlebotomy with hemoglobin monitoring before each session. After 26 weeks, a total of 24 U (units) had been removed, his serum ferritin level was 50 μg/L, and his hemoglobin level was 13 g/dL. The patient reported marked improvement in fatigue, libido, and joint pains. He continues to receive maintenance phlebotomy therapy based on serum ferritin values.

References

Witte DL. Mild liver enzyme abnormalities: Eliminating hemochromatosis as an unrecognized cause. *Clin Chem* 1997 43:8(B):1535-8.

Witte DL, Crosby WH, Edwards, CQ, Fairbanks VF, Mitros FA. Practice parameter for hereditary hemochromatosis. College of American Pathologists. *Clin Chim Acta* 1996; 245:139-200.

Iron Overload and Hereditary Hemochromatosis

Iron overload is classified as primary or secondary, depending on the underlying mechanism. Primary iron overload results from abnormally increased absorption of dietary iron in the small intestine. Secondary overload results mainly from iron accumulated as a consequence of ineffective erythropoiesis, multiple blood transfusions ,or prolonged excessive intake of dietary iron.[1]

Hereditary hemochromatosis is a type of primary iron overload. The excess iron that is absorbed is deposited in the parenchymal cells of the liver, heart, joints, pancreas, and other endocrine organs causing inflammation and subsequent fibrosis and destruction, which results in organ failure and ultimately, chronic diseases.[1,2]

Epidemiologic Factors

Hereditary hemochromatosis is an autosomal recessive disorder previously considered to be rare. The classic diagnosis was clinical, based on the presence of bronze diabetes with cirrhosis. Recent estimates place the prevalence of the homozygous genotype at 1 in 250 persons, and about 1 in nine is a carrier, making hereditary hemochromatosis the most common known genetic disorder in the United States.[1, 3] This condition is under diagnosed among whites. In addition, because it most often affects white men of northern European descent, the disease may not be considered in other populations or ethnic groups (e.g., African Americans, Hispanics) even when symptoms and clinical findings are consistent with the diagnosis.[1, 4-6]

Pathologic Mechanisms

The body has no mechanism for excreting iron absorbed from the diet except through incidental losses. Thus, the level of body iron can be regulated only through absorption of iron from food. The amount of iron absorbed from the diet is influenced by the following factors: the amount of iron stores in the body, the rate and effectiveness of erythropoiesis (functional iron), the amount and chemical form of iron in the diet, and the presence of absorption enhancers and inhibitors in the diet. Persons with normal hemoglobin levels and iron stores (as reflected by serum ferritin values) absorb just enough to meet their daily needs and to balance losses (1 mg per day).[7] In contrast, persons with hemochromatosis continue to absorb high amounts of dietary iron even when their body already has enough or too much iron.

When total body iron exceeds storage capacity (five to ten times the normal quantity), tissue and organ damage begins.[1] At this stage, iron overload has occurred. This condition, if left untreated, can result in arthritis, cirrhosis, diabetes, heart disease, psychological and sexual dysfunction, and premature death.[1]

Clinical Signs and Symptoms

The clinical manifestations of hereditary hemochromatosis usually do not appear until a person reaches 40 to 60 years of age, when sufficient iron has accumulated to cause organ damage. Yet some persons have clinical manifestations by age 20, and others who are homozygous for the disease may never have clinical signs.[2] About 50% of men and 13% to 20% of women with untreated hereditary hemochromatosis will have clinical manifestations of iron overload by the age of 40.[1, 8-9] After age 40, an estimated 67% to 94% of men and 41% of women with hereditary hemochromatosis eventually show signs and symptoms of the disease.[9]

The development of the clinical manifestations of iron overload may be influenced by genetic and environmental factors including menstruation, diet, and blood donation.[1] Use of alcohol and other hepatotoxic drugs lowers the ability of the liver to safely store iron and may accelerate the development of the hepatic sequelae of iron overload.[2]

A common early sign of progressive iron overload is asymptomatic elevation of liver enzyme levels, particularly alanine aminotransferase and aspartate aminotransferase, which later may be accompanied by recurrent right-sided abdominal pain and hepatomegaly. Arthropathy is also common, and occasionally acute episodes of inflammatory arthritis occur, at least some of which are caused by deposits of calcium pyrophosphate dihydrate.[2] Other early signs and symptoms include impotence, amenorrhea, irritability, depression, and fatigue.[2] Because these clinical conditions are not specific to iron overload, the disorder may not be considered in differential diagnosis. Consequently, the underlying cause is not recognized and treated and organ damage progresses.

Liver disease which is present in 30 to 94% of patients with iron overload is the most common complication of hemochromatosis, and cirrhosis is the most common severe sequelae.[1, 10] An autopsy study of patients with cirrhosis showed hemochromatosis as the underlying cause in 7.5% of the deaths.[11] Once cirrhosis is present, risk of liver neoplasm is increased 200 fold in patients with hemochromatosis compared with persons without the disorder, and liver neoplasms account for nearly one third of all deaths among affected patients.[1, 11, 12] Therefore, it is essential that hemochromatosis be considered in the evaluation of any liver abnormality. Other damage to tissues and organs includes gray or bronze skin pigmentation, diabetes mellitus, hypopituitarism, hypogonadism, cardiomyopathy, joint deformity (as arthritis progresses), chronic abdominal pain, and severe fatigue.[1]

The degree of iron overload at the time of diagnosis of hereditary hemochromatosis has prognostic implications.[1, 12] Patients with no evidence of tissue or organ damage have subclinical disease. With proper management, their long-term prognosis, including life expectancy, should not differ from that of healthy persons.[13] The prognosis for persons with significant hepatic fibrosis, diabetes, or cardiomyopathy due to iron overload is poorer.

Diagnostic Considerations

Early diagnosis of hereditary hemochromatosis based on abnormal laboratory values allows prevention and early treatment of clinical manifestations. The presence of several clinical signs of iron overload (e.g., cirrhosis, diabetes, and hyperpigmentation of the skin) should not be a requirement for diagnosis, because these signs indicate late-stage disease. The diagnosis should be broadened to include manifestations of abnormal iron metabolism, such as persistent elevation in transferrin saturation and evidence of increased body iron load regardless of clinical complications. Increasingly, the diagnosis is being made in patients with abnormal laboratory values.[10] The most common tests used in assessing a patient iron status and for iron-overload are described in Table 35.1.

Patients with persistent elevation of transferrin saturation have phenotypic evidence of hemochromatosis. Further evaluation is necessary to determine whether such patients have iron overload and associated organ damage. An elevated serum ferritin concentration not related to an acute-phase response is correlated with excess iron stores and is more predictive of organ damage than an elevated transferrin saturation. The presence and amount of iron may be confirmed by quantitative phlebotomy or liver biopsy.

Quantitative phlebotomy is the removal of a unit (500 ml) of whole blood (200-250 mg of iron) once or twice weekly until iron deficiency develops (as reflected by hemoglobin and serum ferritin levels). The total amount of blood that must be removed to produce iron deficiency provides an estimate of total body iron load and thus, an estimate of excess body iron. The amount of blood needed to confirm iron overload is controversial; most diagnosticians require at least ten units or 3-5 g.[2]

Liver biopsy has long been considered the "gold standard" for the diagnosis of hemochromatosis, because it can detect fibrosis and cirrhosis. Many specialists prefer liver biopsy over phlebotomy, particularly when clinical or laboratory evidence of hepatic involvement is

Table 35.1a. Common Tests Used in Assessment of Iron Status and Detection of Iron Overload (continued on next page).

Test	Description	Normal Values	Value Indicating Overload	Notes
Transferrin Saturation	Most sensitive test for detecting hemochromatosis. Iron is transported in the body by the protein transferrin. Saturation (the extent to which transferrin has vacant iron-binding sites) is calculated by dividing serum iron concentration by total iron binding capacity. High saturation indicates high level of body iron.	>15-40%	≥60% in men; 50% in women	A fasting test eliminates short-term effects of diet on saturation. Infection and inflammation can depress saturation. Compared with normal population heterozygotes for hereditary hemochromatosis have elevated levels but not as high as those in homozygotes. Saturation ≤15%:
Serum Ferritin Concentration	Ferritin is an intracellular iron storage protein. Its concentration in serum indicates the level of iron stored in the body (concentration 1 µg/L = 10 mg of stored iron).	20 to 400 µg/L in men; 20 to 200 µg/L in women of childbearing age; 20 to 300 µg/L in post-menopausal women	> 400 µg/L in men; >200 µg/L in women of childbearing age and > 300 µg/L in Post-menopausal women	A high concentration may also indicate infection or inflammation, especially liver disease. Level of <20 µg/L indicates iron deficiency; <12 µg/L indicates iron depletion
Hemoglobin	Hemoglobin content in circulating red blood cells.	13.6 mg/L in men; 12 mg/L in women:	Normal or low	High level does not occur with iron overload. Iron deficiency may occur due to anemia from chronic inflammation and illness

Table 35.1b. Common Tests Used in Assessment of Iron Status and Detection of Iron Overload (continued from previous page).

Test	Description	Normal Values	Value Indicating Overload	Notes
Quantitative Phlebotomy	Removal of blood until iron deficiency develops. The amount of blood removed indicates total body iron load	Variable, usually >2 to 3 U in 2 wk result in drop in hemoglobin	About 10 U whole blood	Also used to treat iron overload.
Liver Biopsy	The amount of iron in the liver (hepatic iron concentration) is measured by atomic absorption spectrophotometry of hepatic parenchymal cells or extimated histologically with perls' stain.	Hepatic iron concentration <80 mol/g dry weight	Hepatic iron concentration ≥80 mol/g dry weight	Biopsy used to evaluate prognosis on the basis of extent of iron infiltration into tissues (fibrosis and cirrhosis).
	Hepatic iron index equals the hepatic iron concentration divided by the patients age.	Hepatic iron index ≤1.1	Hepatic iron index ≥1.9	Used to differentiate hemochromatosis from other liver diseases. Liver iron levels are affected by age, menstruation, blood donation, and pathologic blood losses.
	Perls' staining using a grading system to describe the amount of parenchymal iron on a scale from 0-4	Perls' stain grade 0-1 stainable hepatic parenchymal iron	Grade 3-4 stainable liver iron	Young homozygotes will have normal or near-normal stainable iron

present. In patients less than 40 years of age who have a serum ferritin concentration of less than 750 ng/mL and normal liver enzyme levels, phlebotomy therapy can be started without biopsy. In all other cases, biopsy remains essential for diagnosis and optimal management. The amount of iron can be measured chemically or estimated histologically with Perls' stain.[1]

A recently discovered genetic mutation, the HFE gene, is associated with a large number of cases of severe hereditary hemochromatosis.[13] However, other genes may be involved, and hemochromatosis can develop in a person who is "normal" or heterozygous for the HFE gene. A "positive" gene test does appear to indicate increased risk. Thus, homozygous patients who have normal iron measures should undergo monitoring for serum ferritin every 2 years to detect iron loading.

Management

Iron overload is treated with successive phlebotomies in both patients with and those without clinical manifestations. The approach has two phases:

1. Removal of excess iron ("de-ironing") by taking 1 U (unit) or 500 ml of blood, once or twice weekly until iron deficiency anemia develops (Hemoglobin 11 g/dL in women and 12 g/dL in men). This step ensures that all stored iron is mobilized.

2. Maintenance of normal iron status by periodic phlebotomy, typically 3 to 5 U of whole blood per year. The frequency of phlebotomy is unique to each patient and should be guided by monitoring of serum ferritin concentration (<50 μg/L) and maintaining a normal hemoglobin level. Phlebotomy during the maintenance phase prevents re-accumulation.

Once the diagnosis is made, patients need information and support. Patient advocacy groups such as the Iron Overload Diseases Association* can assist in providing information. All patients should be advised that their first-degree relatives should undergo screening for hemochromatosis. A genetics counselor may helpful to patients who are trying to understand the disease.

Strict dietary restrictions are not indicated. However, patients interested in limiting the amount of iron in their diet should be provided information on dietary sources of iron as well as inhibitors and enhancers of iron absorption. Referral to a dietitian may be helpful.

Hemochromatosis may exacerbate viral hepatitis, alcoholism and other liver diseases. Alcohol may be consumed in moderation unless there is evidence of liver disease. Persons with both hepatitis C and iron overload respond poorly to treatment with interferon, possibly because iron reduces the effectiveness of the drug.[14] Patients who have iron overload are also at increased risk for infection *Vibrio vulnificus* and *Yersinia entercolitica*. *V. vulnificus* infection is associated with eating raw shellfish, particularly oysters, and nearly 40% of infected persons die.[15]

Screening

Iron overload disease meets many of the criteria for population-based screening: The disorder is common; a sensitive screening test (i.e., transferrin saturation) allows detection during a long presymptomatic phase; and a safe, effective treatment is available, which can eliminate morbidity and premature mortality and reduce health care costs.[1, 16, 17] The transferrin saturation test can be readily included in blood chemistry tests done during routine adult physical examinations. The test also can be used to detect iron deficiency.[17]

Although data supporting universal screening are compelling, several important concerns exist. First, transferrin saturation is quite variable (biologically and analytically), which calls into question the predictive value of the test. Second, many physicians are unfamiliar with the diagnosis and management of hemochromatosis. Third, the extent to which iron overload contributes to the overall burden of disease in the United States remains to be determined. Fourth, patients may need protection from possible discrimination by employers and health and life insurance companies. Many social, legal, and ethical issues of genetic diseases and their testing are unresolved. Recently, an expert committee of the Centers for Disease Control and Prevention and the National Institutes of Health reached a consensus that gene testing for hemochromatosis should only be used only for research purposes and should not be applied clinically until its prognostic significance is clarified.[18]

The ideal age for screening is long before a person has accumulated enough iron to result in organ damage. However, young adults seldom seek medical care except for employment physical examinations, prenatal care, and treatment of acute symptoms. These settings provide good opportunities for screening. Women may need to undergo screening again after menopause, when iron excretion declines. Screening of asymptomatic persons is prudent but must be done through collaboration of the local laboratories and caregivers.

317

The College of American Pathologists recommends screening for iron overload with the transferrin saturation test in all persons 18 years of age or older as part of a routine medical care (e.g., during an employment physical examination, curative services, or gynecologic care).[1] Screening is also advised in all persons, regardless of age, who have one or more of the following risk factors: a family history of iron overload disease, any of the clinical manifestations of iron overload (e.g., impotence, severe fatigue, hypogonadism, amenorrhea, cardiomyopathy, diabetes mellitus, liver disease, or arthritis), and abnormalities found during a routine health examination or testing for iron deficiency (Table 35.1). Pregnant women should not undergo an initial screening for iron overload; first-time screening should occur no sooner than 3 months postpartum, when measures of iron status have stabilized.

If the transferrin saturation is elevated (>50% for women and >60% for men), it should be repeated to enhance specificity. Before the second test, the patient should fast overnight and avoid iron or vitamin C supplements for at least 24 hours. Liver enzyme levels, serum ferritin concentration, and complete blood cell count should be assessed at that time. Physical examination for liver, heart, and endocrine disease should be performed.

When the transferrin saturation is persistently elevated and cannot be explained by the presence of other medical conditions (e.g., liver disease from another cause or secondary iron overload), a presumptive diagnosis of hereditary hemochromatosis may be made. A patient who has a persistently elevated transferrin saturation, with or without high iron stores (elevated serum ferritin level) or clinical signs of iron overload, should be referred to a physician familiar with iron overload disease for further diagnosis and management. If the transferrin saturation is not elevated on follow-up testing but the serum ferritin concentration is, evaluation for causes of inflammation is warranted.

A detailed description of screening, diagnosis, treatment, and follow-up of hereditary hemochromatosis can be found in the practice parameters developed by the College of American Pathologists.[1]

Conclusion

Diagnosis of iron overload is often delayed until clinical manifestations have appeared and it is too late to prevent organ damage. Therefore, basic and continuing medical education about the disease is urgently needed. Physicians and their specialty groups will be important leaders for change. Further studies on the prevalence and penetrance of hereditary hemochromatosis, the capability of current laboratory tests to detect this disease and the cost-effectiveness of screening for the disease are also needed.

References

1. Witte DL, Crosby WH, Edwards, CQ, Fairbanks VF, Mitros FA. Practice parameter for hereditary hemochromatosis. College of American Pathologists. *Clin Chim Acta* 1996; 245:139-200.

2. Rouault TA. Hereditary hemochromatosis. *JAMA* 1993;269:3152-4

3. McLaren C, Gordeuk VR, Looker AC, et al. Prevalence of heterozygotes for hemochromatosis in the white population of the United States. *Blood* 1995;86(5):2021-7

4. Centers for Disease Control and Prevention. Iron overload disorders among Hispanics—San Diego, CA, 1995. *MMWR* 1996;45(45):991-3

5. Edwards CQ, Kushner JP. Screening for hemochromatosis. *N Engl J Med* 1993;328:1616-20

6. Barton J, Edwards CQ, Bertoli LF, et al. Iron Overload in African Americans. *Am J Med* 1995;99(6):616-23

7. Bothwell TH. Overview and mechanisms of iron regulation. Nutr Rev 1995;53(9):237-45

8. Edwards CQ, Griffen LM, Kushner JP. The morbidity of hemochromatosis among clinically unselected homozygous: preliminary report. In: Hershko C, Konjim AM, Alsen P, eds. Progress in iron research. New York: Plenum, 1994;303-8

9. Bradley L, Haddow JE, Palomaki GE. Population screening for hemochromatosis: expectations based on a study of relatives of symptomatic probands. *J. Med Screening*. 1996;3:171-7

10. Adams PC, Valberg LS. Evolving expression of hereditary hemochromatosis. Seminars in Liver Disease. 1996;16:47-54

11. McSween RN, Scott AR. Hepatic cirrhosis: a clinico-pathological review of 520 cases. *J. Clin Path* 1973;26:936-42

12. Neiderau C, Fischer R, Purschel A, Stremmel W, Haussinger, D, Strohmeyer G. Long-term survival in patients with hereditary hemochromatosis. *Gastroenterology* 1996;110:1107-19

13. Feder JN, Gnirke A, Thomas W, et al. A novel MHC class I-like gene is mutated in patients with hereditary hemochromatosis. *Nat Genet* 1996;13:399-409

14. Rubin RB, Barton AL, Banner BF, Bonkovsky HL. Iron and chronic viral hepatits: emerging evidence for an important interaction. *Dig Dis* 1995;13:223-38

15. Hlady WG, Klontz KC. The epidemiology of *Vibrio* infections in Florida, 1981-1993. *J Infect Dis* 1996;173(5):1176—83

16. Phatak PD, Gunman G, Woll JE, Robson A, Helps CE. Cost-effectiveness of screening for hereditary hemochromatosis. *Arch Int Med* 1994;154:769-776

17. Bradley L, Haddow JE, Palomaki GE. Population based screening for haemochromatosis: a unifying analysis of published intervention trials. *J Med Screening* 1996:3;178-84

18. Cogswell ME, McDonnell SM, Khoury M, Franks A, Burke W. Population-based screening for hemochromatosis: where do we go from here? Ann Intern Med (in press).

—*by Sharon M. McDonnell, MD, MPH,*
and David Witte, MD, PhD.

Chapter 36

Niemann-Pick Disease

What Is Niemann-Pick Disease?

Niemann-Pick disease (NP) is an inherited metabolic disorder in which harmful quantities of a fatty substance accumulate in the spleen, liver, lungs, bone marrow, and, in some patients, the brain. The clinical designations applied to NP are somewhat erratic. Patients are currently subdivided into 4 categories. In the first, called type A, enlargement of the liver and spleen are apparent early in infancy and profound brain damage is evident. These children rarely live beyond 18 months. In the second group, called type B, enlargement of the liver and spleen characteristically occur in the pre-teen years. Most of these patients also have pulmonary difficulties, but the brain is not affected. The fatty material that accumulates in types A and B is called sphingomyelin. This lipid is a major component of the membrane of all cells in the body. The metabolic defect in types A and B is insufficient activity of an enzyme called sphingomyelinase that initiates the biodegradation of sphingomyelin that arises from normal cell turnover.

The term NP also includes two other variant forms called types C and D. Patients with these types have only moderate enlargement of their spleens and livers. They have brain involvement that can be extensive leading to inability to look up and down, difficulty in walking and swallowing, as well as progressive loss of vision and hearing. The disorder may appear early in life or its onset may be delayed into

National Institute of Neurological Disorders and Stroke (NINDS), NIH April 1996.

the teen years. Both types are characterized by an inability to mobilize cholesterol in the nerve cells in the brain where it accumulates and causes malfunction of these cells. The only difference between these two subtypes is that type D arises in people with a common ancestral background in Nova Scotia.

Is There Any Treatment?

There is currently no effective treatment for patients with type A. Bone marrow transplantation has been attempted in a few patients with type B, and encouraging results have been reported. Since type B resembles type 1 Gaucher's disease to a considerable degree, one might anticipate that enzyme replacement, and ultimately gene therapy, will eventually be helpful for these patients. Patients with types C and D are frequently placed on a low-cholesterol dietary regimen.

What Is the Prognosis?

Patients with type A die in infancy. Type B patients may live a comparatively long time, but many require supplemental oxygen because of lung involvement. The life expectancies of patients with types C and D are quite variable. Some patients die in childhood while others who appear to be less drastically affected live into adulthood.

The NINDS is conducting a study to identify the gene that is involved in patients with type C (and D). NINDS is also conducting trials of therapeutic agents in a mouse model of type C that NINDS scientists discovered.

Additional Reading

These articles, available from a medical library, may provide more in-depth information on NP:

"Niemann-Pick Disease Types A and B: Acid Sphingomyelinase Deficiencies." Chapter 84 in The Metabolic and Molecular Bases of Inherited Disease, 7th edition, McGraw Hill, Inc., New York, pp. 2601-2624 (1995).

"Niemann-Pick Disease Type C: A Cellular Cholesterol Lipidosis." Chapter 85 in The Metabolic and Molecular Bases of Inherited Disease, 7th edition, McGraw-Hill, Inc., New York, pp. 2625-2639 (1995).

"The metabolism of sphingomyelin. II. Evidence of an enzymatic deficiency in Niemann-Pick disease." Proceedings of the National Academy of Science, USA, 55; 366-369 (1966).

Additional Information

Information may also be available from the following organizations.

National Niemann-Pick Foundation
3734 E. Olive Ave.
Gilbert, AZ 85234
Phone (602) 497-6638
Fax (602) 497-6346
E-mail: stevekenyon@nnpdf.org
URL: http://www.nnpdf.org

Ara Parseghian Medical Research Foundation
760 E. River Road, Suite 115
Tucson, AZ 85718
(520) 577-5106
URL: http://www.parseghian.org/index.html

National Tay-Sachs and Allied Diseases Association, Inc.
2001 Beacon Street, Suite 204
Brighton, MA 02135
(800) 906-8723
Fax: (617) 227-0134
URL: http://www.ntsad.org

Chapter 37

Primary Hyperoxaluria

General Information

Hyperoxaluria (and its accompanying oxalosis) has several forms: Primary Hyperoxaluria Type 1 and Type II, a poorly defined Type III, Acquired Hyperoxaluria, and Absorptive or Enteric Hyperoxaluria. The common factor among all of these forms of Hyperoxaluria is an excessive excretion of oxalate in the urine. Oxalosis is the excessive accumulation of oxalate in the body. Oxalate is a very hard substance that is normally eliminated by the body. In the case of oxalosis, the oxalate is not removed from the body and is deposited in tissues and organs. Hyperoxaluria may lead to kidney failure.

Primary Hyperoxaluria Type I

Primary Hyperoxaluria (also known as PHI) is a rare metabolic disease caused by the liver making too much oxalic acid that is excreted in the urine of the affected person. The excess oxalic acid combines with calcium inside the kidneys, causing calcium oxalate stones in the urinary tract. The stones can cause pain in the kidneys, the bladder, and in the ureters as the body attempts to eliminate the foreign objects. While the kidneys continue to function, the excessive oxalate is eliminated through the urine. If the kidneys fail, the disease progresses to oxalosis.

"About Primary Hyperoxaluria," © 1995, reprinted with permission of the Oxalosis and Hyperoxaluria Foundation.

PHI is an inherited disease (autosomal recessive) which is passed on to the children of two healthy parents who each carry a defective gene. In other words, the parents have no apparent problem, yet the chances are that one in four of newborns will be affected by the disease.

In PHI, the disease is caused by a missing liver enzyme that is necessary for the body to eliminate the chemicals that lead to excessive oxalate in the urine. The missing enzyme (alanine glyoxalate - AGT) is normally found in a special area of liver cells (peroxisome). At present, it is not possible to synthesize the missing enzyme.

Primary Hyperoxaluria Type II

PHII is also an autosomal recessive disorder caused by a defective gene in liver cells and other cells. PHII is a milder disease and does not usually present the long-term kidney impairment that is seen with PHI.

Primary Hyperoxaluria Type III

In poorly defined PHIII, the cause remains unknown.

Oxalosis

Oxalosis occurs when the kidneys fail and stop eliminating calcium oxalate crystals from the body through the urine. Because the kidneys stop functioning, oxalate crystals are deposited elsewhere in the body such as the eyes and other major organs. These crystals are sometimes detected by an ophthalmologist during a routine eye exam. In the latter stages of oxalosis, crystals may be deposited in the bones and joints causing painful bone disease. Occasionally, bone disease occurs prior to diagnosis of kidney problems. This represents late diagnosis of previously present asymptomatic, but progressive renal disease.

Acquired Hyperoxaluria

Acquired Hyperoxaluria occurs when a person ingests an unusually large amount of oxalate such as rhubarb or another substance that is converted to oxalate by the liver. These substances include: ethylene glycol (antifreeze), methoxyflourane, Xylitol, Piridoxilate, or Vitamin C in doses in excess of 4 grams per day. Additional causes of Acquired Hyperoxaluria include pyridoxine or thiamine deficiency.

Absorptive Hyperoxaluria

Absorptive Hyperoxaluria occurs in about ten percent of people who have had surgical removal of a portion of the bowel. Some patients who have chronic inflammatory bowel disease, chronic pancreatic disease, chronic biliary tract disease, primary small bowel disease with malabsorption, cirrhosis, bacterial overgrowth syndrome, blind loop syndrome, or jejunoleal bypass surgery may develop Absorptive Hyperoxaluria.

Absorptive Hyperoxaluria causes unabsorbed fatty acids to combine with calcium. This causes too much oxalate to be absorbed by the intestines. Typical treatment includes a low oxalate and low fat diet. Organic marine hydrocolloid (brand name: Ox-absorb) has been helpful in some patients. An inherited form of Absorptive Hyperoxaluria without any known bowel disease has been reported.

Effects

In any form of Hyperoxaluria, calcium oxalate crystals or calcium oxalate kidney stones can produce severe kidney pain (renal colic), urinary tract obstruction, and blood in the urine (hematuria). The small crystals can also collect in the kidneys (nephrocalcinosis) because the kidneys filter and concentrate wastes from the blood. The stones in the kidneys can cause progressive kidney damage and eventual kidney failure.

Symptoms and Signs

The first sign of Hyperoxaluria is commonly kidney stones, blood in the urine, or even kidney failure. This typically appears from infancy to mid-twenties. Hyperoxaluria occasionally appears after the mid-twenties, but this is less common. The severity of the disease varies widely from a complete absence of symptoms and late development of kidney stones to an extremely serious and progressive disease. It is generally believed that the earlier kidney failure occurs, the more severe the disease. It is extremely important that treatment begin as early as possible to increase the chances of preserving kidney function. Therefore, early diagnosis is critical. Siblings of patients should be tested immediately.

Diagnosis

Hyperoxaluria is diagnosed by measuring the oxalic acid level in the urine of affected people. The most accurate measurement can be obtained by gas chromatography of urine or by double enzyme method. Enzyme studies on a liver biopsy can provide a specific diagnosis. Prenatal diagnosis cannot yet be confidently obtained except by fetal liver biopsy; however this test has risks. The severity of the disease varies and is not predictable, but is related to the overall supersaturation of urine components, especially urine oxalate and calcium levels.

Treatment

The primary treatment for Hyperoxaluria is large fluid intake, large daily doses of Vitamin B6 (pyridoxine), phosphate and/or citrate and magnesium supplements, and often an oxalate restricted diet. In patients who maintain kidney function, a significantly increased fluid intake helps keep the kidneys flushed out and limits crystal formation. In patients who have lost kidney function, aggressive dialysis is an appropriate treatment until a living-related kidney can be transplanted.

It is recommended that a kidney be transplanted as soon as possible after renal failure occurs since dialysis does not adequately remove oxalate. Previously, kidney transplants were considered inappropriate for Primary Hyperoxaluria patients; however, kidney transplantation with treatment to help prevent recurrence is now a successful method of treatment. Recently, combined kidney and liver transplants have been performed with promising results. If successful, the combined kidney-liver transplant is curative.

Liver transplantation replaces the missing enzyme and is therefore a cure for the disorder, and can prevent destruction of a new kidney. A liver transplant has considerable risk and no backup such as dialysis is possible if the liver transplant fails. The long term success of combined transplants has not been determined, though it may be appropriate when a living related donor is not available. Life expectancy cannot be accurately predicted because these advances in treatment occurred in the 1980s and 1990s and there has been insufficient time to evaluate the long-term success of these new treatments; although results have been encouraging.

Other Treatment Issues

In spite of recent advances, some physicians may discourage parents from treating their children. Recent successes in treatment are not known by all physicians; although they do know of treatment failures. Some physicians still consider kidney transplants inappropriate for Hyperoxaluria patients. The Oxalosis and Hyperoxaluria Foundation (OHF) can provide families and physicians with the latest medical information and emotional support. OHF's Medical Advisory Board has the medical expertise and information resources to help you and your medical professionals evaluate your case and plan an appropriate treatment.

Future for Primary Hyperoxaluria

We believe that genetic research is our best hope to find a permanent cure for Primary Hyperoxaluria. There have been some initial successes in research such as the location of one PHI genetic marker. However much more research is needed before a treatment can be developed.

Oxalate crystals also form in people without the metabolic defect that causes PHI; and in fact, these crystals produce the most common type of kidney stones from which millions of people suffer. Thus finding a cure for PHI may help people well beyond the victims of this orphan disease.

Additional Information

Oxalosis and Hyperoxaluria Foundation
12 Pleasant Street
Maynard, MA 01754
888-721-2432 PIN# 5392
978-461-0614
Fax: 978-461-0614
E-mail: info@ohf.org
URL: http://www.ohf.org

OHF Midwest Foundation Office
5727 Westcliffe Dr.,
St. Louis, MO 63129
314-846-3645
314-846-6779
E-mail: secy@ohf.org

Chapter 38

Tyrosemia

Hereditary tyrosemia is a genetic inborn error of metabolism associated with severe liver disease in infancy. The disease is inherited in an autosomal recessive fashion which means that both parents must be carriers of the gene for the disease. In such families, there is a one out of four risk that pregnancies will produce an affected infant.

The clinical features of the disease tend to fall into two categories. In the so-called acute form of the disease, abnormalities appear in the first month of life. Babies may show poor weight gain, enlarged liver and spleen, distended abdomen, swelling of the legs, and increased tendency to bleeding, particularly nose bleeds. Jaundice may or may not be prominent. Despite vigorous therapy, death from hepatic failure frequently occurs between three and nine months of age. Children with this form of disease are excellent candidates for liver transplantation.

Some children have a more chronic form of tyrosinemia with a gradual onset and less severe clinical features. In these, enlargement of the liver and spleen are prominent, the abdomen is distended with fluid, weight gain may be poor, and vomiting and diarrhea occur frequently. Affected patients usually develop cirrhosis and its complications. In older patients, there is an increased risk of liver cancer. These children also require liver transplantation.

The liver tests are often abnormal. Low serum albumin and clotting factors are frequently found. The transaminases may be mildly to moderately elevated, but the bilirubin is increased to a variable extent. Because of the biochemical defect, abnormal products may be measured in the urine which confirm diagnosis. These are parahydroxy phenylactic acid and parahydroxy phenylpyruvic acid. In addition, succinylacetone and succinylacetoacetate are found in the urine. There may be hypoglycemia (low blood sugar) and evidence of loss of certain substances in the urine including sugar, protein, and amino acids.

The basic biochemical defect is an abnormality in a key enzyme in the metabolism of an essential amino acid, phenylalanine. The enzyme is fumarylacetoacetate hydrolase (FAH) which is markedly reduced in affected patients. As a consequence, toxic metabolic products in the pathway by which phenylalanine is utilized build up and damage a variety of tissues, although the major findings occur in the liver and kidneys.

Prenatal diagnosis is possible and can be performed by measuring succinylacetone in the amniotic fluid or fumarylacetoacetate hydrolase (FAH) in amniotic fluid cells. This allows for genetic counseling and consideration of termination of pregnancy in affected infants.

Although treatment has not been shown to be of benefit, it is customary to place affected infants on diets low in phenylalanine, methionine, and tyrosine. This will lead to normal blood amino acid levels which may be of some value. Strict attention to excellent nutrition, adequate vitamin and mineral intake, prevents nutritional deterioration and helps keep the patient as well as possible for transplantation. The most effective form of therapy at the present time is liver transplantation.

Additional Information

American Liver Foundation
75 Maiden Lane, Suite 603
New York, NY 10038
1-800-GO LIVER (465-4837)

The American Liver Foundation is a national voluntary health organization dedicated to preventing, treating, and curing hepatitis and other liver and gallbladder diseases through research and education.

The information contained in this chapter is provided for information only. This information does not constitute medical advice and it should not be relied upon as such. The American Liver Foundation (ALF) does not engage in the practice of medicine. ALF, under no circumstances, recommends particular treatments for specific individuals, and in all cases recommends that you consult your physician before pursuing any course of treatment.

Chapter 39

Wilson's Disease

What Is Wilson's Disease?

Wilson's Disease is a genetic disorder that is fatal unless detected and treated before serious illness develops from copper poisoning. Wilson's Disease affects one in thirty thousand people worldwide. The genetic defect causes excessive copper accumulation. Small amounts of copper are essential as vitamins. Copper is present in most foods, and most people get much more than they need. Healthy people excrete copper they don't need, but Wilson's Disease patients cannot.

Copper begins to accumulate immediately after birth. Excess copper attacks the liver and brain resulting in hepatitis, psychiatric, or neurologic symptoms. The symptoms usually appear in late adolescence. Patients may have jaundice, abdominal swelling, vomiting of blood, and abdominal pain. They may have tremors, difficulty walking, talking, and swallowing. They may develop all degrees of mental illness including homicidal or suicidal behavior, depression, and aggression. Women may have menstrual irregularities, absent periods, infertility, or multiple miscarriages. No matter how the disease begins, it is always fatal, if is not diagnosed and treated.

Reprinted with permission "What Is Wilson's Disease," © 1998 Wilson's Diseases Association, and "Exploring Therapeutic Options for Wilson's Disease" by Sandra J. Ackerman, National Center for Research Resources (NCRR), *Reporter* September/October 1997.

The first part of the body that copper affects is the liver. In about half of Wilson's Disease patients, the liver is the only affected organ. The physical changes in the liver are only visible under the microscope. When hepatitis develops, patients are often thought to have infectious hepatitis or infectious mononucleosis when they actually have Wilson's Disease hepatitis. Any unexplained abnormal liver test should trigger thought about Wilson's Disease.

How Is Wilson's Disease Diagnosed?

The diagnosis of Wilson's Disease is made by relatively simple tests which almost always make the diagnosis. The tests can diagnose the disease in both symptomatic patients and people who do not show signs of the disease. It is important to diagnose Wilson's Disease as early as possible, since severe liver damage can occur before there are any signs of the disease. Individuals with Wilson's Disease may falsely appear in excellent health.

Blood, ceruloplasmin, urine copper, eye test for Kayser-Fleischer rings, and liver biopsies are used to make the diagnosis.

Is Wilson's Disease an Inherited Disorder?

Wilson's Disease is transmitted as an autosomal recessive disease, which means it is not sex-linked (it occurs equally in men and women). In order to inherit it, both parents must carry a gene which each passes to the affected child. Two abnormal genes are required to have the disease. The responsible gene is located at a precisely known site on chromosome 13. The gene is call ATP7B.

Many cases of Wilson's Disease occur due to spontaneous mutations in the gene. A significant number of others are simply transmitted from generation to generation. Most patients have no family history of Wilson's Disease.

People with only one abnormal gene are called carriers. They do not become ill and should not be treated. More than thirty different mutations have been identified thus far.

Therefore, it has been difficult to devise a simple genetic screening test for the disease. However, in a particular family, if the precise mutation is identified, a genetic diagnosis is possible. This may help in finding symptom-free relatives so that they may be treated before they become ill or handicapped. Someday a genetic test may help in prenatal diagnosis.

How Is Wilson's Disease Being Treated?

Wilson's Disease is a very treatable condition. With proper therapy, disease progress can be halted and often symptoms can be improved. Treatment is aimed at removing excess accumulated copper and preventing its reaccumulation. Therapy must therefore be continued for life.

Patients may become progressively sicker from day to day so immediate treatment can be critical. Delay of even a few days may cause irreversible worsening.

The newest FDA-approved drug is zinc acetate (Galzin). Zinc acts by blocking the absorption of copper in the intestinal tract. This action both depletes accumulated copper and prevents it reaccumulation. Zinc's effectiveness has been shown by 15 years of considerable experience overseas. A major advantage of zinc therapy is its lack of side effects. Other drugs approved for use in Wilson's Disease include pencillamine (Cuprimine, Depen) and trientine (Syprine). Both of these drugs act by chelation or binding of copper, causing its increased urinary excretion.

Tetrathiomolybdate is under investigation for initial treatment of Wilson's Disease in the hope that it will not cause neurological worsening, as may occur with pencillamine. Although its side effects are not clearly established, indications are that it is quite safe.

Patients with severe hepatitis may require liver transplant. Patients being investigated or treated for Wilson's Disease should be cared for by specialists in Wilson's Disease or in consultation with such specialists by their primary physicians.

Stopping treatment completely will result in death, sometimes in three months. Decreasing dosage can result in unnecessary disease progression.

Exploring Therapeutic Options for Wilson's Disease

A young woman with symptoms of an advanced neurological ailment was referred to geneticist Dr. George Brewer, professor of internal medicine and genetics at the University of Michigan Medical Center in Ann Arbor. Once healthy, the woman could not speak, feed herself, or walk without assistance because of tremor in her limbs. Two years ago she was told she had multiple sclerosis, and her condition had grown steadily worse since then. But Dr. Brewer paid particular attention to the state of the young woman's liver and issued a diagnosis of his own: Wilson's disease. When the patient received specific treatment for this rare disease, her condition stabilized, and she started on the long road to recovery.

Wilson's disease is an inherited disorder of metabolism in which the body is unable to excrete excess copper. "Most of us take in about one milligram of copper per day in our diet, and that's about 25 percent more than we need," says Dr. Brewer. Under normal circumstances, a protein in the liver binds the excess copper and shepherds it along an excretory pathway into the bile. In Wilson's disease patients this crucial protein is defective. As a result, says Dr. Brewer, excess copper builds up in liver and brain, leading to jaundice or liver failure. Copper may also cause neurological disorders that interfere with swallowing, speech, and movement, or cause psychiatric symptoms that include impaired cognitive performance, depression, and uncontrollable anger.

Because it can produce such a wide variety of clinical signs, Wilson's disease often is misdiagnosed—with tragic results. Without timely treatment, much of the damage to the brain, in particular, is irreversible. And because it is so rare, affecting only an estimated 5,000 to 6,000 people in the United States (about one in 40,000), Wilson's disease has not been a top priority for pharmaceutical companies, researchers, or funding agencies. This makes the new treatment, which Dr. Brewer developed with assistance from the NCRR-supported General Clinical Research Center at the University of Michigan, all the more noteworthy.

The treatment, which became available commercially in early 1997, consists of zinc in a salt form called zinc acetate, to be taken orally (trade name Galzin®). "The zinc induces cells of the intestinal tract to produce a protein called metallothionein, which has a very high affinity for copper," Dr. Brewer explains. "When these intestinal cells die—in approximately six days—they take the bound copper along with them for elimination in the stool." Zinc treatment is effective over long periods of time, even a lifetime, and poses no major side effects.

Up to now the two conventional treatments for Wilson's disease have been the drugs penicillamine and trientine, which bind excess copper in the blood and cause it to be excreted in the urine. However, both drugs carry a significant risk in the early stages of treatment because they temporarily raise levels of copper in the brain as they mobilize the metal for excretion. Even this brief overabundance can cause lasting neurological damage.

Developing a safer treatment for Wilson's disease was not Dr. Brewer's primary goal when he first received NCRR funding to study the clinical effects of zinc 20 years ago. Instead, he hoped to develop a new therapy for sickle-cell anemia. "We had reason to think that increasing zinc levels would be beneficial in sickle-cell disease," he says. Part of the problem in that disease is that the red cell membrane becomes sticky and stiff. The cell loses its characteristic shape and eventually becomes irreversibly damaged. "When we gave zinc to sickle-cell patients, we saw a reduction in the number of these damaged cells." As treatment proceeded, Dr. Brewer raised the levels of zinc he was administering—until he began to see adverse effects in the form of copper depletion. "One patient became clinically copper deficient," he says, "and another seven had lowered levels of ceruloplasmin," a blood protein that transports and maintains copper in various tissues of the body. These effects reversed themselves quickly once the treatment was modified, but the incident drew Dr. Brewer's attention to other possible therapeutic uses for zinc. His work on Wilson's disease has been supported by NCRR since 1981, with the zinc acetate treatment receiving approval by the Food and Drug Administration (FDA) in early 1997.

Pharmacological treatment of Wilson's disease dates back only to the 1950s and was first developed in the form of injections, giving way to oral penicillamine by the end of the decade. Nondrug treatment, including diet modification, has been less successful, says Dr. Brewer. "Low-copper diets have been a part of treatment for a long time," he says, "but almost all foods contain some copper." Nevertheless, when measured with today's sensitive instruments, foods thought to contain very high levels of copper contain much less than had been previously realized. In contrast to old lists of prohibited foods, which included items ranging from beans to chocolate to mushrooms, the restricted list for Wilson's disease patients today is likely to contain only two main items, shellfish and liver, both very high in copper.

With these few dietary constraints and zinc acetate treatment, a patient can live a healthy life. But identifying Wilson's disease is not a simple matter. Often by the time patients are properly diagnosed, they have developed acute symptoms from excess copper in the brain and liver. "We have proved zinc acetate to be effective for maintenance therapy of Wilson's disease," says Dr. Brewer "We also advocate it for people who are presymptomatic"—for example, siblings of a Wilson's disease patient, who have a 25-percent chance of developing the disease themselves.

"But we haven't pushed zinc acetate as an initial treatment, because it is slow-acting and produces little effect in the first week to 10 days." Instead, as an initial treatment in the disease state, Dr. Brewer administers ammonium tetrathiomolybdate. "It's very strong and quick-acting, but it doesn't move copper into the brain on the way out of the body," he explains. Tetrathiomolybdate therapy has not yet entered the long process leading to FDA approval, but has shown good results in almost 60 patients so far.

The two new treatments have strong clinical implications. Regarding the young woman who spent two years struggling with a diagnosis of multiple sclerosis while actually enduring the symptoms of Wilson's disease, Dr. Brewer is now cautiously optimistic. "Over one to two years the liver can carry out quite a bit of recovery," he says, "and in the brain, treatment gets rid of inflammation and swelling and allows sick neurons to come back to life. Two years from now that young woman will probably have only a minor disability." Although the number of people receiving this treatment will always be small, for each of them it is the gift of life.

Additional Reading

Brewer, G. J., Johnson, V., and Kaplan, J., The treatment of Wilson's disease with zinc XIV. Studies of the effects of zinc on lymphocyte function. *Journal of Laboratory Clinical Medicine*, in press.

Brewer, G. J., Johnson, V., Dick, R. D., et al., Treatment of Wilson disease with ammonium tetrathiomolybdate. *Archives of Neurology* 53:1017-1025, 1996

Brewer, G. J., Practical recommendations and new therapies for Wilson's disease. *Drugs* 50:240-249, 1995.

Part Eight

Other Diseases of the Liver

Chapter 40

Biliary Atresia

What Is Biliary Atresia?

Biliary atresia is a serious disease of the very young infant. It results in inflammation and obstruction of the ducts that carry bile from the liver into the intestine. When bile cannot flow normally, it backs up in the liver (a situation called biliary "stasis"). This causes "jaundice," or a yellowing of the skin, and cirrhosis. Cirrhosis occurs when healthy liver cells are destroyed, in this case by disease, and replaced with scar tissue. This scarring interferes with blood flow through the liver, causing more cell damage and scarring.

What Are the First Signs of Biliary Atresia?

The symptoms of biliary atresia are usually evident between two and six weeks after birth. The baby will appear jaundiced, and may develop a large, hardened liver and a swollen abdomen. The stools are usually pale grey and the urine appears dark.

Some babies may develop intense itching, or "pruritus," which makes them extremely uncomfortable and irritable. The exact cause of this itching is not yet known, although researchers have found a connection between it and the backup of bile.

This chapter contains text from "Biliary Atresia," © 1995, and "Children's Liver Research Agenda," © 1997, reprinted with permission of the American Liver Foundation 1-800-GO-LIVER.

What Causes Biliary Atresia?

The cause of biliary atresia has not yet been discovered.

Approximately 1 in 8,000 to 1 in 15,000 infants will develop biliary atresia, a bile duct disorder in which rapid and progressive scarring leads to obstruction of the flow of bile between the liver and the intestine. Eventually even the ducts within the liver become obliterated. More infants and children come to liver transplantation for biliary atresia than for any other single liver disease. Finding a cause still remains a major challenge today.

Various viruses (such as cytomeglalovirus or rubella virus) have been linked to individual cases of biliary atresia—but these infections occur commonly in infants, and the link so far between any single virus and biliary atresia appears to be only coincidental. More recent attention has focused on the rotavirus, which can cause scarring of bile ducts similar to that seen in biliary atresia in newborn mice. There are also a number of other recently proposed theories about the cause(s) of biliary atresia. One reason for thinking there may be more than one process or disease that leads to duct scarring is the observation that about 20-35% of infants with biliary atresia are born without a spleen or with multiple spleens and may also have other defects present at birth as well. This group of infants may have a defect in one or more genes that help control the development of unformed organs.

Sixty-five percent of infants with biliary atresia have no other associated abnormalities. Although there are some families where several brothers and sisters have the disease, there are many reported cases where only one of identical twins has the disorder, while the other is healthy. This suggests that for most infants biliary atresia is not an inherited disorder, although perhaps a susceptibility to develop biliary atresia can be inherited. Autoimmune disorders we now know are much more likely to occur in susceptible individuals with certain "tissue types." These are inherited "markers" on all cells in the body that the immune system uses to distinguish between its own cells and someone else's—as in the case of an organ transplant. Work is in progress to determine if the immune system helps initiate the damage to the ducts, which then become scarred and close.

Biliary atresia is not a hereditary condition (although in some very rare cases, more than one infant in a family may be affected). Many parents experience feelings of guilt, but they should be reassured that nothing they have done caused their child's illness.

How Is Biliary Atresia Diagnosed?

There are many liver diseases which cause symptoms similar to those of biliary atresia. Consequently, many tests may have to be performed before biliary atresia can be diagnosed conclusively.

Every effort should be made to search for any of the causes of jaundice which might be confused with biliary atresia. This involves blood and urine tests; liver function tests; blood counts and a test for clotting function. A painless examination using ultrasound (ECHO) is often done to study the liver and determine the size of the bile ducts and gallbladder.

Other tests which are often used are specialized x-ray techniques or radioactive scans of the liver which can be helpful in focusing on the true abnormality. A liver biopsy, in which a tiny sample of the liver is removed with a needle, allows the physician to examine the liver tissue microscopically.

What about Treatment?

The most successful treatment for biliary atresia to date is a type of surgery which creates drainage of bile from the liver when the ducts have become completely obstructed. This operation is called the Kasai procedure (hepatoportoenterostomy) after Dr. Morio Kasai, the Japanese surgeon who developed it.

In the Kasai procedure, the surgeon removes the damaged ducts outside of the liver (extrahepatic) and replaces them with a length of the baby's own intestine, which acts as a new duct.

The aim of the Kasai procedure is to allow excretion of bile from the liver into the intestine via the new duct. The operation accomplishes this about 50% of the time. In those who respond well, jaundice usually disappears after several weeks.

In the remaining 50% of cases where the Kasai procedure does not work, the problem often lies in the fact that obstructed bile ducts are "intrahepatic" or inside the liver, as well as outside. No procedure has yet been developed to correct this problem except for transplantation.

What Happens after Surgery?

The aim of treatment after surgery is to encourage normal growth and development. If bile flow is good, the child is given a regular diet. If bile flow is reduced, a low fat diet is recommended as bile is required to aid in the absorption of fats and vitamins. Multiple vitamins,

343

vitamin B complex, and vitamins E, D, and K can be given as supplements.

Is the Kasai Procedure a Cure for Biliary Atresia?

Unfortunately, despite bile flow, the Kasai procedure is not a cure for biliary atresia. For reasons which are still unknown, liver damage often continues and, eventually, cirrhosis and its complications appear.

What Are the Complications?

Patients with cirrhosis have changes in blood flow through the liver which may produce abnormalities, such as easy bruising of the skin, nosebleeds, retention of body fluid, and enlarged veins, called varices, in the stomach and esophagus. Increases in pressure in these veins can make them leaky and internal bleeding results. This can usually be stopped. In some cases, a procedure may be required whereby a hardening (sclerosing) agent is injected into these veins.

As the disease progresses, other complications may occur. While all infants tend to be sleepy after eating, those with biliary atresia may experience excessive sleepiness after eating protein, due to increased nitrogen products in the bloodstream. The child may also suffer from an increased risk of infection.

What Can Be Done about These Complications?

Following the Kasai operation, infection in the bile ducts (cholangitis) is common. This is usually treated initially using intravenous antibiotics and may be continued with oral antibiotics.

If retention of body fluid occurs, it can be treated with diuretics and potassium replacement.

Jaundice or itching can often be treated successfully with medications (phenobarbital, cholestyramine, and ursodeoxycholic acid).

What Is the Outlook for a Baby with Biliary Atresia?

The extent and type of liver damage differ in each baby with biliary atresia. Some infants respond to the Kasai procedure; others do not. If bile continues to flow, long-term survival is possible. However, it is presently impossible for a physician to determine in advance which baby is likely to respond to treatment.

Is Liver Transplantation the Solution?

Liver transplantation is an option which is becoming increasingly useful to victims of certain liver diseases. The survival rates for transplant recipients have increased dramatically with improved surgical techniques and the development of new drugs which help to overcome the problem of organ rejection. Ultimately, about two-thirds of patients with biliary atresia will have a liver transplant.

In children with biliary atresia, liver transplantation is generally not attempted until the Kasai procedure has been performed. If this operation is not successful, and before complications of the resulting cirrhosis become severe and life threatening, liver transplantation may be attempted. It has been successful in numerous cases. However, as in all organ transplantation, success depends greatly upon the timely availability of suitably matched organs for donation, the time factor involved (a donated liver must be used within 16 hours for the operation to be successful), and other factors which are only now being investigated. The use of reduced-size and living-related transplants are aiding in the timing and availability of suitable donor organs.

What Can the Family Do?

Watching a young infant suffer from biliary atresia is a devastating experience. It can also be frustrating, because so little is known about the disease. Feelings of anger and helplessness are not uncommon. What does one do when there is so little one can do?

Many parents have found it helpful to learn as much as they can about the disease. Talk to your physician, inquire about specialists, and request any literature on the subject.

Perhaps the biggest comfort for parents is to discuss the problem with others who have or are going through a similar tragedy. Finding out that they are not alone, that others feel the way they do, and learning how other parents are coping with their child's disease, is often a great comfort.

Where Can Parents Turn for Support?

The American Liver Foundation recognizes that parents of children with biliary atresia need help in coping with the immense strain of this chronic illness. To meet this need, the American Liver Foundation is continually organizing and coordinating mutual help groups through its chapters to provide emotional support for families, making referrals to specialists where appropriate, and keeping people aware of the latest research developments. A listing of American Liver Foundation Chapters is available in Chapter 60 of this book.

Will There Ever Be a Cure for Biliary Atresia?

There can be no cure for biliary atresia until the cause of the disease can be determined. Researchers are focusing on trying to find this cause, but a great deal of work still needs to be done. More research into how the liver works is also vital.

Research is the key that will unlock this mystery. The American Liver Foundation is the only national voluntary health agency dedicated to funding research and helping people understand more about the liver and liver disease.

Additional Information

American Liver Foundation
75 Maiden Lane, Suite 603
New York, NY 10038
1-800-465-4837 (GO-LIVER)
Fax: 212-483-8179
E-mail: webmail@liverfoundation.org
URL: http://www.liverfoundation.org

Chapter 41

Budd-Chiari Syndrome

Budd-Chiari syndrome is clotting of the hepatic vein, the major vein that leaves the liver. Most patients with Budd-Chiari syndrome have an underlying condition that predisposes to blood clotting. About 10% have polycythemia vera, a condition in which abnormal amounts of red blood cells are present. About 10% of patients with Budd-Chiari syndrome take birth control pills which also may predispose them to blood clotting.

The most common symptom in Budd-Chiari syndrome is ascites, or fluid accumulation in the abdomen. Patients can also have abnormal blood tests indicative of liver disease. Some individuals with Budd-Chiari syndrome may be jaundiced (yellow skin). The examining doctors often first suspect cirrhosis as a cause of the symptoms in patients with Budd-Chiari syndrome.

Patients with Budd-Chiari syndrome who have deteriorating liver function and complications usually need to undergo liver transplantation. Other surgical procedures have been used with variable degrees of success. In some cases, the underlying condition that caused the syndrome excludes transplantation as a treatment option.

Chapter 42

Cystic Disease of the Liver

An important task of the liver is producing and excreting bile. This yellow-green bitter tasting fluid flows into the intestine through the bile ducts. The bile ducts in the liver are like the branches on a tree, that come together just below the stomach. A side branch leads to a sack for storing bile, called the gallbladder.

Gallbladder disease is a common type of illness involving the biliary tree. Less common, but significant, is cystic disease of the biliary tree. This can take several forms:

- cysts in the main trunk (choledochal cysts),

- cysts (or lakes) in the small branches within the liver (Caroli's syndrome), or

- cysts in the liver separate from the biliary tree (polycystic liver disease).

Choledochal Cyst

In this condition, the main trunk (the common bile duct) of the biliary tree is structurally abnormal, probably from the time of birth. Eventually (usually by age 2 or 3 but sometimes not until adolescence or adulthood) the bile accumulates in the duct. It forms a sack or cyst which then presses on the bile duct and prevents bile from reaching

Reprinted with permission, © 1997 American Liver Foundation, 1-800-GO-LIVER.

the intestine. Bile backs up into the liver and the patient becomes jaundiced (yellow). Occasionally this accumulation of bile becomes infected, causing abdominal pain and fever. In some patients the cyst can be felt by the doctor examining the abdomen. In most patients the diagnosis can be confirmed by using sonic pictures (ultrasound) or by injecting a radioactive substance which gives an "image" of the abnormal duct (nuclear medicine). Treatment is surgical. The abnormal bile duct is removed and a piece of intestine used to replace it. In most cases, surgery permanently corrects the disease. Rarely, infection in the newly formed biliary tree recurs. If the condition is not correctly diagnosed the blockage of bile may result in scarring in the liver (cirrhosis).

Caroli's Syndrome

Caroli's syndrome (intrahepatic ductal ectasia) is another rare congenital (from birth) disease. It is probably inherited. In this syndrome, the small branches of the biliary tree in the liver are abnormal. Small lakes alternate with narrowed segments of bile ducts, instead of the normal smooth contour. These abnormalities may be present throughout the liver, or limited to only a small area. If the bile duct becomes infected, the patient develops fever, abdominal pain, and rarely, jaundice. This complication may not occur until middle age or may first appear in childhood. This disease is usually diagnosed by using radioisotopes to "image" the biliary tree and by injecting dye directly into the biliary tree. This may be done by inserting a needle through the skin into the liver (percutaneous transhepatic cholangiogram) or using a tube to pass dye through the intestine up into the bile duct (endoscopic retrograde cholangiography).

Congenital Hepatic Fibrosis

In patients with this condition, there is abnormal growth of fibrous tissue (scar) around the small branches of the bile ducts in the liver. As a result, the liver becomes enlarged and hard and blood can no longer flow freely through the liver. The spleen becomes enlarged and the blood must return to the heart through weak veins along the tube to the stomach (esophageal varices). These veins may burst and cause bleeding into the stomach and bowels. Patients with this condition are usually discovered in childhood, either because of the large liver or because of bleeding. This diagnosis is proven by liver biopsy and x-ray of blood vessels. There is no specific treatment for this condition but many patients require rerouting of blood from the intestines (shunt operation) to prevent more intestinal bleeding.

Polycystic Liver Disease

In some patients, large lakes (cysts) separate from the biliary tree form in the liver. In severe cases, the liver looks like a sponge. These cysts may cause pain, but do not affect liver function. In most patients, the kidneys are similarly affected with cysts, which may cause high blood pressure and kidney failure. The tendency to form cysts is probably present at birth in these patients, but usually the cysts do not enlarge and give problems until adulthood. This condition may be detected using ultrasound or CAT scan and x-rays of the kidney (intravenous pyelogram). Polycystic disease is inherited and once it has been detected in one member of a family, all the patient's relatives should be tested for it. There are two major categories of polycystic disease of the liver and kidney. In the more benign, the cysts are mostly in the liver and kidney function is near normal. These patients have a normal life expectancy. However those patients who have kidney damage need treatment for the equivalent of polycystic kidney disease.

All these conditions are rare and many people have never heard of them. They will probably be diagnosed with greater frequency in the future with the help of new tools such as ultrasonography. Several of these conditions are inherited. To help patients and their children, we need to know more about what causes these diseases and how to diagnose and treat them.

Chapter 43

Fatty Liver

The Liver

The liver is the largest organ in the body. It is found high in the right upper abdomen, behind the ribs. It is a very complex organ and has many functions. They include:

- Storing energy in the form of sugar (glucose)

- Storing vitamins, iron, and other minerals

- Making proteins, including blood clotting factors, to keep the body healthy and help it grow

- Processing worn out red blood cells

- Making bile which is needed for food digestion

- Metabolizing or breaking down many medications and alcohol

- Killing germs that enter the body through the intestine

The liver shoulders a heavy workload for the body and almost never complains. It even has a remarkable power to regenerate itself. Still it should not be taken for granted. Certain conditions that develop, such as fatty liver and steatohepatitis, may be signs of liver injury that can lead to permanent liver damage.

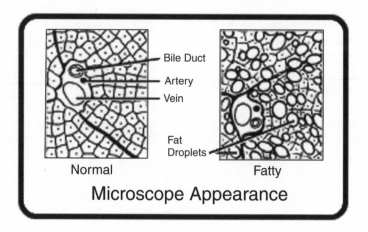

Figure 43.1. *Liver Tissue Samples*

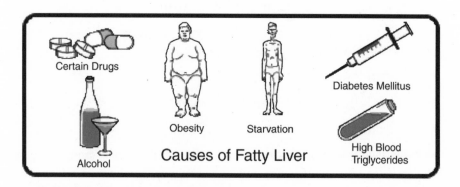

Figure 43.2. *Causes of Fatty Liver*

What Is Fatty Liver?

Fatty liver is just what its name suggests: the build-up of fat in the liver cells. Although this is not a normal condition, fat in the liver usually causes no damage by itself. However, on some occasions it can be a sign that other more harmful conditions are at work. Fatty liver may be associated with or may lead to inflammation of the liver. This can cause scarring and hardening of the liver. When scarring becomes extensive, it is called cirrhosis, and this is a very serious condition. Therefore, it is important that a physician thoroughly examine a patient with fat in the liver.

Cause

It would seem logical that eating fatty foods would cause a fatty liver, but this is not the case. The liver does play an important role in the metabolism or breakdown of fats. Something goes wrong in this process of metabolism, but it is still not known what does cause fat to build-up in the liver. It is known that fat accumulates in the liver with a number of conditions. The most common is obesity. Fatty liver is also associated with diabetes mellitus, high blood triglycerides, and the heavy use of alcohol. It may occur with certain illnesses such as tuberculosis and malnutrition, intestinal bypass surgery for obesity, excess vitamin A in the body, or the use of certain drugs such as valproic acid (trade names: Depakene/Depakote) and corticosteroids (cortisone, prednisone). Sometimes fatty liver occurs as a complication of pregnancy.

Symptoms and Diagnosis

There are usually no symptoms that are noticeable to the patient. In fact, fatty liver is frequently uncovered during a routine physical examination. There may be a rise in certain liver enzymes found in the blood, and sometimes the liver is slightly enlarged. Fatty liver may also be discovered while the physician is evaluating a patient for other illnesses. For example, an ultrasound exam of the abdomen done for other reasons may show fat in the liver. To be certain of a diagnosis of fatty liver, the physician may recommend a liver biopsy. Under local anesthesia, a slender needle is inserted through the right lower chest. A small piece of liver tissue is taken out with the needle and examined under a microscope.

What Is Steatohepatitis?   .

The term hepatitis means inflammation of and damage to the liver cells. Steato (pronounced stee-at´-toe) refers to fat. Therefore, steatohepatitis is inflammation of the liver related to fat accumulation. Heavy alcohol use can lead to fatty liver and inflammation, usually called alcoholic hepatitis. Steatohepatitis resembles alcoholic hepatitis, but it can and does occur in people who seldom or never drink alcohol. In this instance, it is often called nonalcoholic steatohepatitis or NASH. Both alcoholic hepatitis and steatohepatitis can lead to serious liver damage and cirrhosis.

Studies have shown that many people who are significantly overweight have developed, or will develop, steatohepatitis. It can also occur with rapid weight loss. Steatohepatitis has been connected to estrogen hormones in some women. In the case of diabetes mellitus, researchers believe steatohepatitis may develop only in those patients whose diabetes is not properly controlled.

Treatment

In most instances, treatment of fatty liver and steatohepatitis requires control of the underlying conditions. This may include reduction of high blood triglycerides, good control of diabetes, or not drinking alcohol. In some cases, surgical reversal of intestinal bypass for obesity is required.

Since being overweight is by far the most critical factor, weight loss is the key to ridding the liver of fat. This is especially necessary if damage to the liver is occurring, and early signs of scarring are present on biopsy. High blood triglycerides and diabetes are also worse with obesity. So, when steatohepatitis is present with these conditions, people gain even greater benefits from losing weight. Losing weight can be difficult. However, it must be done because the alternative may be eventual cirrhosis and the need for a liver transplant.

Currently, studies are underway on certain drugs such as Actigall. This drug appears to reduce liver damage in cases of steatohepatitis. At this time, however, it is not certain how helpful these drugs will be. To repeat the point, losing weight is by far the most important treatment.

Liver Transplantation

Liver transplantation is now an accepted form of treatment for chronic, severe liver damage. Advances in surgical techniques and the use of new drugs to suppress rejection have dramatically improved the success rate. Steatohepatitis is one of the more uncommon reasons for a liver transplant. However, every transplant center does a few each year as a result of this disease. Survival rates at transplant centers are well over 90% with a good quality of life after recovery.

Summary

Fatty liver is simply the build-up of fat in the liver. Fat in the liver usually does not cause liver damage. However, certain other conditions and diseases can be associated with the development of fatty liver. Research is ongoing to uncover what processes may take place to trigger fat build-up in the liver. This condition is usually reversible when the underlying causes are treated or removed. Patients who follow the advice of their physicians can expect to reverse and control a fatty liver or steatohepatitis.

Note: This material does not cover all information and is not intended as a substitute for professional care. Please consult with your physician on any matters regarding your health.

Chapter 44

Gallstones

What Are Gallstones?

Gallstones form when liquid stored in the gallbladder hardens into pieces of stone-like material. The liquid, called bile, is used to help the body digest fats. Bile is made in the liver, then stored in the gallbladder until the body needs to digest fat. At that time, the gallbladder contracts and pushes the bile into a tube—called a duct—which carries it to the small intestine, where it helps with digestion.

Bile contains water, cholesterol, fats, bile salts, and bilirubin. Bile salts break up fat, and bilirubin gives bile and stool a brownish color. If the liquid bile contains too much cholesterol, bile salts, or bilirubin, it can harden into stones.

The two types of gallstones are cholesterol stones and pigment stones. Cholesterol stones are usually yellow-green and are made primarily of hardened cholesterol. They account for about 80 percent of gallstones. Pigment stones are small, dark stones made of bilirubin. Gallstones can be as small as a grain of sand or as large as a golf ball. The gallbladder can develop just one large stone, hundreds of tiny stones, or almost any combination.

Gallstones can block the normal flow of bile if they lodge in any of the ducts that carry bile from the liver to the small intestine. That includes the hepatic ducts, which carry bile out of the liver; the cystic duct, which takes bile to and from the gallbladder; and the common

National Institute of Diabetes and Digestive and Kidney Diseases (NIDDK), NIH Publication No. 99-2897, January 1999.

bile duct, which takes bile from the cystic and hepatic ducts to the small intestine. Bile trapped in these ducts can cause inflammation in the gallbladder, the ducts, or, rarely, the liver. Other ducts open into the common bile duct, including the pancreatic duct, which carries digestive enzymes out of the pancreas. If a gallstone blocks the opening to that duct, digestive enzymes can become trapped in the pancreas and cause an extremely painful inflammation called pancreatitis.

If any of these ducts remain blocked for a significant period of time, severe—possibly fatal—damage can occur, affecting the gallbladder, liver, or pancreas. Warning signs of a serious problem are fever, jaundice, and persistent pain.

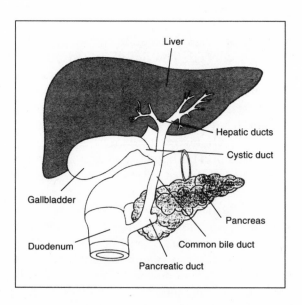

Figure 44.1. *The Biliary System. The gallbladder and the ducts that carry bile and other digestive enzymes from the liver, gallbladder, and pancreas to the small intestine are called the biliary system.*

What Causes Gallstones?

Cholesterol Stones

Scientists believe cholesterol stones form when bile contains too much cholesterol, too much bilirubin, or not enough bile salts, or when the gallbladder does not empty as it should for some other reason.

Pigment Stones

The cause of pigment stones is uncertain. They tend to develop in people who have cirrhosis, biliary tract infections, and hereditary blood disorders such as sickle cell anemia.

Other Factors

It is believed that the mere presence of gallstones may cause more gallstones to develop. However, other factors that contribute to gallstones have been identified, especially for cholesterol stones.

- **Obesity.** Obesity is a major risk factor for gallstones, especially in women. A large clinical study showed that being even moderately overweight increases one's risk for developing gallstones. The most likely reason is that obesity tends to reduce the amount of bile salts in bile, resulting in more cholesterol. Obesity also decreases gallbladder emptying.

- **Estrogen**. Excess estrogen from pregnancy, hormone replacement therapy, or birth control pills appears to increase cholesterol levels in bile and decrease gallbladder movement, both of which can lead to gallstones.

- **Ethnicity.** Native Americans have a genetic predisposition to secrete high levels of cholesterol in bile. In fact, they have the highest rates of gallstones in the United States. A majority of Native American men have gallstones by age 60. Among the Pima Indians of Arizona, 70 percent of women have gallstones by age 30. Mexican-American men and women of all ages also have high rates of gallstones.

- **Gender.** Women between 20 and 60 years of age are twice as likely to develop gallstones as men.

- **Age.** People over age 60 are more likely to develop gallstones than younger people.

- **Cholesterol-lowering drugs.** Drugs that lower cholesterol levels in blood actually increase the amount of cholesterol secreted in bile. This in turn can increase the risk of gallstones.

- **Diabetes.** People with diabetes generally have high levels of fatty acids called triglycerides. These fatty acids increase the risk of gallstones.

- **Rapid weight loss.** As the body metabolizes fat during rapid weight loss, it causes the liver to secrete extra cholesterol into bile, which can cause gallstones.

- **Fasting.** Fasting decreases gallbladder movement, causing the bile to become over-concentrated with cholesterol, which can lead to gallstones.

Who Is at Risk for Gallstones?

- Women
- People over age 60
- Native Americans
- Mexican-Americans
- Overweight men and women
- People who fast or lose a lot of weight quickly
- Pregnant women, women on hormone therapy, and women who use birth control pills

What Are the Symptoms?

Symptoms of gallstones are often called a gallstone "attack" because they occur suddenly. A typical attack can cause

- Steady, severe pain in the upper abdomen that increases rapidly and lasts from 30 minutes to several hours
- Pain in the back between the shoulder blades
- Pain under the right shoulder
- Nausea or vomiting

Gallstone attacks often follow fatty meals, and they may occur during the night. Other gallstone symptoms include

- Abdominal bloating
- Recurring intolerance of fatty foods
- Colic

- Belching
- Gas
- Indigestion

People who also have the following symptoms should see a doctor right away:

- Sweating
- Chills
- Low-grade fever
- Yellowish color of the skin or whites of the eyes
- Clay-colored stools

Many people with gallstones have no symptoms. These patients are said to be asymptomatic, and these stones are called "silent stones." They do not interfere in gallbladder, liver, or pancreas function and do not need treatment.

How Are Gallstones Diagnosed?

Many gallstones, especially silent stones, are discovered by accident during tests for other problems. But when gallstones are suspected to be the cause of symptoms, the doctor is likely to do an ultrasound exam. Ultrasound uses sound waves to create images of organs. Sound waves are sent toward the gallbladder through a handheld device that a technician glides over the abdomen. The sound waves bounce off the gallbladder, liver, and other organs, and their echoes make electrical impulses that create a picture of the organ on a video monitor. If stones are present, the sound waves will bounce off them, too, showing their location.

Other tests used in diagnosis include

- **Cholecystogram or cholescintigraphy.** The patient is injected with a special iodine dye, and x-rays are taken of the gallbladder over a period of time. (Some people swallow iodine pills the night before the x-ray.) The test shows the movement of the gallbladder and any obstruction of the cystic duct.

- **Endoscopic retrograde cholangiopancreatography (ERCP).** The patient swallows an endoscope—a long, flexible, lighted tube connected to a computer and TV monitor. The doctor guides the endoscope through the stomach and into the small intestine. The doctor then injects a special dye that temporarily stains the ducts in the biliary system. ERCP is used to locate stones in the ducts.

- **Blood tests.** Blood tests may be used to look for signs of infection, obstruction, pancreatitis, or jaundice.

Gallstone symptoms are similar to those of heart attack, appendicitis, ulcers, irritable bowel syndrome, hiatal hernia, pancreatitis, and hepatitis. So accurate diagnosis is important.

What Is the Treatment?

Surgery

Surgery to remove the gallbladder is the most common way to treat symptomatic gallstones. (Asymptomatic gallstones usually do not need treatment.) Each year more than 500,000 Americans have gallbladder surgery. The surgery is called cholecystectomy.

The standard surgery is called laparoscopic cholecystectomy. For this operation, the surgeon makes several tiny incisions in the abdomen and inserts surgical instruments and a miniature video camera into the abdomen. The camera sends a magnified image from inside the body to a video monitor, giving the surgeon a close-up view of the organs and tissues. While watching the monitor, the surgeon uses the instruments to carefully separate the gallbladder from the liver, ducts, and other structures. Then the cystic duct is cut and the gallbladder removed through one of the small incisions.

Because the abdominal muscles are not cut during laparoscopic surgery, patients have less pain and fewer complications than they would have had after surgery using a large incision across the abdomen. Recovery usually involves only one night in the hospital, followed by several days of restricted activity at home.

If the surgeon discovers any obstacles to the laparoscopic procedure, such as infection or scarring from other operations, the operating team may have to switch to open surgery. In some cases the obstacles are known before surgery, and an open surgery is planned. It is called "open" surgery because the surgeon has to make a 5 to 8 inch incision in the abdomen to remove the gallbladder. This is a major surgery and may require a 2 to 7 day stay in the hospital and several more weeks at home to recover. Open surgery is required in about 5 percent of gallbladder operations.

The most common complication in gallbladder surgery is injury to the bile ducts. An injured common bile duct can leak bile and cause a painful and potentially dangerous infection. Mild injuries can sometimes be treated nonsurgically. Major injury, however, is more serious and requires additional surgery.

If gallstones are in the bile ducts, the surgeon may use ERCP in removing them before or during the gallbladder surgery. Once the endoscope is in the small intestine, the surgeon locates the affected bile duct. An instrument on the endoscope is used to cut the duct, and the stone is captured in a tiny basket and removed with the endoscope. This two-step procedure is called ERCP with endoscopic sphincterotomy.

Occasionally, a person who has had a cholecystectomy is diagnosed with a gallstone in the bile ducts weeks, months, or even years after the surgery. The two-step ERCP procedure is usually successful in removing the stone.

Nonsurgical Treatment

Nonsurgical approaches are used only in special situations—such as when a patient's condition prevents using an anesthetic—and only for cholesterol stones. Stones recur after nonsurgical treatment about half the time.

- **Oral dissolution therapy.** Drugs made from bile acid are used to dissolve the stones. The drugs, ursodiol (Actigall) and chenodiol (Chenix), work best for small cholesterol stones. Months or years of treatment may be necessary before all the stones dissolve. Both drugs cause mild diarrhea, and chenodiol may temporarily raise levels of blood cholesterol and the liver enzyme transaminase.

- **Contact dissolution therapy**. This experimental procedure involves injecting a drug directly into the gallbladder to dissolve stones. The drug—methyl tert butyl—can dissolve some stones in 1 to 3 days, but it must be used very carefully because it is a flammable anesthetic that can be toxic. The procedure is being tested in patients with symptomatic, noncalcified cholesterol stones.

- **Extracorporeal shockwave lithotripsy (ESWL).** This treatment uses shock waves to break up stones into tiny pieces that can pass through the bile ducts without causing blockages. Attacks of biliary colic (intense pain) are common after treatment, and ESWL's success rate is not very high. Remaining stones can sometimes be dissolved with medication.

Don't People Need Their Gallbladders?

Fortunately, the gallbladder is an organ that people can live without. Losing it won't even require a change in diet. Once the gallbladder is removed, bile flows out of the liver through the hepatic ducts into the common bile duct and goes directly into the small intestine, instead of being stored in the gallbladder. However, because the bile isn't stored in the gallbladder, it flows into the small intestine more frequently, causing diarrhea in some people. Also, some studies suggest that removing the gallbladder may cause higher blood cholesterol levels, so occasional cholesterol tests may be necessary.

Points To Remember

- Gallstones form when substances in the bile harden.

- Gallstones are common among women, Native Americans, Mexican-Americans, and people who are overweight.

- Gallstone attacks often occur after eating a fatty meal.

- Symptoms can mimic those of other problems, including heart attack, so accurate diagnosis is important.

- Gallstones can cause serious problems if they become trapped in the bile ducts.

- Laparoscopic surgery to remove the gallbladder is the most common treatment.

Additional Information

National Digestive Diseases Information Clearinghouse
2 Information Way
Bethesda, MD 20892-3570
E-mail: nddic@info.niddk.nih.gov

Chapter 45

Gilbert's Syndrome

Gilbert's Syndrome is a relatively common and benign congenital (probably hereditary) liver disorder, found more frequently in males. It is characterized by a mild, fluctuating increase in serum bilirubin, a yellow pigment excreted by the liver into bile.

It is estimated that from 3 to 7% of the adult population has Gilbert's Syndrome.

Bilirubin is produced from hemoglobin (the red pigment of red blood cells) in the bone marrow, the spleen, and elsewhere and is carried to the liver in the blood. It undergoes chemical changes in the liver and then is excreted into bile and passes out of the body after further chemical changes in the intestines. Small amounts of bilirubin are normally present in the blood. However, when there is excessive breakdown of red blood cells or interference with bile excretion, the amount is increased and may produce jaundice.

The onset of Gilbert's Syndrome usually occurs in the teens or early adulthood (20's and 30's); there are rarely significant symptoms, but occasionally mild jaundice may appear, and the white of the eye becomes yellow. It may show up as an incidental laboratory finding. The serum bilirubin increases with fasting or an intercurrent illness such as influenza.

Except for the elevated serum bilirubin level, conventional liver function tests are normal and so is cholangiography (x-ray of the bile ducts).

Many patients are initially misdiagnosed or transformed into "hepatic neurotics" with a variety of nonspecific symptoms. The major goal of the clinician is to distinguish this benign disorder from more serious causes of liver dysfunction. The diagnosis of Gilbert's Syndrome is established primarily by documenting the persistence of an increased serum bilirubin when other liver function tests are repeatedly normal. A liver biopsy may occasionally be necessary to rule out other abnormalities. Other diagnostic procedures that may be useful include:

1. the effect of reduced caloric intake on plasma bilirubin concentration

2. intravenous administration of nicotinic acid which appears to increase bilirubin formation in the spleen, or

3. administration of radioactive bilirubin to estimate the percentage of the dose remaining in plasma after four hours

Gilbert's Syndrome does not require treatment and will not interfere with a normal lifestyle.

For Additional Information

American Liver Foundation
75 Maiden Lane, Suite 603
New York, NY 10038
1-800-GO LIVER (465-4837)
Fax: 212-483-8179
E-mail: webmail@liverfoundation.org
URL: http://www.liverfoundation.org

The American Liver Foundation is a national voluntary health organization dedicated to preventing, treating, and curing hepatitis and other liver and gallbladder diseases through research and education.

Chapter 46

Primary Biliary Cirrhosis

What Is Primary Biliary Cirrhosis?

Primary Biliary Cirrhosis (PBC) is a rare chronic liver disease that slowly destroys the bile ducts. Liver inflammation over a period of years causes scarring which leads to cirrhosis. The cause of PBC is unknown, and because of the varying symptoms, diagnosis can sometimes be overlooked. Women are affected 10 times more than men. PBC is usually diagnosed in patients between the ages of 35 to 60 years.

Those with PBC usually look extremely healthy, and many are 10 to 30 pounds overweight. The slight bronze pigmentation of the skin very is often present and makes the individual look tanned. The outward appearance doesn't tell the story of what is going on inside their bodies.

PBC is considered an autoimmune disease. When diagnosed, it may be associated with one or more autoimmune diseases such as Rheumatoid Arthritis, Sjogren's Syndrome, Raynauds, Lupus, or Scleroderma.

Upon diagnosis, patients are advised to avoid alcohol. Many doctors recommend PBC patients start a low fat–low sodium diet, drink at least 64 ounces of water daily, take calcium with vitamin D, lower

---

This chapter includes the following copyrighted articles reprinted with permission of the Primary Biliary Cirrhosis Support Group; "What is Primary Cirrhosis" by Linda Moore, "Waiting for the Other Shoe to Drop" by Dr. Marilyn Blau Klainberg, and "PBC Disease Stages."

caffeine intake, avoid stress, and exercise if possible. Walking is often recommended for exercise.

The number of patients being diagnosed at the asymptomatic stage has risen dramatically over the past few years due to widespread laboratory screening. Typically, the blood lab pattern is an above normal alkaline phosphatase level with a low or normal bilirubin. Unlike other liver diseases, bilirubin does not increase until final disease stage.

Medical tests used to confirm PBC:

- A liver biopsy helps confirms the diagnosis and stage of the disease.

- Blood lab tests that show liver dysfunction:

  - Liver function tests Mitochondrial antibodies (Positive AMA is found in about 95% of PBC patients)
  - Serum cholesterol and lipoproteins may be increased.
  - Haptoglobin & ACE levels may be altered

Many patients remain without symptoms for years, and the initial symptoms vary among PBC patients. Symptoms may be present in any combination and include:

- Chronic fatigue is usually the first symptom the patient notices, causing him or her to visit their doctor. The fatigue associated with PBC appears to be totally different from any other sort of fatigue. In early stages, many patients have commented they could sleep for hours. As the disease progresses, the fatigue continues to grow worse and sleeping becomes more difficult. At this time there is little research into the cause and treatment of the liver disease fatigue. It is not due to depression, and some researchers believe it is an abnormality of the axis between the pituitary and the adrenal glands. Support and understanding from family members, friends, and the doctor is very important, making it somewhat bearable.

- Intense and unrelenting itching of the skin

- Gradual darkening or changes in skin texture, and various skin rashes.

- Small yellow or white bumps under the skin, usually around the eyes

- Dry Eye Syndrome

- Dry mouth, sometimes referred to as cotton mouth.

- Thyroid Problems

- Arthritic aches and pains in bones, muscles, and joints are common. These pains can be severe and debilitating. Some PBC patients report severe pain when just touching leg , feet, and hip bones.

As the PBC progresses, other symptoms usually appear. These symptoms may include any combination of the following:

- Osteoporosis or other metabolic bone disease

- Enlarged abdomen from fluid accumulation

- Easy bruising or bleeding

- Jaundice (yellowing of the skin and eyes)

- Increased bilirubin

- Internal bleeding in upper stomach and esophagus

- Hepatic Encephalopathy causing personality changes: dulling of mental functions, neglect of personal appearance, forgetfulness, and trouble concentrating, changes in sleeping habits, confusion, breath odor, and muscle stiffness. (Some patients refer to Hepatic Encephalopathy as "Fuzzy Brain.")

- Fever, nausea, and vomiting

- Reflux and stomach ulcers

- Weight increase or decrease

- Swelling of the hands, legs, and ankles

- Sexual problems (impotence in men, absence of periods in women, lack of desire.)

- Trembling hands

- Difficulty in sleeping and changes in sleeping habits. As the disease progresses, many patients note they have difficulty sleeping more than 3–5 hours at any one time. Some wake up at all hours of the night even though they feel extreme fatigue. Many require 2 or 3 naps during the day. The majority of PBC patients notice the itching intensifies when they lay down to sleep, and those who have liver pain say it is more severe in a sleeping position.

- Abdominal pain or pressure in the upper right quadrant.

PBC advances slowly over a period of years. Many patients lead normal lives for years without symptoms, depending on how early diagnosis is made. There is no cure for PBC, but patients are having positive results in slowing the disease progress with Actigall and Methotrexate. Some patients require vitamin A, vitamin K, and vitamin D replacement therapy to add back fat-soluble vitamins which are lost in fatty stools. In early diagnosis, a calcium supplement is usually prescribed to help prevent osteomalacia and osteoporosis.

When medical treatments, such as URSO, Actigall, and methotrexate no longer control the disease, the patient should be evaluated for a liver transplant. The end stage of PBC is liver failure. Many signs indicate liver failure: increased bilirubin, jaundice, malnutrition, gastrointestinal bleeding, intractable itching, bone fractures, and heptic coma. Transplant is recommended before most of these symptoms occur. The transplant outcome for PBC patients is excellent.

As with any other chronic illness, support and understanding is very important in helping the PBC patient cope with day to day living.

PBC Disease Stages

Stage 1: Portal Stage

Normal sized triads; portal inflammation, subtle duct damage

Stage 2: Periportal Stage

Enlarged triads; periportal fibrosis and/or inflammation

Stage 3: Septal Stage

Active and/or passive fibrous septae

Stage 4: Biliary Cirrhosis

Nodules present; garland or jigsaw pattern
Although 4 typical stages of evolution have been defined, the disease initially is focal with considerable overlap between stages in any one case.

First is inflammation of the medium-sized bile ducts and chronic inflammation of the portal tracts. Granulomas may be found. With progression of PBC, the portal tracts become distorted, inflammation spreads into the parenchyma, bile ducts proliferate intensely, and periportal fibrosis develops.

Progressive scarring continues with less bile duct proliferation and less inflammation. Fibrous bands link the portal tracts, and zone 1 cholestasis and Mallory hyaline can become evident. The end product is a firm, regular, intensely bile-stained cirrhosis, difficult to distinguish from other cirrhotic processes in the absence of granulomas and the pathognomonic bile duct lesions.

Laboratory Findings

Early findings feature cholestasis with alkaline phosphatase elevated disproportionately greater than serum bilirubin and aminotransferases. In fact, the serum bilirubin is often normal early in the course of the disease. Serum bile acid concentration and gamma-glutamyl transpeptidase activity are elevated. Serum cholesterol concentration and total lipids usually are increased. Serum lipoproteins are increased, mainly because lipoprotein-X is present. Serum albumin is normal early in the course of the disease, but the globulins usually increase the serum IgM often to very high values. Antibodies against a component of the inner membrane of mitochondria (in 85 to 95% of patients) are important diagnostically, but they can also be found in some patients with HBsAg-negative chronic active hepatitis, making this differentiation difficult.

Prognosis

The course of PBC varies greatly. It may not diminish the quality or the duration of life. Of patients who present without symptoms, 50% show evidence of liver disease over the ensuing 15 years. Slow progression suggests prolonged survival. A rising serum bilirubin, associated with autoimmune disorders, and advanced histologic changes indicate a poor prognosis.

PBC is one of the best indications for liver transplantation.

Waiting for the Other Shoe to Drop—Living with PBC

I am delighted to be here today! You know the old joke, I am delighted to be anywhere. It sure beats a hospital or other options. There are conditions and situations which may be considered much worse than PBC, and therefore it is more productive to discuss strategies for living with PBC.

I am married, a mother of four, grandmother of seven and an Assistant Professor of Nursing at a small University in Long Island. As I share my thoughts with you today, please remember that I am new to this disease, a year ago, before being diagnosed, I had never heard of PBC. My story is probably similar to yours, yet it was shocking to me as a healthcare professional and of course personally. Today, I am trying to help educate my colleagues and others in the health care profession about PBC. Aside from being identified as a rare disease, since PBC primarily affects women, I sometimes personally wonder what effect that has had on the knowledge base of health care providers.

I was newly diagnosed at stage three, 11 months ago after many years of undiagnosed symptoms. For many years my physician told me my fatigue was due to aging, menopause, being overweight, and overworked. My elevated liver enzymes, he assumed were due to a fatty liver which I had had for many years. Fatty liver can be one of the symptoms of PBC I later discovered. I also had an elevated AMA [antimitochondrial antibody] which my doctor attributed to the fact that my mother had an auto immune disease (MS). Not until my AMA nearly went off the charts at 2000 did he acknowledge that there might be something else wrong and referred me for further testing. A positive AMA gave confirmation of PBC.

Although there is no generally acceptable cure for PBC, as it is one of many auto-immune diseases, there are strategies for living and coping with it. I will look at and present PBC through the eyes of a nurse.

Persons with PBC need to address osteoporosis, adhere to a low fat diet, take vitamins to prevent deficiencies, be aware of the impact upon the liver of certain prescriptions and over the counter medications, and limit or totally avoid alcohol intake. It is also important to be aware of the signs and symptoms of encephalopathy (fuzzy brain). Individuals with PBC must try to live as normally and healthily as possible. How can this be done?

Where to Begin

Always remember that symptoms and problems of other diseases also occur in people with PBC. People with PBC are prone to other autoimmune diseases such as thyroid disease, arthritis, diabetes, and sjogrens. So remember not to conclude or let your health care professional attribute everything to PBC alone. Also share with your family and friends how you are feeling so they can be of help to you. Do not try to shelter family or friends as you usually look well. Do not expend your energies beyond their limits. Inform all healthcare providers, which includes other physicians (eye doctors), pharmacists, and dentists that you have PBC. For some it may seem uncomfortable but it could save your life and prevent medications or even anesthesia which could have damaging effects on the liver.

Fighting Fatigue

The fatigue associated with PBC is totally different from any other sort of fatigue. You must learn to rest. Pacing oneself is imperative — you may need to change jobs and must remember when to stop and take a break. Recognize that tiredness is a physical symptom. Share this with your families, children, and spouses. It is not giving up, just slowing up. But you also must keep as active as you can. You need to be fit!

Fluids

Increase water intake, this is particularly important in preventing or slowing down hepatic encephalopathy (fuzzy brain). Hepatic encephalopathy causes lethargy, drowsiness, agitation and occurs when toxic levels of ammonia and other protein by-products reach the brain because the liver cannot filter them adequately.

Try to have two to three bowel movements daily to prevent ammonia buildup. Note if stools are bright red or black restrict sodium, decrease caffeine intake. Caffeine is often hidden in products which we do not suspect. Read the label.

Dry mouth — keep a bottle of water near. Dry eye — in simple cases over the counter remedies are available, but be sure to check with an opthamologist or your medical doctor. Persons with PBC are prone to other autoimmune diseases, such as Sjogrens in which dry eye is significant.

Dry eye does not automatically mean you have Sjogrens. Vaginal dryness is often a problem for women, it may be due to normal menopause. The use of products like Replens is not just for comfort in sexual relations alone, but for the relief of general discomfort in the vaginal area. Dryness in this area just like other areas can lead to burning or infection due to irritation caused by the dryness.

Diet/Meals

Eat a healthy balanced diet, eat foods low in fat. Avoid foods particularly high in saturated fat as they are difficult for the liver to process. However, unsaturated fats such as fish oils that are found in oily fish like salmon are advised. A good way to determine if fats are saturated or unsaturated is put them in the refrigerator and if they congeal (harden) they are saturated oils.

Meals should be small and eaten often during the day. Restrict salt as fluid retention is part of the cirrhosis. Try to eat a diet high in fiber (fruits, cereals, whole grain breads, and pasta—whole wheat pasta) and a diet low in sugar as adult diabetes may be a problem for persons with PBC.

Alcohol

Carefully read labels of over-the-counter medications and certain food products to avoid alcohol. Inform your pharmacist so that they can help you with prescribed or over-the-counter medications. Inform friends and family that you are alcohol sensitive.

Osteoporosis

The use of estrogen is controversial. Some physicians feel the estrogen patch works well as it does not affect the liver. Some feel that oral estrogen although it is processed by the liver is acceptable. Many recommend products like Fosamax, Calcimar internasal, and parentally or slow released fluoride preparation.

Calcium is taken by tablets, in high calcium foods, or calcium enriched foods.

Weight bearing exercises are important to strengthen bone. Walking, in a mall, on a treadmill, or outside, wherever you prefer, is a great weight bearing exercise. The important thing is to do it.

Weight bearing exercising in a pool is easier on the joints. Many public pools offer in-pool activities. Although Yoga is not necessarily considered a weight bearing exercise I usually recommend it as good for stretching and preparing for other exercises.

Itching

First, not everyone with itching has PBC and not everyone with PBC has itching, but as the liver becomes more affected there will be an increase in itching. There are many medications which can be prescribed such as Questran and some over-the-counter anti-itching medications such as Sarna, which work fairly well but there are other things you can try. Short showers with tepid not hot water work for some people. Hot water makes one feel more itchy as it brings the blood to the area. Also, a diet which is not too spicy may be helpful. Try to keep linens clean and sleep in loose fitting light sleepwear. Skin integrity is very important. Scratching allows bacteria to easily invade the protection of the skin.

Complementary Medicine

Medications

Be aware of medications which foster the immune system such as Echinacea. You do not want to increase the immune system it is busy enough!

Stress Management

Stress Management is very important. Learn relaxing breathing techniques.

Nutrition

Supplement your diet with vitamins A, D, and E. Baby vitamins may be easier for some people to digest, but read the label to be sure it is adequate for adults.

Medicaid

"Buy in" or "buyback" is available in some states. Contact a social worker, elder attorney, or your local homecare provider for assistance.

Laughter as Medicine

The most important thing to do is to remember to laugh, find reasons to laugh! It is truly the best medicine, and people like to be around you more. Laughter has been proven to relieve stress, reduce pain, and is generally thought to be therapeutic. Remember to live in the moment. We are all mortal and might as well enjoy life now not later. Find the humor in work, relationships, disability, and the medical profession.

Chapter 47

Primary Sclerosing Cholangitis (PSC)

The Liver

The liver is the largest organ in the body. It is found high in the right upper abdomen, behind the ribs. It is a very complex organ and has many functions. They include:

- Storing energy in the form of sugar (glucose)

- Storing vitamins, iron, and other minerals

- Making proteins, including blood clotting factors, to keep the body healthy and help it grow

- Processing worn out red blood cells

- Making bile which is needed for food digestion

- Metabolizing or breaking down many medications and alcohol

- Killing germs that enter the body through the intestine

The liver cells excrete bile into tiny tubes within the liver called bile ducts. These tubes come together like the tiny veins on a leaf. They drain the bile into the common bile duct, a larger single tube leading into the intestine. There the bile aids digestion and gives stool its brown color. As you can see, the liver is a very important organ.

Reprinted with permission, © 1998 Chek Med Systems, Inc.

What Is Primary Sclerosing Cholangitis (PSC)?

Primary sclerosing cholangitis is a disease primarily of the bile ducts, both inside and outside the liver. The ducts of the gallbladder and pancreas may also be involved. The walls of the bile ducts become inflamed (cholangitis). The inflammation causes scarring and hardening (fibrosis) that narrows the bile ducts. Because bile cannot drain properly through the ducts, it accumulates in the liver causing damage to liver cells. Eventually, so much bile is accumulated, it seeps into the bloodstream. Finally, with long term cell damage, the liver develops cirrhosis (hardening or fibrosis) and it can no longer function properly.

Cause of Primary Sclerosing Cholangitis (PSC)

The exact cause of PSC is unknown. However, the most likely cause appears to be changes in the way the immune system works. When the immune system is working properly, it protects the body from infections caused by foreign invaders like bacteria and viruses. Sometimes, however, it recognizes certain body parts or organs as foreign. The body then goes to war against itself, damaging the body part it thinks is foreign.

PSC often starts between the ages of 30 and 50, and it occurs most often in men. It was once considered a rare disease, but recent studies show it is more common than previously thought. About 70% of the patients with PSC also have an inflammatory bowel disease, especially ulcerative colitis in which the colon becomes inflamed and ulcerated. Medical experts believe genetic factors may link PSC and ulcerative colitis.

Symptoms of Primary Sclerosing Cholangitis (PSC)

PSC usually progresses very slowly. Early on there may be no symptoms. Usually the only findings are abnormal laboratory test results. For example, a liver enzyme called alkaline phosphatase may be above normal ranges in the blood. When symptoms do develop, they may be intermittent or persistent. Gradually, they may worsen. The symptoms are caused by two things: the bile is not being drained properly through the bile ducts, and the liver is not doing its job. Bile ducts can become infected, causing chills, fever, and upper abdominal tenderness. Itching may occur when bile seeps into the bloodstream. As the disease progresses, chronic fatigue, loss of appetite, weight loss, and jaundice (yellowing of skin and eyes) may occur. Finally, in the advanced stages of cirrhosis, extensive swelling can occur in the abdomen and feet. Liver failure may take many years to develop.

Diagnosis

The physician may suspect PSC from the patient's medical history, especially a history of inflammatory bowel disease, and from abnormal blood tests. The diagnosis is usually made by cholangiography, an x-ray called ERCP that involves injecting dye into the bile ducts. The test is performed under sedation. A lighted, flexible endoscope is inserted through the mouth, stomach and then into the small intestine. A thin tube is place through the scope into the bile ducts, and the dye is injected to highlight the bile ducts on the x-ray. If there is narrowing of the bile ducts, the diagnosis of PSC is confirmed.

As the disease progresses, a liver biopsy is usually needed to determine how much damage has occurred. Under local anesthesia, a slender needle is inserted through the right lower chest to extract a small piece of liver for microscopic analysis.

Treatment

At the present time there is no cure for PSC, but effective treatment is available. There are a number of ways to treat symptoms and the various stages of the disease. Itching, from too much bile in the bloodstream, can be controlled with drugs such as Questran. Bile is usually reabsorbed into the bloodstream from the large intestine, and goes back to the liver to be reused. Questran binds up bile in the intestine, allowing it to be eliminated with the stool instead. This helps to reduce the build-up of bile in the body. Actigall is a drug that favorably changes the make-up of bile in the liver. This, in turn, seems to reduce the amount of liver damage that occurs. Results of early medical studies seem to indicate that this drug may increase survival. Sometimes the bile ducts become infected and must be treated with antibiotics. If ulcerative colitis is also present, it is treated with the appropriate medicines. Swelling of the abdomen and feet, due to fluid retention from cirrhosis, can be treated with a salt-restricted diet and diuretics (fluid pills). Presently, there are exciting studies being done to test the effectiveness of other drugs on the body's immune system, since this seems to be the underlying problem.

In some cases, endoscopic or surgical procedures may be used to open major blockages in bile ducts. Through an endoscope, the physician places a tiny tube with a balloon on the end into the narrowed bile duct. The balloon is inflated to expand the duct so bile can flow through it once again. Sometimes stents (plastic tubing) can be placed in the narrowed ducts to keep them open. Often PSC progresses to a point where liver transplantation must be considered.

Liver Transplantation

Liver transplantation is now an accepted form of treatment for chronic, severe liver disease. Advances in surgical techniques and the use of new drugs to suppress rejection have improved the success rate of transplantation. The outcome for PSC patients is excellent. Because of the disease's slow progress, it is possible to plan elective transplant surgery. Survival rates at transplant centers are well over 90 percent, with a good quality of life after recovery.

Summary

Primary sclerosing cholangitis is a slow, progressive disease. Once diagnosed, treatment is directed at managing symptoms and opening narrowed bile ducts. A great deal of research is underway aimed at preventing damage to the bile ducts, improving symptoms, and prolonging life. By working closely with the physician, there is good reason to expect a favorable long-term outlook.

Note: This material does not cover all information and is not intended as a substitute for professional care. Please consult with your physician on any matters regarding your health.

Chapter 48

Reye's Syndrome

What Is Reye's Syndrome?

Reye's syndrome (RS) is primarily a children's disease, although it can occur at any age. It affects all organs of the body but is most harmful to the brain and the liver—causing an acute increase of pressure within the brain and, often, massive accumulations of fat in the liver and other organs. RS is defined as a two-phase illness because it generally occurs in conjunction with a previous viral infection, such as the flu or chicken pox. The disorder commonly occurs during recovery from a viral infection, although it can also develop 3 to 5 days after the onset of the viral illness. RS is often misdiagnosed as encephalitis, meningitis, diabetes, drug overdose, poisoning, sudden infant death syndrome, or psychiatric illness. Symptoms of RS include persistent or recurrent vomiting, listlessness, personality changes such as irritability or combativeness, disorientation or confusion, delirium, convulsions, and loss of consciousness. If these symptoms are present during or soon after a viral illness, medical attention should be sought immediately. The symptoms of RS in infants do not follow

This chapter contains text from "Reye's Syndrome," National Institute of Neurological Disorders and Stroke (NINDS), NIH June 1996, updated April 7, 1998, "Reye Syndrome: The Decline of a Disease," by Evelyn Zamula, *FDA Consumer* November 1990, "On the Teen Scene: Using Over-the-Counter Medications Wisely," *FDA Consumer* November 1991, revised May 1995, Publication No. (FDA) 95-3199, and "Reye's Syndrome," © 1997, reprinted with permission of the American Liver Foundation, 1-800-GO-LIVER.

a typical pattern; for example, vomiting does not always occur. The cause of RS remains a mystery. However studies have shown that using aspirin or salicylate-containing medications to treat viral illness increases the risk of developing RS. A physician should be consulted before giving a child any aspirin or anti-nausea medicines during a viral illness, which can mask the symptoms of RS.

Reye's Syndrome Defined

The Centers for Disease Control and Prevention established case definitions for regional surveillance and outbreak investigations in the late 1960's. Criteria for a case included mental status changes, such as delirium or coma, and a liver biopsy (tissue sample) showing fat accumulation in the liver (or high levels of liver enzymes and ammonia in the blood). There also needed to be no other more reasonable explanation for the brain or liver abnormalities.

How the Illness Progresses

The course of the illness is variable. Reye's syndrome can be mild and self-limiting, or it can progress rapidly, causing death within hours of onset, usually from brain swelling. But the progression may also stop at any stage, with complete recovery in 5 to 10 days and the quick return of normal liver function.

Doctors classify stages of Reye's syndrome based on the level of the patient's consciousness and corresponding physical signs: Stages 0 to 2 are pre-comatose, with lethargy or delirium, and sometimes combativeness, but with the child still responding to stimuli. Coma progressively deepens in stages 3 to 5; the child is unresponsive to stimuli, and heart and lung functions begin to shut down.

The earlier the diagnosis and treatment, the better the chance for survival. Intense supportive care in a hospital experienced in dealing with Reye's syndrome also improves odds. Children who survive but experience the most severe stages of the illness—especially infants—are sometimes left with neurological abnormalities, often mental retardation or disorders of voice and speech.

Fatality rates when national surveillance began on a regular basis in 1976 were as high as 40 percent, declined to between 20 and 30 percent from 1978 to 1987, but rose in 1988 and 1989. CDC experts speculate that this higher death rate may reflect decreasing interest in the syndrome—because of its rarity—resulting in the reporting of only the most serious cases.

The Aspirin Connection

Investigators in the United States looked for some common factor among children who developed the syndrome. They found it in aspirin taken during flu or chicken pox.

In 1980, results of studies conducted in Ohio, Michigan, and Arizona demonstrated an association between Reye's syndrome and aspirin use during a preceding respiratory tract or chicken pox infection.

"It was those initial studies that we reviewed in 1980 that first led CDC to report in its Morbidity and Mortality Weekly Report [*MMWR*] that there was an association," states Lawrence B. Schonberger, M.D., an epidemiologist with the agency. In 1981, CDC reported in *MMWR* results of a fourth study that revealed the same association. In 1982, the Surgeon General of the U.S. Public Health Service issued a warning against giving aspirin to children with flu or chicken pox.

The public was quick to pick up on the association. "A kind of natural study was occurring, because once people heard about the results [of the studies], they started to lower the use of aspirin in their children," says Schonberger. "If aspirin had nothing to do with it [Reye's syndrome], then one might anticipate that there would be no clear decrease in the incidence of Reye's syndrome."

That's not what happened. Aspirin use in children under 10 declined by at least 50 percent from 1981 to 1988, and the number of Reye's syndrome cases went down correspondingly. In the opinion of Peter C. Rowe, M.D., assistant professor of pediatrics, Children's Hospital of Eastern Canada, Ottawa, Ontario, the declining use of aspirin and the decreasing incidence of Reye's syndrome represent a "natural ecological experiment."

Other Government Actions

The federal government made other moves. To confirm the preliminary findings of the state studies, in 1985-1986 the government sponsored the "Public Health Service Study of Reye's Syndrome and Medications." Twenty-seven children who developed Reye's syndrome after a preceding respiratory illness or chicken pox were matched with 140 children who had had the same illnesses at the same time, but did not develop Reye's syndrome. More than 96 percent of the Reye's syndrome cases, compared with 38 percent of the controls (the children who did not develop Reye's syndrome), had received aspirin (or other salicylates) to treat the preceding illness. The study was prematurely ended because not enough Reye's syndrome children who had not been exposed to aspirin could be found to justify the expense of continuing the investigation, in itself an indication of a public health triumph.

In 1986, FDA adopted a preliminary rule requiring aspirin manufacturers to add warnings to product labels about the possible association between aspirin use and the development of Reye's syndrome. The permanent rule became final in 1988, and the labeling reads: Children and teenagers should not use this medicine for chicken pox or flu symptoms before a doctor is consulted about Reye's syndrome, a rare but serious illness reported to be associated with aspirin.

The number of Reye's syndrome cases, which reached a high in 1980 with 555 cases, has steadily decreased, compared with years in which there has been similar types of influenza activity. The decline has been most dramatic among children from 5 to 10 years of age. In 1989, a heavy influenza B year, 27 cases of Reye's syndrome were reported to CDC, almost half of them fatal. According to CDC, since 1985, 40 to 65 percent of reported Reye's syndrome patients have been older than 10. Because this age group often self-medicates, recent educational efforts have been geared to reach them.

Other Factors

Some questions about the relationship between aspirin and Reye's syndrome still remain. Although figures show that 90 to 95 percent of Reye's syndrome patients in the United States have taken aspirin during a preceding viral illness, it is estimated that less than 0.1 percent of children having a viral infection and treated with aspirin develop the syndrome.

Reye's syndrome has always been a puzzling disease. Research on possible causes has been hampered because no one can come up with a simple specific diagnostic test for the syndrome. The waters are further muddied by the existence of at least 19 viruses, including the chicken pox and flu viruses, that cause infectious illness which can precede Reye's syndrome development. Some experts have proposed that Reye's syndrome develops from the interaction of a viral illness, genetic susceptibility to the disease, and exposure to chemicals, such as salicylates, pesticides, and aflatoxin. Others speculate that unidentified viruses or other infectious agents are involved.

That some children may be more susceptible to Reye's syndrome than others has been shown by cases appearing among children in the same family and by recurrent episodes of the illness in the same child. It is possible that more than one type of Reye's syndrome exists, or that some of these cases may not be Reye's syndrome at all.

Reye's Syndrome Symptoms

In most cases, children seem to be recovering from a viral illness when the following symptoms occur:

- nausea
- vomiting, usually very severe
- fever
- lethargy
- stupor or coma, sometimes followed by convulsions
- wild delirium and unusual restlessness noted in about half of patients.

Treatment

There is no cure for RS. Successful management, which depends on early diagnosis, is primarily aimed at protecting the brain against irreversible damage by reducing brain swelling, reversing the metabolic injury, preventing complications in the lungs, and anticipating cardiac arrest. It has been learned that several inborn errors of metabolism mimic RS in that the first manifestation of these errors may be an encephalopathy with liver dysfunction. These disorders must be considered in all suspected cases of RS. Some evidence suggests that treatment in the end stages of RS with hypertonic IV glucose solutions may prevent progression of the syndrome.

Prognosis

Recovery from RS is directly related to the severity of the swelling of the brain. Some people recover completely, while others may sustain varying degrees of brain damage. Those cases in which the disorder progresses rapidly and the patient lapses into a coma have a poorer prognosis than those with a less severe course. Statistics indicate that when RS is diagnosed and treated in its early stages, chances of recovery are excellent. When diagnosis and treatment are delayed, the chances for successful recovery and survival are severely reduced. Unless RS is diagnosed and treated successfully, death is common, often within a few days.

Products Containing Salicylates

The following products don't have aspirin in their brand names but they contain aspirin or other salicylates and shouldn't be taken by teens or children who have symptoms of flu or chickenpox unless told to do so by a doctor. (Ingestion of salicylates during these illnesses increases childrens' and teens' risk of Reye's syndrome.)

- 4-Way Cold Tablets
- Alka-Seltzer Effervescent Antacid and Pain Reliever (also the extra-strength version)
- Alka-Seltzer Plus Night-Time Cold Medicine
- Anacin
- Anacin Maximum Strength Analgesic Coated Tablets
- Ascriptin A/D Caplets (also the regular and extra-strength versions)
- Aspergum
- BC Powder
- BC Cold Powder Multi-Symptom Formula
- BC Cold Powder Non-Drowsy Formula
- Bayer Children's Cold Tablets
- Bufferin (all formulations)
- Coricidin
- Coricidin Demilets
- Dristan Tablets
- Excedrin
- Excedrin Extra-Strength Analgesic Tablets and Caplets
- Medilets
- Pepto-Bismol
- Triminicin
- Ursinus Inlay-Tabs
- Vanquish Analgesic Caplets

In addition, many products to treat arthritis contain aspirin. (This list contains many common products, but is not all-inclusive. So be sure to read the label before purchasing any OTC medication.)

Additional Information

National Reye's Syndrome Foundation
P.O. Box 829
Bryan, OH 43506
(419) 636-2679 or (800) 233-7393
E-mail: reyessyn@mail.bright.net
URL: http://www.birhgt.net/~reyessyn

The Food and Drug Administration
CDER-HED-210
5600 Fishers Lane
Rockville, MD 20857
(301) 827-4573 or (888) 463-6332

Chapter 49

Type I Glycogen Storage Disease

Glycogen Storage Disease has been divided into at least 10 different types based on the deficiency of a particular enzyme which controls blood sugar levels.

Type I Glycogen Storage Disease is a deficiency of the enzyme glucose –6–phosphatase which helps in maintaining a normal blood glucose (sugar concentration) during fasting. Patients with this particular disorder show a large number of abnormalities which exhibit themselves in growth failure, a greatly enlarged liver, and a distended (swollen) abdomen. The abnormal blood chemical condition is indicated by low blood sugar concentration and higher than normal levels of lipids and uric acid.

The Different Forms of Glycogen Storage Disease

An absence or a deficiency of any of the enzymes (catalysts) that are important to the making or breaking down of glycogen can result in glycogen storage disease. The enzyme may be important in all of the cells of the body or found specifically in muscle or liver. Thus the many forms of glycogen storage disease can be described as affecting primarily the liver or the muscles.

This chapter contains text from "Association for Glycogen Storage Disease: Could Someone You Know Be Affected?," © Association for Glycogen Storage Disease, reprinted with permission, and "Type I Glycogen Storage Disease," © 1997 American Liver Foundation, 1-800-GO-LIVER, reprinted with permission.

Liver Forms

The most frequent liver form in the United States, Canada, and Europe is often called von Gierke's disease (Type 1) and it is due to an absence or deficiency of glucose –6–phosphatase. This is the catalyst for the final step in the production for glucose (dextrose) by the liver. These individuals cannot maintain their blood glucose levels and therefore are at risk for hypoglycemia (low blood sugar). Without treatment they grow slowly, have very large livers, have excessive fat in the blood, and increased uric acid which can lead to gout.

The next most frequent liver form of glycogen storage disease (GSD) with prominent symptoms is often called short-chain glycogen storage disease (Type III). The clinical symptoms may be indistinguishable from von Gierke's disease or they may be very mild. Many of these individuals also have muscle problems.

Type IV GSD which forms long-chain glycogen storage disease is associated with cirrhosis (scarring) of the liver. These children rarely live past 5 years of age.

There are other liver forms which tend not to be as prominent clinically.

Muscle Forms

Without question the most dramatic and tragic muscle type of glycogen storage disease is generalized glycogen storage disease or Pompe's disease (Type II). The infantile form appears normal at birth, but within 3 or 4 months becomes progressively weaker and dies before the second year of life. The later onset forms have a slower progression and have symptoms similar to muscular dystrophy.

The other types with muscle involvement tend to be without symptoms unless they exercise vigorously which can lead to serious trouble.

Genetics

Most of the glycogen storage diseases are transmitted as an autosomal recessive condition. That means that girls and boys are equally affected and the parents are not affected. The affected individual receives the GSD genetic trait from each parent. One quarter of the children of such a union will be affected. The only exception to this mode of genetic transmission is that for Type IX which is sex-linked. This means that 50% of the male offspring of a carrier mother with the gene will be affected and 50% of his sisters will be carriers or heterozygous.

Treatment

There are several approaches available for the treatment of von Gierke's disease or Type I, in which hypoglycemia is a difficult problem.

In the past, these patients have been treated by frequent feedings during the daytime and occasional feedings during the normal sleeping hours which required waking the patient. This was the accepted form of therapy until 1966 to 1967, but the patients continued to show various difficulties in physical development and blood chemistry.

Starting in 1967, surgeons began performing a surgical procedure, called a portacaval shunt, which bypassed the blood around the liver. In some patients this procedure resulted in improvement in observable physical condition and improved biochemical levels in the blood. In 1974 it was found that patients also did exceedingly well if the blood glucose level was maintained within the normal range by frequent daytime feedings and by continuous infusion of a solution high in glucose concentration into the stomach during the night. Maintenance of the blood glucose level either in total intravenous feedings or by continuous infusion of high glucose-containing foods into the stomach could reverse all of the physical and chemical signs of this disease.

A practical management technique for maintaining the blood glucose level has been devised in which a naso-gastric tube is inserted into the stomach each evening and through this tube is infused a solution containing a high concentration of glucose so the blood sugar level remains between 75 and 120. In the daytime the tube is removed and the patient eats a high starch feeding approximately every 2-1/2 to 3-1/2 hours. Using this technique, most of the physical and biochemical abnormalities are completely reversed.

One study in which a total of 14 patients were followed, nine for a period of greater than 5 years, has shown this to be an effective form of treatment. Although younger children will have to use the tube each evening, doctors feel that this may not be necessary past puberty.

A high protein diet benefits most individuals with short-chain GSD (Type III). The high protein diet may be of substantial benefit to other muscle forms of GSD.

As noted, Type IV or long-chain GSD is the one form of GSD where liver transplant currently offers the only hope.

For More Information

The Association for Glycogen Storage Disease

Hollie Swain
Box 896
Durant, IA 52747
(319) 785-6038

American Liver Foundation

75 Maiden Lane, Suite 603
New York, NY 10038
1-800-GO LIVER (465-4837)
Fax: 212-483-8179
E-mail: webmail@liverfoundation.org
URL: http://www.liverfoundation.org

Part Nine

Liver Transplantation

Chapter 50

What Every Patient Needs to Know

Chapter Contents

Section 50.1

Liver Transplant Overview

Reprinted with permission "Liver Transplant,"
© 1998 Chek Med Systems, Inc.

The liver is the largest organ in the body. It is found high in the right upper abdomen, behind the ribs. It is a very complex organ and has many functions. They include:

- Storing energy in the form of sugar (glucose)
- Storing vitamins, iron, and other minerals
- Making proteins, including blood clotting factors, to keep the body healthy and help it grow
- Processing worn out red blood cells
- Making bile which is needed for food digestion
- Metabolizing or breaking down many medications and alcohol
- Killing germs that enter the body through the intestine

The liver also has a remarkable power to regenerate itself. However, there are illnesses that can cause permanent and irreversible damage to the liver. Liver transplantation has become a standard treatment for a patient whose liver no longer functions well enough to maintain life. This revolutionary treatment has moved from research and the first actual transplant in the 1960s, to a standard form of therapy in the 1990s. There are two main reasons why liver transplants have become so successful. There have been major advances in surgical techniques, and new drugs are now available to prevent rejection of the new liver.

Reasons for Liver Transplantation

Medical treatment for liver diseases and liver damage is always the first choice of therapy. The only reason to perform a liver transplant is

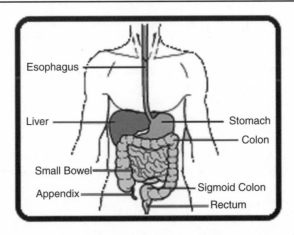

Figure 50.1. *The Digestive System*

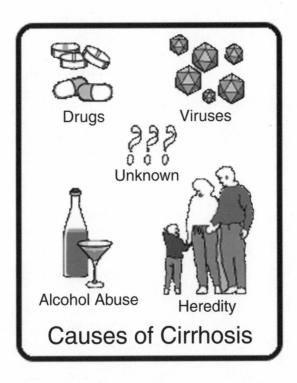

Figure 50.2. *Cirrhosis is severe and advanced scarring of the liver. It leads to end stage liver disease.*

that all other forms of treatment have been unsuccessful, and the patient's liver can no longer support life. This is called end stage liver disease. There have been over 60 different liver diseases treated with liver transplantation. However, there are several conditions that are more commonly treated with this procedure. They are frequently conditions that cause chronic or continuing liver inflammation. As the inflammation heals, fibrous tissue forms, much like a scar forms when a cut in the skin heals. Severe and advanced scarring of the liver is called cirrhosis. Cirrhosis is not reversible and leads to end stage liver disease. The following conditions are the most common causes of end stage liver disease:

- Chronic viral hepatitis B and C
- Alcohol related liver disease
- Autoimmune hepatitis
- Primary sclerosing cholangitis
- Primary biliary cirrhosis
- Steatohepatitis
- Liver disorders inherited or present at birth
- Drug induced liver damage

In children, the most common cause of liver failure is biliary atresia. This is a condition in which the bile ducts fail to develop. These ducts carry bile from the liver to the intestine. If there are no ducts, the bile backs up in the liver and causes damage. Biliary atresia is usually present at birth.

Special Considerations

Alcoholism is a common cause of end stage liver disease. Although these patients are not denied a liver transplant, all transplant centers will insist on a thorough psychological evaluation beforehand. They also require treatment of the alcoholism, proven abstinence for at least six months, and good prospects that the patient will continue to abstain from alcohol. A transplanted liver will become severely damaged by alcohol just like the old one.

Most patients infected with hepatitis B and some with Hepatitis C recover completely with no further liver damage. However, some will develop chronic hepatitis leading to cirrhosis and end stage liver disease. This is more common with Hepatitis C. A liver transplant under these circumstances is difficult to manage because the new liver almost always becomes infected with these viruses. Ongoing treatment is usually necessary to keep the new liver healthy.

Most cancers of the liver develop in other parts of the body and spread to the liver. These patients are never transplanted because their cancer is not curable. Occasionally, cancer develops first in the liver. This is called a primary cancer or hepatoma. When a primary liver cancer is identified early, a liver transplant will be performed. However, long-term survival is less common in this case than with transplants for other conditions.

Transplant Centers

Transplant centers are very specialized facilities that are usually located at university teaching hospitals or large medical centers. They require a large staff of surgeons and other professionals to evaluate and select patients, and perform surgery and follow-up care. In addition, they must maintain close communications with transplant candidates and the national network that rations the livers as they become available. All transplant centers have equal access to technical skills and drugs to prevent rejection, so survival rates depend a great deal on the underlying disease of the recipient. Primary cancer of the liver has the lowest long-term survival at about 50%-60%. Primary biliary cirrhosis and primary sclerosing cholangitis have survival rates of over 90%. Transplants that are performed for other diseases have survival rates ranging somewhere in between these figures.

Unfortunately, there are more patients who need a new liver than there are donors. Choosing who gets a liver can be difficult, so a fair system of allocation had to be developed. There is an organization called United Network for Organ Sharing (UNOS) in Richmond, VA. UNOS provides a distribution plan to each transplant center, based on population. Donor livers almost always come from individuals who have suffered fatal brain damage due to trauma, rather than disease. Ideally, physicians and patients should be able to plan and perform a transplant before the patient reaches end stage liver disease. However, because of the lack of donor livers, the choice of who gets a new liver now depends on how critically ill the patient is. Other considerations, such as a patient's psychological make-up, are a part of the decision. For example, an unreformed alcoholic will have little chance for a liver transplant. The patient's family situation and support at home are also factors. Often a panel of lay people and medical personnel will help make the choice at each transplant center. Once patients are selected as candidates, they are placed on the active transplant list and given a beeper to wear at all times. This is so they can get to the transplant center at a moment's notice. If for some reason the patient selected is not suitable for the operation at the time a liver becomes available, there is always a back-up candidate for each donor liver.

Surgery

Liver transplantation is a complicated process. There are really three operations involved. The first is the removal of the liver from the donor. If the liver is donated at a different location, it must be transferred to the transplant center under sterile refrigerated conditions within 8 to 20 hours. The second operation is the removal of the diseased liver from the patient, and the third is the operation to insert and connect the new liver. The operations on the recipient are so detailed they require a long time to complete. But, the team of surgeons, nurses, and support staff are now very experienced in the technique. The new liver is attached to the various blood vessels and bile ducts. When the surgery is completed, the patient goes to the recovery area.

Recovery

Recovery begins with several weeks in the hospital. Immediately after surgery, the patient is in intensive care for a time. This is so there can be continual monitoring for any infection, rejection, or poor functioning of the new liver. Rejection occurs because the transplanted liver is recognized as foreign by the body. This is the body's normal reaction to any foreign substance. The body's rejection of the transplant would cause inflammation and damage to the new liver. Because of this, medications must be given to calm the rejection reaction in the body. Long-term treatment against rejection is always necessary.

There are three main medications used to prevent rejection. One is a cortisone drug, usually prednisone (trade names: Deltasone, Orasone). It is often used in a low dose. The side effects are fluid build-up and puffiness of the face. A more serious side effect is a change in the bones. Prednisone causes a loss of calcium that can lead to osteoporosis and damage to joints such as knees, hips, and shoulders. A second drug is called Sandimmune. Sandimmune is difficult to regulate and can produce high blood pressure, kidney damage, and occasionally growth of body hair. A third drug is Prograf. This drug has been dramatic in providing successful transplants with the lowest side effects. But even here, kidney damage can occur. It is easy to see why close follow-up is needed for patients on these drugs. Frequent blood tests are required to monitor the patient's progress and reduce side effects.

As recovery progresses, the patient is released to outpatient status, but must stay close to the transplant center for daily visits and blood testing. Finally as things stabilize, the patient is sent home to the care of his/her personal physician. Usually, follow-up is maintained with the patient's physicians at the transplant center. Once patients have recovered, they can resume normal physical and sexual activities. Even vigorous exercise is possible after full recovery, but this should only be done after discussion with the physician. There are few dietary restrictions. The patient is often advised to restrict salt (sodium) intake. A well-balanced diet with adequate protein is necessary. For reasons that are not clear, obesity frequently becomes a problem with liver transplant patients. To avoid this problem, patients should take control of their calorie intake early on.

As the body becomes familiar with the transplanted liver, the amount of medicine needed to control rejection can be adjusted and usually reduced. However, most liver transplant patients will always have to take at least some medication.

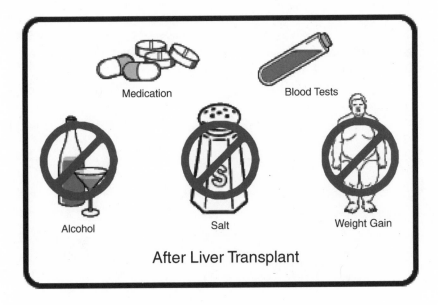

Figure 50.3. Recovery Requirements

Liver Donation

It is very important that more livers become available for donation. All healthy people are encouraged to make arrangements to become liver donors if they are ever in a situation that would make this possible. Generally, there are no restrictions on age, sex, or race. The only matching requirements for livers are that the donor and recipient must be about the same size and have compatible blood types. Some states allow people to register to become organ donors when they apply for or renew a driver's license. Anyone wishing to become an organ donor should carry an organ donor card or an ID card with an organ donor sticker attached. It is important to discuss organ donation with family members, because they must always give consent when the circumstances take place.

Summary

Liver transplantation is an important move forward in the treatment of severe liver disease. It has opened a new world for patients who otherwise were destined to die from their liver disease. The operation is a major one, and there are still problems associated with medications used to prevent rejection. But overall, patients can usually expect a good outcome with return to normal activities.

This material does not cover all information and is not intended as a substitute for professional care. Please consult with your physician on any matters regarding your health.

Section 50.2

Preparing for Your Transplant

The Transplant Experience

1. Your doctor recommends that you be evaluated for a transplant.

2. You are evaluated for a transplant by the medical team at a transplant center.

3. Once you have been accepted as a transplant candidate, you are registered on the UNOS waiting list.

4. You begin mapping your financial strategy.

5. The waiting period begins.

6. The transplant takes place.

7. A plan is developed for post-transplant care.

The Transplantation Network

What Is the United Network for Organ Sharing?

The transplant community is joined under a nationwide umbrella: the United Network for Organ Sharing, or UNOS. From its Richmond, Virginia, headquarters, UNOS members and staff serve transplant patients in a variety of ways.

What Does UNOS Do?

- UNOS manages the national transplant waiting list, matching donors to recipients 24 hours a day, 365 days a year.

- UNOS monitors every organ match to ensure adherence to UNOS policy.

- UNOS members work together to develop equitable policies that maximize the limited supply of organs and give all patients a fair chance at receiving the organ they need—regardless of age, sex, race or religion; lifestyle, financial, or social status.

- UNOS sets professional standards for efficiency and quality patient care.

- UNOS maintains the database that contains all clinical transplant data. These data are used to improve the medicine and science of transplantation, develop organ allocation policy, support transplant professionals in caring for patients, and help patients make informed healthcare decisions.

- UNOS raises public awareness about the importance of organ donation and works to keep patients informed about transplant issues and policy.

How Is UNOS Funded?

UNOS is a non-profit scientific and educational organization. Through federal contracts, UNOS coordinates the Organ Procurement and Transplantation Network (OPTN) and the U.S. Scientific Registry of Organ Transplant Recipients (SR).

These two contracts represent about 15 percent of the organization's total operating budget. UNOS relies mostly upon membership fees, charitable donations, and project-specific grants from foundations and corporations.

Commonly Asked Questions about Transplantation

How Are Patients Added to the UNOS Waiting List?

When a patient's physician determines that an organ transplant may be necessary, the patient is referred to a transplant center for evaluation. The medical team at the transplant center considers the patient's past and present medical condition, and such factors as his or her history of complying with past medical directives, and the emotional support from the patient's family or friends. Transplant candidates are then placed on the UNOS waiting list.

What Qualifications Must Patients Meet to Be Placed on the Waiting List?

Traditionally, each transplant center has used its own criteria to list patients. Recently, UNOS committees, consisting of transplant professionals, recipients, and donor family members, have developed uniform guidelines to determine the minimal qualifications a candidate must meet.

How Are Donor Organs Matched to Patients Awaiting Transplant?

When a patient is added to the transplant waiting list, his or her medical profile is entered in the UNOS computer. The computer adds the patient's name to a "pool" of patient names. When an organ donor becomes available, all patients in the pool are compared to that particular donor. The computer then generates a list of patients who match the donor organ.

Matches are based on many criteria, including medical urgency of the transplant candidate, time spent on the waiting list, biologic compatibility between the donor and the recipient (such as organ size, blood type, and genetic makeup), and the candidate's ability to be transplanted immediately. Donated organs are distributed locally first. If no suitable match exists in the local area, the organ is offered regionally, then nationally.

Can Patients List at More than One Transplant Center?

Yes. This is called "multiple listing" and permits patients to be considered for organs that become available in other areas. Patients should keep in mind that there is no advantage to listing at more than one transplant center in the same OPO local area. Each center has its own criteria for who it accepts as a candidate and reserves the right to decline patients who are listed at other centers. Patients who wish to list at more than one center should inform the centers they contact of their plans.

How Long Does It Take to Receive an Organ?

Patients added to the UNOS waiting list may receive an organ that day, or they may wait years. Factors affecting waiting time include how well the donor and recipient match, the medical urgency status of the patient, and the availability of donors compared to the number of patients waiting in a geographic area. UNOS publishes waiting time statistics by geographic region, sex, age, blood type, and race in its statistical annual report.

Does UNOS Oversee Donation and Transplantation Around the World?

No. However, UNOS provides a list of similar organizations in other countries that may be contacted for transplant information.

Can a Patient from Another Country Receive a Transplant in the U.S.?

Yes. Patients can travel from other countries to the U.S. to receive transplants. Once accepted by a UNOS transplant center, international patients receive organs based on the same policies as those that apply to U.S. citizens.

How Can I Find Out about UNOS Policy Changes and Legislation that Affect Organ Transplantation and Donation?

Publication of information on policy and legislation occurs routinely on the UNOS World Wide Web site (www.unos.org) and in UNOS publications. UNOS also maintains a mailing list of patients and members of the public who wish to receive policy proposals published for public comment. To request these resources, please contact UNOS.

How Can I Receive UNOS Data on Organ Transplantation and Donation?

Phone toll-free (888) TX INFO-1 or visit the UNOS World Wide Web site at www.unos.org.

Terms You Need To Know—A Transplant Glossary

Allograft

An organ or tissue transplanted from one individual to another of the same species; i.e. human to human. Example: a transplanted kidney.

Antibody

A protein substance made by the body's immune system in response to a foreign substance, for example a previous transplant,

408

blood transfusion, virus, or pregnancy. Because the antibodies attack the transplanted organ, transplant patients must take powerful anti-rejection drugs.

Antigen

A foreign substance, such as a transplant, that triggers an immune response. This response may be the production of antibodies, which try to inactivate or destroy the antigen (the transplanted organ).

Anti-Rejection Drugs

Medicines developed to suppress the immune response so that the body will accept, rather than reject, a transplanted organ or tissue. These medicines are also called immunosuppressants.

Brain Death

When the brain has permanently stopped working, as determined by the physician. Artificial support systems may maintain functions such as heartbeat and respiration for a few days, but not permanently. Donor organs are usually taken from persons declared brain dead.

Coalition on Donation

A non-profit alliance of health and science professionals, transplant patients, and voluntary health and transplant organizations. The Coalition works to increase public awareness of the critical organ shortage and create a greater willingness and commitment to organ and tissue donation.

Compliance

The act of following orders, adhering to rules and policies. Example: taking medications as directed.

Crossmatch

A blood test for patient antibodies against donor antigens. A positive crossmatch shows that the donor and patient are incompatible. A negative crossmatch means there is no reaction between donor and patient and that the transplant may proceed.

Cyclosporine

A drug used following organ transplantation to prevent rejection of the transplanted organ by suppressing the body's defense system.

Durable Power of Attorney

A document in which individuals may designate someone to make medical decisions for them when they are unable to speak for themselves.

ESRD

End-Stage Renal Disease/chronic kidney failure. A condition in which the kidneys no longer function and for which patients need dialysis or a transplant.

Graft

A transplanted organ or tissue.

HLA (Human Leukocyte Antigens)

Molecules found on cells in the body that characterize each individual as unique. Human leukocyte antigens (HLA) are inherited from one's parents. In donor-recipient matching, HLA determines whether an organ from one individual will be accepted by another.

HLA System

There are three major genetically controlled groups: HLA-A, HLA-B, and HLA-DR. In transplantation, the HLA tissue types of the donor and recipient are important in determining whether the transplant will be accepted or rejected. Genetic matching is routinely performed on kidneys and pancreases only.

Immune response

The body's natural defense against foreign objects or organisms such as bacteria, viruses, or transplanted organs or tissue.

Immunosuppression

The artificial suppression of the immune response, usually through drugs, so that the body will not reject a transplanted organ or tissue.

Drugs commonly used to suppress the immune system .after transplant include prednisone, azathioprine (Imuran), cyclosporine (Sandimmune, Neoral), OKT3 and ALG, mycophenolate mofetil (CeliCept), and tacrolimus (Prograf, FK506).

Informed Consent

A process of reaching an agreement based on a full understanding of what will take place. Informed consent has components of disclosure, comprehension, competence, and voluntary response.

NOTA (National Organ Transplant Act)

Passed by Congress in 1984, NOTA outlawed the sale of human organs and initiated the development of a national system for organ sharing and a scientific registry to collect and report transplant data.

Organ Preservation

Donated organs require special methods of preservation to keep them viable between procurement and transplantation. Without preservation, the organ will deteriorate. The length of time organs and tissues can be kept outside the body vary depending on the organ, the preservation fluid, and the temperature.

Organ Preservation Time

- Heart—4-6 hours
- Liver—12-24 hours
- Kidney—48-72 hours
- Heart-Lung—4-6 hours
- Lung—4-6 hours
- Pancreas—12-24 hours

Organ Procurement

Recovery or retrieval of organs and tissues for transplantation.

Organ Procurement Organization (OPO)

OPO's serve as the vital link between the donor and recipient and are responsible for the retrieval, preservation, and transportation of organs for transplantation. As a resource to the community they serve, they engage in public education on the critical need for organ donation. Currently, there are 69 OPO's around the country. All are UNOS members.

OPO Local Area

Each OPO provides its organ procurement services to the transplant programs in its area. An OPO's local service area can include a portion of a city, a portion of a state, or an entire state.

When an organ becomes available, the list of potential recipients is generated from the OPO's local service area. If a patient match is not made in that local area, a wider, regional list of patients waiting is generated.

Panel Reactive Antibody (PRA)

The percentage of cells from a panel of donors with which a potential recipient's blood serum reacts. The more antibodies in the recipient's blood, the more likely the recipient will react against the potential donor. The higher the PRA, the less chance of receiving an organ that will not be rejected. Patients with a high PRA have priority on the waiting list.

Rejection

Rejection occurs when the body tries to destroy a transplanted organ or tissue because it sees the graft as a foreign object and produces antibodies to destroy it. Immunosuppressive (anti-rejection) drugs help prevent rejection.

Retransplantation

Due to organ rejection or transplant failure, some patients need another transplant and return to the waiting list. Reducing the number of retransplants is critical when examining ways to maximize a limited supply of donor organs.

Required Request

Hospitals must tell the families of suitable donors that their loved one's organs and tissues can be used for transplant. This law is expected to increase the number of donated organs and tissues for transplantation by giving more people the opportunity to donate.

Sensitization

When there are antibodies in the blood of the potential recipient, usually because of pregnancy, blood transfusions, or previous rejection of an organ transplant. Sensitization is measured by panel reactive antibody (PRA). Highly sensitized patients are less likely to match with a suitable donor and more likely to reject an organ than unsensitized patients.

Status

A code number used to indicate the degree of medical urgency for patients awaiting heart or liver transplants.

Survival Rates

Survival rates indicate what percentage of patients are alive or grafts (organs) are still functioning after a certain amount of time. Survival rates are used in developing UNOS policy. Because survival rates improve with technological and scientific advances, developing policies that reflect and respond to these advances will also improve survival rates.

Tissue Typing

The examination of human leukocyte antigens (HLA) in a patient. Tissue typing (genetic matching) is done for all donors and recipients in kidney transplantation to help match the donor to the most suitable recipient.

U.S. Scientific Registry of Transplant Recipients

A database of post-transplant information. Follow-up data on every transplant are used to track transplant center performance, transplant success rates, and medical issues impacting transplant recipients. Under contract with the Health Resources and Services Administration (HRSA), UNOS facilitates the collection, tracking, and reporting of transplant recipient and donor data.

Waiting List

After evaluation by the transplant physician, a patient is added to the national waiting list by the transplant center. Lists are specific to both geographic area and organ type: heart, lung, kidney, liver, pancreas, intestine, heart-lung, and kidney-pancreas.

Each time a donor organ becomes available, the UNOS computer generates a list of potential recipients based on factors that include genetic similarity, organ size, medical urgency, and time on the waiting list. Through this process, a "new" list is generated each time an organ becomes available that best "matches" a patient to a donated organ.

Xenograft

An organ or tissue procured from an animal for transplantation into a human.

Xenotransplantation

Transplantation of an animal organ into a human. Although xenotransplantation is highly experimental, many scientists view it as an eventual solution to the shortage of human organs.

Section 50.3

The Transplant Process

Registration

Choosing a Transplant Center

As of November 12, 1997, there were 275 transplant centers in the U.S. These centers are fully accredited and must meet a variety of stringent professional standards. When determining which transplant center(s) to list with, many patients simply choose the facility closest to them.

There are many considerations, in addition to the patient's relationship with the transplant team, which must be considered when choosing a transplant center:

- **Convenience:** travel time and costs associated with travel

- **Cost:** cost of living in that area before and after transplant

- **Follow-up Care:** routine check-ups, possible emergency care

- **Moral Support:** availability of family and friends for help and moral support.

Evaluating Outcome Performance

To help patients evaluate transplant center performance, UNOS publishes a Report of Center Specific Graft and Patient Survival Rates. This report provides actual and expected graft and patient survival rates per transplant program. This information helps patients compare outcomes of the transplant programs they are considering with the national average. This report is available by calling UNOS at 888 TX INFO-1.

Multiple Listing

A patient may wish to register at more than one transplant center. However, each center determines who it accepts as candidates and reserves the right to decline patients who are listed at other centers. Patients should inform the centers they contact of their multiple listing plans.

Questions a Patient Should Ask

Patients should ask the following questions when evaluating a transplant center and its staff:

- What are my choices besides transplantation?
- What are the benefits and risks of transplantation?
- What does the evaluation and testing process include?
- How does it affect whether I am put on the list?
- What are the organ and patient survival rates for my type of transplant at this hospital?
- How many of my type of transplant do you perform each year?
- How long have you been doing them?
- What are your criteria for accepting organ offers?
- What part of the transplant cost is covered by my insurance?
- What financial coverage is accepted by the hospital?
- How much will I have to pay?
- What happens if my financial coverage runs out?
- Who are the members of the transplant team and what are their jobs?
- How many attending surgeons are available to do my type of transplant?
- Who will tell me about the transplant process?
- Is there a special nursing unit for transplant patients?
- Can I tour the transplant center?
- Will I be asked to take part in research studies?

- Does the hospital do living donor transplants? Is a living donor transplant a choice in my case? If so, where will the living donor evaluation be done?

- What are the organ recovery costs if I have a living donor?

How Organ Matching Works

The Transplant Waiting List

All patients accepted onto a transplant program's waiting list are registered with UNOS. UNOS maintains a centralized computer network linking all organ procurement organizations and transplant centers. Organ placement specialists operate the network 24 hours per day, seven days a week.

The Matching Process

When an organ becomes available, the local procurement organization coordinates the surgical recovery team, accesses the UNOS computer, enters information about the donor organs, and runs the match program. This computer program generates a list of patients ranked according to objective medical criteria such as blood type, tissue type, size of the organ, and the patient's medical urgency. Other factors are time spent on the waiting list and distance between the donor and the transplant center. The specific criteria differ for each type of organ.

The list of patients waiting in the local area is checked first (except for kidneys, which are sent to perfectly matched patients, regardless of where they live, if such a match exists). If no match is made with the patients listed locally, the organ is checked against the regional list of patients waiting. If no match is made on the regional list, the organ is made available to patients nationwide.

The computerized matching process can locate best possible matches between donor organs and the patients who need them, but the final decision rests with the patient's transplant team.

The Five Steps in Organ Matching

1. An organ is donated. When an organ becomes available, the OPO managing the donor sends information to UNOS. The OPO procurement team reports medical and genetic information, including organ size and condition, blood type, and tissue type.

2. UNOS generates a list of potential recipients. The UNOS computer generates a list of potential transplant candidates who have medical and biologic profiles compatible with the donor's. The computer ranks candidates by this biologic information, as well as clinical characteristics and time spent on the waiting list.

3. The transplant center is notified of an available organ. Organ placement specialists at the OPO or the UNOS Organ Center contact the centers whose patients appear on the local list.

4. The transplant team considers the organ for the patient. When the team is offered an organ, it bases its acceptance or refusal of the organ upon established medical criteria, organ condition, candidate condition, staff and patient availability, and organ transportation. The transplant team has only one hour to make its decision.

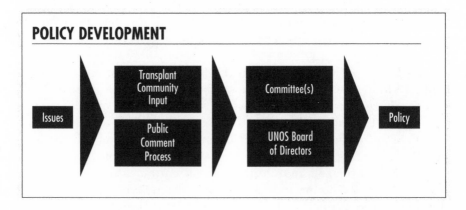

POLICY DEVELOPMENT

Issues → Transplant Community Input / Public Comment Process → Committee(s) / UNOS Board of Directors → Policy

Figure 50.4. How Policies Are Made. The organ distribution and matching process is based on policies developed by UNOS members. As the science of transplantation continues to advance, UNOS policies also evolve. The goal of UNOS policy-making is to create a system that gives every transplant candidate a fair chance at receiving the organ he or she needs. Organ transplantation is the only discipline in American medicine in which patients have a formal role in the policy-making process.

5. The organ is accepted or declined. If the organ is not accepted, the OPO continues to offer it for patients at other centers until it is placed.

The Organ Offer

When an organ is offered, the transplant team must consider several factors to decide the best medical care for each individual patient. It is not unusual for a transplant team to say "no" to a particular organ. This is a normal part of the matching process. After being turned down for one patient, the organ is offered to the next patient on the list. These offers continue until the organ is placed.

Facts about UNOS

- Organ sharing policies forbid favoritism based upon political influence, race, gender, religion, or financial or social status. Sharing is based upon medical and scientific criteria.

- UNOS' Scientific Registry contains data on every solid organ transplant since October 1, 1987. This is the most comprehensive data analysis system for a single mode of therapy anywhere in the world.

- UNOS data are available on request to anyone who asks. However, to protect the privacy of all transplant patients and ensure anonymity, each patient's name is replaced with a code number at registration.

- UNOS data enable scientists and physicians to exchange information vital for the progress of transplantation and help patients make informed decisions about their care.

Section 50.4

Developing Your Financial Strategy

Social Services Available for Transplant Patients

No matter where you are in the transplant process, you do not have
to face your concerns alone. Your transplant team recognizes that living with a transplant will affect your lifestyle in many ways. Your
transplant team will help you resume many of your former activities
and become involved in new ones.

Transplant Social Workers

Every transplant program is staffed with social workers who are
ready to help you. Transplant social workers can counsel you and your
family and provide a variety of helpful resources. They can also help
you develop your financial plan.

Through an informal interview, your social worker will determine
your needs and help you understand and cope with basic problems
associated with your illness, such as:

- inability to pay your medical bills;

- lack of funds to meet daily needs;

- lack of reliable transportation to and from the transplant facility;

- referrals for re-employment services;

- help in caring for children or other family members.

You have a right to request that the information you share with
your social worker be kept confidential—as long as the information
is not vital to your medical care.

Financial Coordinators

Although the social worker may have knowledge about government funding and disability programs, financial issues are only a part of his or her responsibilities. The financial coordinator has detailed knowledge of financial matters and hospital billing methods.

Social workers and financial coordinators work together to determine how you can best afford the cost of your transplant.

The Costs of Transplantation

Transplant costs include:

- transplant evaluation and testing;

- transplant surgery;

- follow-up care, lab tests, and medication.

Even before the transplant, these costs add up quickly.

One of the biggest expenses is related to time spent in the hospital's intensive care unit (ICU). The ICU is staffed by critical care nurses and is equipped to monitor and treat critically ill patients. Patients are generally taken to the ICU after the transplant operation, but some are also treated in the ICU before the transplant.

If you are traveling any distance to receive your transplant, remember to consider the cost of food, lodging, and transportation. The cost of food and lodging for your family while you are in the hospital can vary greatly from city to city. Some centers offer families lodging at reduced or no cost, while other centers do not. More than likely, these expenses will not be covered by insurance.

In addition, there may be lost earnings if your employer does not pay for the time you or your spouse spend away from work.

Other costs directly associated with transplantation include:

- fees for transplant surgeons and operating room personnel;

- anesthesia;

- recovery and in-hospital stay;

- extensive lab tests;

- charges for evaluating and accepting a patient for transplant;

- recovery of the organ from the donor;

421

- transportation to and from the transplant center—not only for the transplant, but for patient evaluation and check-ups;

- laboratory tests;

- child care;

- physical or occupational therapy and other rehabilitation;

- and the cost of anti-rejection drugs and other medications, which can easily exceed $10,000 per year for the rest of the recipient's life.

Estimated Charges for Liver Transplantation

In 1996 dollars the estimated cost of a liver transplant was $314,500 with estimated annual follow-up charges being $21,900 (1996 dollars). Your transplant could cost much less or much more, depending on how many of the services are included in your bill and the area in which your transplant takes place. Some transplant patients and families find that even with good sources of funding, they may have difficulty covering all of the costs associated with transplantation. The following sections will help you explore your options for covering all of your transplant costs.

Financing Transplantation

Few patients are able to pay all of the costs of transplantation from a single source. For example, you may be able to finance the transplant procedure through insurance coverage and pay for other expenses by drawing on savings accounts and other private funds or by selling some of your assets. Most likely, you will have to rely on a combination of funding sources. Its a good idea to keep your transplant center social workers and financial coordinators informed of your progress in obtaining funds.

The most common funding sources are:

- Insurance;

- Extending Insurance Coverage through COBRA

- Medicare Coverage;

- Tricare (HMO)-CHAMPUS (Civilian Health and Medical Program of the Uniformed Services)

- Charitable Organizations;

- Advocacy Organizations; and

- Fund Raising Campaigns.

Insurance

You or your family may have health insurance coverage through an employer or a personal policy. Many insurance companies offer at least optional coverage for transplant costs. However, the terms and extent of insurance coverage vary widely. Read your policy carefully and contact the insurance company if you have questions.

Usually, insurance companies will pay about 80 percent of your hospital charges. This means that you are responsible for the remaining 20 percent from other sources until you reach your "out-of-pocket" limit. Be sure to pay your premiums so that your policy will not lapse.

Most insurance policies have some sort of lifetime maximum amount, or "cap". After a patient has reached this amount, the insurance company does not have to pay any additional benefits. The amount of the cap varies greatly, depending on the individual policy. The cap may apply to just one procedure or treatment or to all combined procedures and treatments. Even after the actual transplant, the ongoing cost of care may exceed the cap, so it is important to be familiar with the amount and terms of your insurance cap and how your insurance dollars are spent.

Some insurers consider certain transplant procedures "experimental" or "investigational" and do not cover these cases. If you have any doubts about how your coverage is determined, contact your insurance company. If you still have questions, contact the office of your state insurance commissioner. Some potential insurers may consider you "uninsurable" if you have certain medical conditions. This may be a particular problem if you work for a small business or are self-employed. More that 25 states have "risk pools, " which are state programs that provide benefits to people who are otherwise declared uninsurable.

In other states, you may qualify for a "community rate" plan, which some insurers offer as a non-profit service. You must still pay insurance premiums to participate in these plans. These premiums may be more expensive than the average insurance premium. Your state insurance commissioner can tell you if these options are available to you.

Many companies require prior authorization (approval) for organ transplant procedures. Make sure you are not in a waiting period for coverage for conditions you may have had before joining the insurance plan. Delays in insurance payments can cause you unnecessary stress, so make arrangements with your insurance company prior to the transplant. Transplant center social workers and financial coordinators will help you with the information you need to complete this process.

You may want to seek help from an advocacy or charitable organization or a legal advisor to negotiate with your insurer. For example, if the company does not wish to cover your transplant, you may be able to prove that it has covered similar procedures in the past, or that a transplant would be more cost-effective than your current care (especially in the case of dialysis). If you can, you may have a better chance of getting coverage for your particular case.

Extending Insurance Coverage through COBRA (Consolidated Omnibus Budget Reconciliation Act)

If you are insured by a group health plan (medical, dental or vision) through your place of work and you must leave your job or have your work hours reduced, you and your family may qualify for extended coverage through COBRA.

COBRA stands for the Consolidated Omnibus Budget Reconciliation Act of 1985. This is a federal law that requires certain group health plans to allow participating employees and their dependents to extend their insurance coverage for up to 36 months when benefits would otherwise end. This requirement is limited to companies employing 20 or more people. While you may receive extended coverage through COBRA, you would still be fully responsible for premium payments to your group health plan. Learn more by contacting your employer's employee benefits office.

Qualifying for Extended Coverage

As an employee covered by a group health plan, you may continue your coverage for up to 18 months in the following cases:

- you leave your job voluntarily or involuntarily (for reasons other than misconduct), or

- your working hours are reduced beyond the minimum amount to qualify for health benefits.

If you are considered disabled under Social Security guidelines at the time you leave your job, you may choose to continue your health coverage for up to 29 months, after which you become eligible for

Medicare. You have to show that you are insurable in order to continue your coverage.

If you leave your job because of your disability, you may be able to keep your life insurance if your policy has a disability waiver. You may do this as long as you notify your insurer and provide proof of your disability.

Deadline for Choosing Extended Coverage

By law, you have 60 days from the day you leave your job to decide whether to continue participating in your health plan through COBRA. When you leave your job, your employer must notify you of your right to continue, how much your premium will be, and where payment should be made. If you do not respond within 60 days, you cannot extend your benefits.

If you work for an employer with less than 20 employees, you may be able to convert your policy to an individual policy at the end of your coverage period. If you are eligible to continue coverage through COBRA, you should receive information from your employer telling you how to participate. If you have additional questions, check with your employer.

Coverage may end before the maximum time limit in any of the following cases:

- the premium is not paid;

- the company holding the policy stops offering an employee group health plan;

- a covered beneficiary joins another group health plan;

- or a covered beneficiary becomes eligible for Medicare.

This is only a brief summary and is not intended to provide complete information.

Portability and Accountability Act of 1996

On August 21, 1996, the Health Insurance Portability and Accountability Act of 1996 (HIPAA) was enacted. The HIPAA changed the continuation of coverage requirements under the Consolidated Omnibus Budget Reconciliation Act of 1985 (COBRA). It also required that qualified beneficiaries be notified of certain HIPAA changes to COBRA that may affect their COBRA rights. The new requirements were generally effective as of January 1, 1997, regardless of whether the qualifying event occurred before, on, or after that date.

Under COBRA, if the qualifying event is a termination or a reduction in hours, qualified beneficiaries are allowed to continue coverage for up to 18 months, subject to timely premium payments. In addition to changing some of the COBRA requirements, HIPAA restricts the extent to which group health plans may impose limits on pre-existing conditions, enabling workers to change jobs without a lapse in coverage of these conditions, in many cases.

When you leave your health plan, your employer must provide proof of when you were covered under the employer's group plan.

Medicare Coverage

State and federal government funding is another possibility for coverage under two programs:

* Medicare, operated by the federal government, and
* Medicaid, administered by each state with federal assistance.

These programs are often considered an "insurance of last resort," particularly Medicaid, as they are generally offered to patients and families with no other resources to meet their expenses. You may qualify for Medicare as part of your Social Security disability benefits. Some states do not cover transplants through Medicaid.

Medicare is a federally-funded health insurance program available to retirees, the disabled, and other qualifying individuals, such as dependents of Medicare beneficiaries. Medicare offers two basic plans: Part A and Part B.

Part A covers basic hospital care and some types of follow-up treatment. It is funded by tax money and is offered free to those who qualify. Part B covers additional services such as doctor bills. It is supported partly by federal funds and partly by premiums paid by those who wish to participate.

Medicare, like most private insurance plans, does not pay 100 percent of your costs. In most cases, it pays hospitals and health providers according to a fixed fee schedule, which may be less than the actual cost. You must pay deductibles and various other expenses. Many people choose to buy a private insurance policy, often called a supplemental or "Medigap" policy, to pay for expenses Medicare does not cover. Check with a local insurance agent for further information on the availability of these policies.

Medicare currently offers coverage for kidney, heart, lung, heart-lung, and liver transplants. This coverage includes payment for a number of the direct costs of the transplant operation. Patients who receive transplants as of July 1, 1995, are eligible for 36 months of immunosuppressive drug coverage through the Omnibus Budget Reconciliation Act (OBRA) of 1993.

To receive full Medicare benefits for a transplant, you must go to a Medicare approved transplant program. These programs meet Medicare criteria for the number of transplants they perform and the overall quality of patient outcomes. Nearly all kidney transplant programs meet these criteria. Medicare has also approved more than 60 heart programs and more than 30 liver programs nationwide and certifies additional programs as they qualify.

You may have to meet certain patient selection criteria to be eligible for Medicare coverage. These criteria may include your age and the medical condition for which you need a transplant.

If you have additional questions regarding Medicare eligibility, Medicare benefits for transplants, or Medicare-approved transplant programs, contact the office of your local Medicare provider or your local Social Security office.

CHAMPUS (Civilian Health and Medical Program of the Uniformed Services)

Government funding for families of active duty, retired or deceased personnel may be available through the Civilian Health and Medical Program of the Uniformed Services (CHAMPUS). CHAMPUS shares the cost of heart, lung, heart-lung, liver, kidney and combined liver-kidney transplants for patients with end-stage organ disease. Patients must receive pre-authorization from the CHAMPUS medical director and meet CHAMPUS selection criteria. Pre-authorization is based on a narrative summary submitted by the attending transplant physician.

Veterans of the Armed Forces who first became ill while in service or who are indigent as defined by the Veterans Administration (VA) may be eligible to receive a transplant at a VA Medical Center. Some veterans may also receive medications funded by the VA. For further information, contact your local VA office or your nearest VA Medical Center.

For more information regarding CHAMPUS transplantation benefits, contact the health benefits advisory at your nearest military healthcare facility or call the CHAMPUS Benefits Service Branch.

Charitable Organizations

Charitable organizations offer different types of support. Some provide information about diseases of certain organs or about a particular type of transplant and encourage research into these diseases and treatments.

Other groups provide limited financial assistance through grants and direct funding. However, it is very unlikely that one group can cover all of the costs for an individual patient. An organization may have limits on using available funds and may only be able to help with direct transplant costs, food and lodging, or medication costs.

Many groups can help you explore other funding sources, ask an insurance company to reconsider a case or help you sort out difficulties with Medicaid funding.

Advocacy Organizations

Advocacy organizations advise transplant patients on financial matters. They should be able to provide supporting information and background documentation to prove they are legally recognized to help those in need. Ask them to provide you with copies of the following documents:

- their current federal or state certification as a charitable, non-profit organization;

- their current by-laws, constitution, and/or articles of incorporation; and

- their financial statement for the preceding year, preferably one that has been audited by an independent organization.

You should review each document before entering into a commitment with any of these organizations. This is important, because patient financial needs must be met in a timely, agreed upon fashion. It is a good idea to ask the organization for references (for example, the names and phone numbers of other patients they have helped). You may also want to ask members of your transplant team about their knowledge of the organization.

Brochures and other background information should never serve as substitutes for the documents listed above.

If you agree to a financial arrangement, make sure that the funds are available in a manner that suits your needs. Because this is so important, you may want legal assistance in reviewing the written agreement before it is signed. Your bank can also help you review the arrangement.

Review all documents, including insurance policies and funding agreements, very carefully. Inspect the fine print and make sure that all of your questions are answered to your satisfaction. Your needs must come first.

Fund Raising Campaigns

Patients and families often use public fund raising to help cover expenses not paid by medical insurance. This may be a key source for financing transplantation.

Proceed with caution and plan carefully before you begin, as there are many legal and financial issues to consider. For example, if you and your family have been accepted for Medicaid benefits and funds are raised for you, the donated money could be counted as income, and you may then lose your Medicaid eligibility.

Before you begin accepting donations, keep the following points in mind: You must have some place to put the money you receive, such as a trust fund or a special account. Public donations must never be mixed with personal or family money. Also, if donated money has to be counted as income, it is taxable.

There may be legal requirements regarding solicitation of donations from the public. Check with your city and county governments and with your legal advisor before seeking or accepting donations.

Publicly donated money can be handled through a special trust account at a bank, or a local volunteer or service group may be willing to hold the funds in trust for you if the group is legally able to do this.

Another possibility is placing donated funds with one of the advocacy/charitable organizations—again, with a clear, written agreement that the money, will be used to benefit the patient needing the transplant.

It is essential to have timely access to the money for your needs. Also, it is inappropriate to have only a partial release of funds that is less than the amount you will need to take care of an expense.

State and local laws may set additional guidelines for fund raising; therefore, you may wish to seek legal advice or assistance.

Planning and Organizing Fund Raising Campaigns

It is a good idea to ask for assistance in planning, publicizing, and carrying out your fund raising activities.

You may want to contact local newspapers and radio or television stations. Try to enlist the support of local merchants and other sponsors to promote or contribute to your events. This can benefit both you and your sponsors. Your friends and neighbors, your religious congregation, local chapters of volunteer or service groups, and other community groups can help with your fund raising efforts. Local political leaders and other officials may also be willing to assist you.

To honor their contributions and maintain the trust of those who donated money, these funds should only be used for the direct costs of transplant surgery and patient care, as well as for transplant-related costs such as transportation, food, lodging, and patient medication before and after the transplant.

Important Contacts

It is helpful to seek information and assistance from a number of individuals and groups before making financial decisions. Some may be able to provide funding or other direct assistance; others may be useful as patient advocates or information sources. The most common contacts are listed below. You may have other resources available, depending on your needs and circumstances.

- **Transplant center:** social workers, financial coordinators, and hospital administration representatives

- **Legal services:** your lawyer or legal assistance programs

- **Organizations:** patient advocacy/support groups, charitable/ advocacy organizations, your employer, service organizations, and local merchants

- **Community members:** social workers, pharmacists, bank officials, and religious leaders in your community

- **Government agencies/officials:** The Social Security Administration, the Health Care Financing Administration, and your local and state departments of health. Also, your local and state legislators, your governor, and your U.S. senators and congressional representatives.

Transplant Financial Resources

The following organizations may provide financial assistance to transplant candidates or recipients and their families. This is a sample listing and should not be interpreted as a comprehensive list or an endorsement.

AirLifeLine
50 Fullerton Court
Suite 200
Sacramento, CA 95825
800-446-1231

Transports ambulatory patients up to a distance of 500 to 1,000 miles using private pilots and their aircraft. Can transport people for transplant and follow-up appointments. Must be documented medical and financial need. Service is free of charge.

American Liver Foundation
75 Maiden Lane
Suite 603
New York, NY 10038
800-465-4837

Voluntary agency dedicated to fighting liver disease through research, education, and patient self-help groups. The group acts as trustees for trust funds.

American Organ Transplant Association
3335 Cartwright
Missouri City, TX 77459
Tel: (281) 261-2682
Fax: (281) 208-5279
E-mail: infoaota@a-o-t-a.org
URL: http://www.a-o-t-a.org

A private, non-profit group that provides reduced or free airfare and bus tickets to transplant recipients and their families. AOTA publishes a newsletter for its members. Patients interested in AOTA's services must be referred by their physician. The association also assists people with setting up trust funds and fund raising. No administrative fee is charged.

Angel Flight, American Medical Support Flight Team
3237 Donald Douglas Loop South
Santa Monica, CA 90405
888-426-2643

Provides free air transportation on private aircraft for needy people with healthcare problems and for healthcare agencies, organ procurement organizations, blood banks and tissue banks. There are no fees of any kind. Angel Flight is a volunteer organization serving the public since 1983.

Barbara Anne DeBoer Foundation
2069 South Busse Rd.
Mount Prospect, IL 60056
800-895-8478

Offers a variety of programs that include advocacy services, donor awareness information, referral services, medication, and medical center information. Individual fund raising program is designed to utilize resources in patient's community to raise money for transplant procedure. Works with patients and volunteer committees to develop press releases and plan various events and programs. All local funds raised go to medical expenses—no administrative fee is charged.

Children's Organ Transplant Association
2501 COTA Dr.
Bloomington, IN 47403
812-336-8872

A national, non-profit agency raising funds for individuals and families to assist with transplant and related expenses. Works with adults as well as children. All funds raised go to the individual—no administrative fees are collected.

Medicare Hotline
800-638-6833

National Insurance Consumer Hotline
800-942-4242

Call to obtain the phone number of your state insurance department.

National Organization of Social Security Claimants' Representatives
6 Prospect Street
Midland Park, NJ 07432-1634
800-431-2804
Web address: http://www.nosscr.org

Nielsen Organ Transplant Foundation
580 W 8th St.
Jacksonville, FL 32209
904-798-8999

A regional group that provides assistance to a five-county area in Florida: Duvall, Baker, St. John, Nassau, and Clay. Promotes public education regarding organ donation. Offers limited grant funds for transplant-related expenses.

Organ Transplant Fund, Inc.
1102 Brookfield, Suite 202
Memphis, TN 38119
800-489-3863

Assists transplant candidates and recipients nationwide in obtaining transplants and follow-up care, as well as providing essential support and referral services. Provides clients with fund raising expertise and materials and assures that funds raised are properly dispensed. Limited emergency grants are available for medications and transplant-related expenses.

The Transplant Foundation
8002 Discovery Drive, Suite 310
Richmond, VA 23229
804-285-5115
E-mail: NatFoundTX@aol.com
URL: http://www.otf.org

A national, non-profit volunteer organization providing grants to transplant recipients to offset the costs of immunosuppressant medications. The amount of grants and the number of individuals who can receive assistance are determined by total contributions each year. The organization also acts as a resource referral.

Prescription Drug Patient Assistance Programs

Many pharmaceutical manufacturers provide medications for indigent patients through patient assistance programs. Most programs require that patients meet certain income requirements. The Directory of Prescription Drug Patient Assistance Programs describes more than 55 programs and includes who is eligible, what prescription medications are covered and how to receive assistance. To request a free copy,

Pharmaceutical Research and Manufacturers of America
1100 15th St., NW, Suite 900
Washington, DC 20005
202-835-3414
Fax: 202-835-3416
URL: http://www.pharm.org

The following programs were established by pharmaceutical manufacturers of the three most often prescribed immunosuppressive medications:

Burroughs-Welcome Patient Assistance Program
Medication: Imuran
800-722-9294

Novartis Patient Assistance Program
Medication: Cyclosporine
800-257-3273

Prograf/Fujisawa Patient Assistance Program
Medication: Prograf
800-477-6472

Section 50.5

Life after Transplantation

There are several programs and initiatives that can help finance your care after transplantation. This section outlines the following:

- Rehabilitation
- Social Security Coverage for the Disabled
- Americans with Disabilities Act (ADA)
- Federal Rehabilitation Act (FRA)

Rehabilitation

If you have a disability that prevents you from working, You may be a candidate for vocational rehabilitation. The goal of rehabilitation is to prepare people with disabilities for work. It is important to enter rehabilitation as soon as you are released from the hospital in order to protect your disability coverage.

Both public and private agencies provide rehabilitation services. Public providers offer these services to anyone meeting their eligibility criteria. Often, public agencies serve people who did not become disabled as a result of their job.

Private rehabilitation companies often work with people who become disabled because of job-related injuries or illnesses and who are collecting worker's compensation. Their fees are usually paid by insurance carriers.

Patient Services

Each state provides rehabilitation services through its Department of Vocational Rehabilitation. These agencies are funded by the federal and state governments. State agencies accept referrals from any source. They often provide services to those who have never been able to work because of a disability, and they may arrange sheltered or rehabilitation employment for people with special needs.

State agencies sometimes offer employers partial reimbursement for hiring and providing initial training for their rehabilitation clients. Other programs offer employment preparation training and help their clients establish contacts with potential employers.

Disabled persons often find employment through agencies that provide:

- evaluation of rehabilitation potential;
- counseling, guidance, referral, and placement services;
- vocational training;
- services to help families adjust to disability;
- physical and mental restoration services;
- support for rehabilitation efforts;
- recruitment and training for employment opportunities in areas such as rehabilitation, health and welfare, public safety, and law enforcement;
- occupational licenses, tools, and equipment;
- transportation to rehabilitation activities;
- physical and technological aids and devices;
- rehabilitation engineering; and
- resume development.

Application and Eligibility

Whether you contact a rehabilitation service on your own or you are referred by another person or agency, you must complete an application. Your case will be reviewed to determine your eligibility for service and your potential for employment after completing rehabilitation. Generally, you are considered eligible if you have a physical or mental condition that limits your ability to work, but you would be able to work after receiving rehabilitation.

Assessment and Rehabilitation Plan

If you are eligible, the service will assess your job skills, abilities, and attitudes. This includes medical, psychological, and vocational

testing. The agency will then work with you to develop an individualized, written rehabilitation plan to enhance your skills and abilities.
The plan typically includes:

- long-range vocational goals;
- a schedule of specific services to be provided;
- intermediate objectives to achieve vocational goals;
- the process for evaluating a client's participation and progress;
- rehabilitation equipment or devices;
- client assistance (including financial services); and
- post-employment services.

Training and Assistance

Depending on your needs, as specified in the rehabilitation plan, you will receive vocational training and assistance. Basic services may include physical and occupational therapy, use of physical aids or devices such as artificial limbs or wheelchairs, and/or remedial reading or math courses. You will also receive skills training for the specific type of work you can perform. This involves classroom instruction, individual tutoring, and simulated work.

Job Seeking and Placement

You will be counseled in job-seeking skills, such as preparing a resume or handling job interviews. Most agencies will place you with an employer. After placement, the agency will follow up with the employer to insure that the job match is successful. If you encounter difficulties or need additional assistance in your job, you can receive post-employment services. The terms and eligibility of these services will be covered in your rehabilitation plan.

Social Security Coverage for the Disabled

The Social Security Administration provides general financial assistance and medication grants to transplant patients. Supplemental Security Income (SSI) makes monthly payments to disabled individuals with few assets and low incomes. Social Security Disability Income (SSDI) provides assistance for individuals who are working and paying Social Security taxes. If you are considered disabled, you may begin receiving SSDI benefits while you are involved in an approved rehabilitation program. Contact the Social Security Administration at (800) 772-1213 for these programs.

If your medical condition keeps you from working, you may qualify for disability benefits. Disability programs are offered by a number of private and public agencies, and their eligibility requirements and benefits vary considerably. Social Security provides federally mandated benefits to people who meet its definition of disability. If you qualify, you may receive benefits until you are able to work again on a regular basis. Certain members of your family may also qualify for benefits during this time. There are a number of incentives available to help you return to work.

Who Can Receive Benefits

Unlike some programs, Social Security does not credit partial or short-term disability. Under its definition, you are disabled if you are unable to perform any work for which you are qualified. Also, your disability must be expected to last at least a year or result in death. To qualify for benefits, you must have earned enough work credits for the time you were able to work, and you must file a formal application.

You may receive disability benefits at any age. If you are on disability when you reach age 65, your benefits become retirement benefits. The amount you receive remains the same.

Other members of your family may also qualify for benefits. They include: unmarried dependent children (including stepchildren, adopted children or, in some cases, grandchildren); unmarried children with a disability; or your spouse (if he or she is age 62 or older, disabled, or caring for a child of yours who is under age 16).

When you die, your widow or widower may receive your benefits. To qualify, he or she must be age 50 or older and must become disabled within seven years of your death. A widow or widower caring for dependent children may also qualify if he or she becomes disabled.

Applying for Disability

You should apply for disability benefits as soon as you become disabled, even though you cannot collect benefits until your sixth full month of disability. You may be able to qualify retroactively (dating back to the disabling event), but you may find it harder to gather complete information later.

The claims process takes 60 to 90 days. During that time, Social Security will be gathering your medical information and assessing your ability to work.

Filing an Application

You may apply for disability by telephone, mail, or a personal visit to any Social Security office. The Social Security office can help you access the information you need to apply.

Reviewing the Application

The Social Security office will check your application to see if you meet the initial requirements for disability. It will then send your application to your state's Disability Determination Service for a formal evaluation.

Reviewers will gather information from your doctors about your medical condition, history, and treatment as well as your ability to perform normal work activities. You may need to take a physical examination for further assessment. If additional testing is required, Social Security will pay for these expenses.

Social Security disability guidelines differ from those of other programs. Even if another insurer or government agency has ruled that you are disabled, you must still meet Social Security requirements in order to receive Social Security benefits. Social Security may review and consider the findings of the other agency or program.

You will receive written notice from the Social Security Administration about your claim.

Review Periods and Termination of Benefits

Your case will be reviewed periodically to verify your disability. The review period depends on whether your condition is expected to improve. Social Security will stop paying benefits if you are working on a regular basis and are earning an average of $500 or more a month. Your benefits will also end if your medical condition improves and you are no longer considered disabled.

You must report any improvements in your condition or change in work status to Social Security. Before you receive benefits, Social Security will send you information on how and what to report.

Work Incentives

Social Security continues to offer some benefits if you attempt to work. If you earn more than $200 in one month, it will be considered a "trial" month. You may work for up to nine trial months at any time over a five-year period and earn as much as possible without affecting

439

your benefits. After the trial period ends, Social Security will evaluate your work. Generally, if your earnings average $500 a month or less, you will continue to receive benefits. If you earn more than $500 a month on average, you will receive benefits for an additional three-month grace period before they end. Any work expenses related to your disability will be discounted when your earnings are considered.

If you complete a trial work period, but you are still defined as disabled (up to 36 months after the trial period ends), you may receive a monthly benefit for any month your earnings drop below $500. You will not have to complete a new application within this time period to qualify.

Americans with Disabilities Act

The Americans with Disabilities Act (ADA) of 1990 protects disabled workers from discrimination in job hiring, firing, promotion, pay, and other job-related issues if the discrimination is based on a worker's disability. To be protected under the ADA, you must:

- have a disability as defined by the ADA; and

- be able to perform the essential functions of your current job or a job that you are seeking, either with or without "reasonable" accommodation from your employer.

The ADA's Definition of Disability

The ADA broadly defines disability as a physical or mental impairment that restricts one or more major life activities. You are considered disabled if you have a record of such an impairment or if others commonly believe you have a disability. The ADA specifically excludes drug and alcohol abuse among the disabilities it covers, but it does protect those who have stopped using illegal drugs and have enrolled in or completed a drug rehabilitation program.

Employer Responsibilities

Employers are required to make reasonable accommodations as needed for disabled workers. Reasonable accommodations include a number of possible actions:

- improving access to work facilities for disabled persons;

- restructuring job duties or work schedules;

- reassigning disabled workers to other positions;

- buying new devices or modifying existing ones to assist disabled workers;

- and modifying job examinations, training materials or policies.

Note that the ADA specifies only "reasonable" accommodations. If an employer can prove that an accommodation would pose an undue hardship to the business (too difficult or expensive to provide), the employer may not have to provide it. Also, if you have failed to inform your employer of your condition, the company will be under no obligation to accommodate you, because it will have had no prior knowledge of your disability status.

The ADA does not cover all employers. The Act applies to private companies, state and local governments, and employment agencies and labor unions that employ 15 or more workers for more than 20 weeks.

Under ADA regulations, an employer cannot make you take a medical examination before you are considered for employment, although pre-employment drug testing is allowed. The Act does allow a routine medical examination after a job offer has been made and before you begin work, but the examination must be given to all new employees. You may be asked to voluntarily provide a medical history.

In a job interview, you may only be asked about your disability if the company can prove that the questions relate directly to the necessities of the job and meet certain other considerations.

Filing a Claim

If you wish to file a claim regarding a potential ADA violation, contact your local Equal Employment Opportunity Commission office, listed under "United States Government" in the telephone book. By law, an employer cannot retaliate against anyone filing a claim or participating in an investigation.

Federal Rehabilitation Act (FRA)

The Federal Rehabilitation Act (FRA) offers protection against discrimination by organizations that receive more than $2,500 in federal funds.

Many state and local governments have disability laws similar to the ADA and the FRA. Most vary in coverage by jurisdiction. Check with a local attorney to determine if a state or local disability law would provide you with more protection.

Essential Questions to Ask

Questions to Ask Your Transplant Center Financial Coordinator

- What is your average cost for a pretransplant evaluation?

- What is your average cost for the transplant I need? What is the average cost of follow-up care?

- Do you require a deposit or a down payment for my pretransplant evaluation or transplant? If so, how much is required? What if I have no resources?

- If I run out of funds before I get a transplant, what actions will you take? Will I be made inactive on the patient waiting list or removed from it completely?

- When can I expect to be billed? What kinds of payment options do I have?

- Who is my financial coordinator at the hospital? If I have questions or problems, how can I contact him or her?

- Do you know of any local organizations that can assist us with transportation or lodging?

- Do you have, or know of, any support groups for patients or families?

If You Have Private Insurance

- Do you participate in a "managed care" contract or a "centers of excellence" network with my insurer?

If You Have Medicare Coverage

- Is your program Medicare approved for the type of transplant I need?

If You Are Raising Funds

- Have you worked with fund raising or charitable organizations for transplant patients? If so, which one(s)?

Questions to Ask Your Insurance Company

If you have private insurance, you may want to give your policy a "check-up." Don't hesitate to ask your insurance representatives questions. They are there to help you understand your coverage and its limitations. Some of the coverage limitations and conditions may be negotiable, either directly or through your employer.

- Is transplantation a "covered service" under my policy?

- Do you require pre-authorization for a transplant or for any pretransplant treatment? Do I need to supply any information?

- Do you select "centers of excellence" for the type of transplant I need? If so, must I go to one?

- Does the plan cover the cost of travel for me to go to these centers if they are not nearby? What about my family? What about follow-up care?

- Is there a waiting period for coverage? If so, how long is it? Am I currently in the waiting period?

- Are there any permanent exclusions to my policy? If so, what are they?

- Is a second opinion required?

- What percentage of costs are paid by my policy? Does it vary by the type of service provided (i.e., surgery, tests, prescriptions)?

- Are there any deductibles or co-payments? What is my total "out of pocket" cost per year?

- Are there separate deductibles or co-payments for prescriptions, physician/professional services, or surgery? If so, what are they?

- Do you have a maximum amount or "cap" on my coverage? Can this limit be extended?

- Will you pay for my medications after the transplant?

- Is there any time limit on coverage of my medications?

- Are prescription medications included in the maximum? If not, what is the prescription maximum?

- What else is included in the maximum?

- Who should I call for questions or problems with my coverage?

- Are there any rehabilitation incentives?

Questions to Ask Fund Raising Organizations

If you are hoping to raise funds for your transplant procedure, here are some questions to ask any organization that is planning to assist you.

- How are donated funds kept? How are they released?

- How can I find out the status of my funds?

- Are any fees deducted from actual funds?

- If I don't receive a transplant, what will happen to the funds already raised?

- What if the funds exceed the cost of the operation?

- How many patients and families have you worked with?

- Can you offer references from other patients you have helped?

- Who should I call if I have any questions or problems?

- Are you a 501C (3) organization, so that money raised on my behalf is tax deductible by those who contribute?

Questions about Care after Your Transplant

If You Are Receiving Disability Benefits

- Will my benefits end if I am able to return to work? If so, can I resume getting benefits when I need them?

- Do you have incentives to ease my transition back to work?

If You Take Part in Occupational Therapy or Rehabilitation

- How will my program be structured and evaluated?

- Will you help with job placement?

Questions for Your Physician about Medications

- What medications will I need? Will the dosages change?

- What if I miss a dose?

- How should I notify you if I have problems with my medication?

- Are all my medications available from commercial pharmacies? If not, how do I receive them?

Posttransplant Medications

It is possible your body will recognize your new organ as different and attempt to reject it. You can help prevent rejection by taking immunosuppressant drugs, which will help your immune system accept the transplanted organ. You will take these anti-rejection drugs for the rest of your life. In addition to immunosupressants, your doctor will prescribe other medications to treat side effects and prevent complications.

After your transplant, you may be taking many medications a day. It is extremely important for patients to take all their medications correctly.

Here are some helpful hints:

- Learn everything you can about your medications. Consult your physician, transplant coordinator, pharmacist, support groups, and educational seminars.

- Use reminder tools to help you take your medications. For example a pillbox, sandwich bags labeled with days of the week and dosage times, an alarm clock, or a calendar may work for you.

- Fit medication into your schedule. Don't be afraid to work with your transplant team to create a medication schedule that fits your lifestyle.

- Keep track of your medication supply. It is dangerous to run out of medications even for one or two doses.

- Understand your finances and insurance. Let your healthcare providers know if you are having trouble paying for your medications.

- Ask your family and friends to help. Having a support network will help make the job of taking your medications a little easier.

- Find a pharmacy that will help you manage your medications and provide educational resources designed for your needs. Your transplant coordinator or social worker will have a list of pharmacies for you.

Taking your medication the right way plays a key role in staying healthy and taking care of yourself after your transplant.

Chapter 51

Selecting Candidates— Who Qualifies?

Liver transplantation has emerged from its status as an experimental procedure more than a decade ago to its current position as the preferred treatment for end-stage liver disease. Increasing numbers of patients on the waiting list and the traditionally small pool of donor organs have prompted the establishment of formal listing criteria to optimize organ utilization.

There are no age limits when considering patients for liver transplantation. The absence of significant disease in the heart, brain, lungs, and kidney would favor consideration for transplantation regardless of age. A patent portal or superior mesenteric vein is necessary for successful engraftment. If evidence of partial or complete thrombosis is apparent on initial imaging studies, then angiographic confirmation is recommended. Hepatopulmonary syndrome (hypoxemia related to cirrhosis) occurs occasionally and usually subsides following transplantation. Significant pulmonary hypertension, on the other hand, precludes transplantation since cardiac deterioration following engraftment inevitably occurs and is usually fatal. Patients who are HIV positive or who have psychiatric diseases such as depression and psychosis are not suitable candidates. Patients with a remote (greater than 5 years) history of malignancy in a nonhepatic site may be considered for liver transplantation.

"Selecting Candidates for Liver Transplantation—Who Qualifies?", © The Liver Circulation Newsletter, Spring 1998, reprinted with permission.

The timing of liver transplantation in end-stage liver disease is not clearly established. Advanced cirrhosis is complicated by variceal hemorrhage, ascites, encephalopathy, hepatorenal syndrome, and hepatocellular carcinoma. A number of treatment options are available for the therapy of these complications. However, the referral of patients for transplantation after severe decompensation, i.e., in the face of severe malnutrition, aspiration pneumonia, ARDS, persistent gastrointestinal hemorrhage, or renal failure, bodes a poor outcome.

In the United States, the most common indication (20%-30%) for liver transplantation is cirrhosis due to chronic viral hepatitis. Although viral hepatitis B and C recur frequently in the transplanted liver, the administration of high doses of hepatitis B immune globulin at frequent established intervals following transplant has reduced the recurrence rates of hepatitis B significantly, improving both graft and patient survival. The administration of the nucleoside analogue, lamivudine, to patients prior to transplant is expected to reduce viral replication and promises to enhance this benefit. The progression to cirrhosis in about 10%-20% of patients with hepatitis C permits consideration for transplantation in these patients. However, there are no strategies to prevent the recurrence of hepatitis C in the post-transplant period as exist for hepatitis B, and the majority of patients develop recurrent hepatitis C soon after transplantation. However, long-term survival is the rule in these patients although there may be a slow progression to cirrhosis.

Alcoholic liver disease accounts for about 20% of all liver transplants. Although patients with liver failure due to liver disease of any etiology are candidates, patients with active alcoholism and substance abuse should not be considered because recidivism rates are high in this group. On the other hand, a remote history does not preclude consideration. Current recommendations are: abstinence for longer than 6 months, successful completion of a formally approved program for rehabilitation from substance abuse, and the existence of a favorable living environment after subjective evaluation by a psychiatric social worker.

Cirrhosis due to autoimmune, cryptogenic, cholestatic (biliary cirrhosis, primary sclerosing cholangitis, biliary atresia), metabolic, and genetic diseases comprise the remaining indications for liver transplantation.

For acute liver failure, regardless of etiology, liver transplantation is the treatment of choice, provided this can be achieved before the patient develops deep encephalopathy, irreversible brain edema, and herniation. Patients with early stage hepatocellular carcinoma can be successfully transplanted while those with more advanced disease are not usually considered candidates for liver transplantation unless they are first treated successfully under specific chemotherapy protocols.

—Rick Selby, M.D. and
Jacob Korula, M.D.

Chapter 52

The National Organ
Transplant Act (NOTA)

Legislative History of the OPTN and Scientific Registry

By the early 1980s, organ transplantation had brought new hope
to thousands of people suffering from diseases of the heart, liver, kidneys, lungs, and other organs. Nevertheless, many patients were having difficulties obtaining transplants, leading some to seek assistance
through media coverage. During 1983 and 1984, issues related to
human organ transplantation were widely publicized.

As the issues drew Congressional attention, it soon became clear
that a more comprehensive solution to transplantation-related problems was necessary. In October 1984, Congress passed PL 98-507,
known as the National Organ Transplant Act (NOTA), which among
other things, provided for the establishment of a Task Force on Organ Procurement and Transplantation and an Organ Procurement
and Transplantation Network. As required by law, the Secretary of
Health and Human Services assembled a 25-member Task Force to
conduct comprehensive studies of medical, legal, ethical, economic,
and social issues relevant to human organ transplantation. To study
these issues, experts in medicine, immunology, law, theology, ethics,
allied health, the health insurance industry, and public advocacy were
joined by representatives of the Office of the Surgeon General of the
Public Health Service (PHS), the National Institutes of Health (NIH),
the Food and Drug Administration (FDA), the Health Care Financing

"History of the OPTN and the Scientific Registry," Health Resources and
Services Administration (HHS), Office of Special Programs, updated 5/17/99.

451

Administration (HCFA), and staff from the Office of Organ Transplantation, Health Resources and Services Administration (HRSA). Upon completion of the Task Force report, HRSA issued a request in the fall of 1986 for proposals to establish a National Organ Procurement and Transplantation Network (OPTN) under the National Organ Transplant Act. In the same year, new legislation (Omnibus Budget Reconciliation Act, PL 99-509) mandated that all Organ Procurement Organizations (OPO's) and transplant programs be members of the OPTN. On September 30, 1986, UNOS was awarded the OPTN contract; the Scientific Registry contract was awarded one year later. Both contracts with UNOS were competitively renewed for three years in September 1990, 1993 and most recently in December 1996.

Provisions of NOTA were amended in 1988 and 1990, including expansion of OPTN responsibilities to increase the donor organ supply and assist OPO's in nationwide placement of organs not placed locally.

Current Role of the Health Resources and Services Administration (HRSA)

The OPTN and Scientific Registry contracts are administered by HRSA's Division of Transplantation. Under the terms of both contracts, UNOS conducts numerous tasks and projects to meet the federally established goals of the OPTN and the Scientific Registry. Written reports on the progress and completion of these tasks are regularly provided to the HRSA Project Officer and the Director of the Division of Transplantation (DOT). Representatives of the DOT attend all UNOS Board of Directors and committee meetings (except for executive sessions devoted to matters not involving contract funds).

Purpose of the OPTN

From the inception of the OPTN, its purpose has been "to improve the effectiveness of the nation's organ donation, procurement, and transplantation system by increasing the availability of and access to donor organs for patients with end-stage organ failure." More specifically, as specified in the original HRSA Request for Proposals, the goals of the OPTN are to:

- Improve the effectiveness of cadaver organ procurement and distribution.

- Increase patient access to state-of-the-art transplantation technology.

- Improve the system for sharing renal and external organs so as to:

  1. Facilitate donor and recipient matching, based on specific criteria established for each organ;
  2. Improve transplantation outcomes;
  3. Provide a system by which immunologically sensitized patients are afforded the best possible opportunity to be matched with a compatible donor;
  4. Decrease the wastage of organs.

- Assure quality control by collection, analysis, and publication of data on organ donation, procurement, and transplantation.

- Maintain and improve professional skills of those involved in organ procurement and transplantation.

To achieve these goals, the OPTN operates and maintains a national computer list of patients waiting for kidney, heart, heart/lung, lung, liver, pancreas, and intestinal bowel transplants. UNOS also maintains a computer-assisted organ allocation system and an Organ Center, which allows 24-hour transplant program access to the donor/recipient matching system. Data collected by the OPTN pertain to patients waiting for transplants, donors and recipients of donated organs, donor/recipient matching and organ allocation, and donor/recipient histocompatibility.

In order to operate the OPTN, UNOS has adopted corporate bylaws and policies governing membership standards, organ procurement, organ allocation, and data management. The Secretary of HHS has reviewed these bylaws. On September 8, 1994, the HHS published for public comment a Notice of Proposed Rulemaking for the OPTN in the Federal Register. This was followed by publication of a final rule with the opportunity for additional public comment in the April 2, 1998, edition of the Federal Register. The rules establish requirements and procedures for membership in the OPTN, listing transplants candidates on a nationwide computer network, allocating organs, and maintaining records and reporting by member Organ Procurement Organizations (OPO's) and transplant hospitals. Subject to consideration of the comments submitted, some of the policies and bylaws may be promulgated as regulations by the HHS for operation of the OPTN. Until that time, all UNOS policies and bylaws are considered voluntary guidance to OPTN members.

Organ Allocation According to 1998 UNOS Policies— A Brief Description

The UNOS computer list of potential transplant recipients, together with information pertinent to matching them with donors, is known as the Waiting List. UNOS requires that all cadaveric donors be matched against this list before an organ is offered for transplantation. When specific information about a donor is entered into the UNOS computer match program by the local OPO or by UNOS Organ Center staff, the computer rules out each potential recipient with incompatible blood type and body size. The computer then employs a ranking system to calculate priority for each patient still on the list. A list of potential recipients is then printed, with patients ranked in descending point order. A patient's priority score is determined by a number of different variables that are specific for the type of organ to be transplanted. For example, in renal transplantation, waiting list points are assigned according to:

1. Time on the waiting list accrued after meeting enumerating thresholds;

2. Age (if the recipient is under 18);

3. Degree of antigen mismatch;

4. Status as a prior organ donor; and

5. Other indices of immunological compatibility.

Although seemingly straightforward, the details of the allocation process are complex. Because time is crucial once an organ is removed from its donor, current allocation policy requires that organs be offered first to local patients (generally, patients within the host OPO's service area—the only exception to this policy is that mandatory shared kidneys take precedence over non-zero-antigen mismatch local offers) with highest priority. In general, if no suitable local recipients are available, organs are shared regionally and then nationally.

Purpose of the Scientific Registry

In the NOTA, it was stipulated that a Scientific Registry be established to collect data for continuous evaluation of the clinical and scientific status of transplantation in the United States. The specific goals of the Scientific Registry, articulated in the Task Force recommendations, the NOTA, and the HRSA contract, are as follows:

- To collect, in a computer system, data on all transplant recipients and all transplant programs in the U.S.

- To provide a database that enables regular periodic analysis and reporting on the efficacy of transplantation nationwide.

- To provide a national database for basic and clinical research on organ transplantation.

In contrast to the OPTN, which collects data about donors, Waiting List patients, and information pertinent to organ allocation, the Scientific Registry collects post-transplant recipient data—from the time of transplant until graft failure or recipient death, whichever comes first. Using UNOS organ-specific data collection forms, transplant recipient data are collected, processed, and validated.

Validated data are entered into the Scientific Registry. Data collected include comprehensive medical and histocompatibility information about donors, registrants, and recipients, as well as graft and patient survival information.

Subject to disclosure restrictions under various statutory and regulatory policies, data collected and generated by the Scientific Registry are available to members of UNOS, UNOS staff, Board of Directors and committees, the medical community, government officials, private organizations, and the general public. The data have been used in a variety of ways, perhaps the most important of which is to serve as the basis for the development of transplantation policies. With the aid of accurate and timely information about previous transplants and their outcomes, the Federal Government and the transplant community can identify specific factors that maximize the number of transplants, graft survival, and equity in organ allocation. Examples of specific issues that can be addressed with the aid of the Scientific Registry data are:

- The impact of HLA matching on transplant outcomes.

- The impact of various organ preservation methods on outcomes.

- The impact of various donor characteristics (e.g., age, cause of death, medical history) on outcomes.

- Differential waiting times, transplant rates, and outcomes among racial, ethnic, gender, and age groups.

- Differential patient/graft survival rates among transplant programs.

- Transplant outcome as a function of patient status and disease diagnosis.

Brief History of UNOS

UNOS is a private, non-profit corporation. Among its activities, UNOS operates the national OPTN and the Scientific Registry of Transplant Recipients under contract with HRSA. It is unique in that it is a private corporation that, with input from the Federal Government, develops and implements voluntary policy for a sector of the medical community. A primary goal for UNOS is to ensure equitable organ allocation which results in the best graft survival possible.

In January 1977, UNOS was established as an outgrowth of the South Eastern Regional Organ Procurement Foundation (SEOPF), to facilitate the national use of a computer system for matching kidneys and other organs with suitable recipients. In anticipation of changes in both transplantation technology and related legislation, UNOS was incorporated as a private, non-profit voluntary membership organization in 1984. In 1986, in response to NOTA, the HRSA issued a Request for Proposals (RFP) from private organizations to operate the national Organ Procurement and Transplantation Network. UNOS submitted a proposal and was awarded the OPTN contract on September 30, 1986. In response to a later RFP, UNOS was awarded the Scientific Registry contract on September 30, 1987. These contracts were competitively renewed for three years in September 1990, 1993 and again in December 1996.

The UNOS organization consists of the Board of Directors, members, committees, and a staff in Richmond, Virginia.

Role of UNOS in the OPTN and Scientific Registry

When UNOS was awarded the OPTN and Scientific Registry contracts, it changed its operation to accommodate the mandates of Federal law as established by NOTA. In doing so, the corporation adopted the following objectives:

- optimize access to transplantation for all who can benefit from it;

- maximize the number of organs donated, procured, and transplanted through policies and programs that improve quality, efficiency, efficacy and survival;

- establish standards for membership, access to the allocation of organs, organ acceptability, transplant program and OPO performance, and information collection and reporting;

- allocate organs equitably;

- function as a central resource for the collection, processing, storage, analysis, and reporting of data pertaining to donation and transplantation;

- collaborate with scientists and scientific/professional organizations to stimulate improvements in transplant technology;

- provide technological, analytical, and administrative services to members of the transplant community to improve effectiveness and efficiency; and

- educate professionals and the public about transplantation and donation.

Chapter 53

Waiting Time Disparities for Organ Transplant Recipients

The Department of Health and Human Services has released a report showing wide disparities in the length of time patients wait for organ transplants in different geographic areas of the United States. Organ allocation policies in effect during the period covered by the report were a significant cause of the disparities, HHS said. And while some changes in these policies have been made, fundamental improvements are still needed to ensure fair treatment for patients.

The 1997 Report of the OPTN: Waiting List Activity and Donor Procurement is the first publication by the organ transplant network to include data on local waiting times. For the largest category of patients, waiting times ranged from 46 days in Iowa to 721 days in western Pennsylvania.

> "This report contains some of the strongest evidence yet that our nation's organ transplantation system needs improvement," HHS Secretary Donna E. Shalala said. "It makes clearer than ever that patients can be disadvantaged by the simple fact of where they live and at what transplant center they are listed."

> "Our organ transplant system doesn't have to work that way, and it shouldn't, Secretary Shalala said. "Organs donated for transplantation should go to patients on the basis of medical criteria, not geography. Organs should not be denied to patients

HHS NEWS, January 22, 1999, U.S. Department of Health and Human Services.

who need them simply because of arbitrary boundaries that have no medical rationale."

Under HHS regulations published in 1998, transplant professionals would be required to develop new policies for the transplant network to replace current allocation rules. The new policies would help assure that organs would go to patients with greatest medical need, in accordance with sound medical judgment and effective use of the organs. The current rules often require organs to be used in the local area where they have been procured, instead of being provided to patients with higher medical need, even when such patients may be located in nearby areas. HHS' regulations are to take effect on Oct. 21, 1999, and the Institute of Medicine has been asked by Congress to review the effect of the regulations.

The current allocation rules are a primary cause of the disparity in waiting times for organs in different parts of the nation, and these rules result in higher-than-necessary number of deaths among those who are waiting for organs, according to HHS' Health Resources and Services Administration. A reformed system that allocated organs on the basis of medical criteria, without arbitrary geographic constraints, would result in more organs for those with greatest medical need, and thus would result in fewer deaths, according to HRSA.

This report provides numerous examples of the disparities, measured according to several different categories of patients. In some cases there are significant differences in waiting times even between adjacent areas. For example, the median waiting time for liver transplant patients with similar medical status was 439 days in the Baltimore area, compared with 147 days in nearby Washington, D.C.

For patients with blood type O (representing about 47 percent of all liver transplant patients), the median waiting time was 511 days in New York City, while the median waiting time in bordering northern New Jersey was 56 days. Iowa, with the shortest waiting time among all 66 organ procurement areas at 46 days, compared with neighboring Nebraska at 596 days.

> "An organ that could save a life may be literally stopped at the border, and denied to a patient for non-medical reasons," Secretary Shalala said. "Because of organ allocation rules that put geography ahead of medical need, the more urgent patient in one area may be unable to get a liver for transplantation, even when it comes available in the state or the city next door. That's not in the best interest of patients or those who care for them."

Significant differences also existed in organ recovery activity, with some organ procurement organizations reporting significantly higher rates than others. HHS took action last year to require the nation's hospitals to report virtually all deaths to their local organ procurement organization (OPO), thus providing more opportunity for OPO's to contact the families of potential donors and increase organ donation nationwide. In addition, the pending HHS regulation that would require changes in organ allocation policy would also help provide a fairer system for patients, regardless of differences in OPO recovery rates.

Today's study includes data on local waiting times across the country for patients placed on a transplant waiting list during two periods of time: 1993 to 1995 for kidneys, and 1994 to 1996 for pancreas, kidney-pancreas, hearts, livers, and lungs. The report also documents the number of registered patients transplanted, organ recovery rates from 1994 to 1996 for each OPO, and waiting list activity (additions and removals) for each transplant program nationwide.

Median waiting times differ significantly for all organs depending upon where a patient lives or is listed, as well as patient characteristics such as medical urgency, blood type, age, race, and for kidneys, immune sensitization.

In addition to biologic factors, waiting times appear to be influenced by the demographics of an OPO area, rates of donation, OPO donation request and consent procedures, and transplant center registration and organ acceptance policies.

"This report is a step forward, but it is still not the kind of timely and user-friendly information that patients and their physicians really need," said HRSA Administrator Claude Earl Fox, M.D., M.P.H. "Our goal is for future reports to present more current information in a form that is more understandable for patients, their families, and their physicians, including waiting time data for each transplant center."

The report released totals 2,400 pages in seven separate volumes. It was produced by the United Network for Organ Sharing, a private, nonprofit organization based in Richmond, Va., under contract with HRSA, the HHS agency responsible for administering the organ transplantation system. The pending HHS regulation also requires more current information from the organ transplant network.

This report includes an executive summary and six additional organ-specific volumes with tables on OPO-specific median waiting times, number of patients transplanted, and donor procurement activity, as well as waiting list activity (with additions and removals) for each transplant center. A graphical analysis is presented on median waiting time data. Because greatly variable circumstances surround waiting times, many OPOs accepted the offer to include a narrative explaining the issues affecting their waiting times and donor procurement activity. Each volume has a user's guide containing frequently asked questions, and background on statistical methods, data collection and analysis and the multiple issues that impact waiting times.

The new report should be used in conjunction with The 1997 Report of Center Specific Graft and Patient Survival Rates, released by HHS in December 1997, which provides historical data on actual and expected survival rates for nearly 100,000 transplants. It showed overall survival rates for transplants at an all-time high, with three-year patient survival rates ranging from 75.9 percent for lung recipients, to 81.2 percent for heart-lung, to more than 90 percent for kidney, liver, heart and pancreas.

The executive summary of The 1997 Report of the OPTN: Waiting List Activity and Donor Procurement can be accessed from UNOS' World Wide Web site at www.unos.org. Organ-specific volumes may be ordered by calling UNOS at 804-330-8541. For specific volumes of the report, purchasers will be required to pay shipping and handling charges.

Other reports, including The 1997 Report of Center Specific Graft and Patient Survival Rates and The Annual Report of the OPTN and Scientific Registry, are also available on the UNOS Web site.

Chapter 54

Bioartificial Liver

Bioartificial Liver Helps Keep Patients Alive

Physicians have long appreciated the need for a medical device that would provide long-term support for patients with liver disease in the same way that kidney dialysis machines assist patients with kidney disease. Such a device would help patients awaiting liver transplants survive until a donor organ became available and could also help the millions of people with chronic liver diseases—such as alcoholic cirrhosis and hepatitis—survive life-threatening flare-ups of their conditions.

But developing artificial liver support has been a daunting task because compared to the kidney, which has a limited number of physiological functions that can be simulated mechanically, the liver is extremely complex. The liver is involved in numerous physiological processes, including protein synthesis, detoxification, carbohydrate metabolism, lipid metabolism, immune response, temperature regulation, hormone metabolism, and other processes that are not yet completely understood.

To help patients with acute liver failure to survive until a donor organ becomes available, researchers at Cedars-Sinai Medical Center in Los Angeles have developed an innovative device called the bioartificial liver (BAL) with support from the National Institute of Diabetes and Digestive and Kidney Diseases. BAL was tested in a

"Research Highlight," *NCRR Reporter*, November/December 1997, National Center for Research Resources (NCRR).

phase I study at the NCRR-supported General Clinical Research Center (GCRC) at the Cedars-Sinai Medical Center, which is a satellite of the GCRC at Harbor-University of California, Los Angeles. Initial experience with more than 30 patients who had complete liver failure suggests that the BAL, a washing-machine-sized device that is wheeled to the patient's bedside to deliver treatments that typically last about six hours, is effective at "bridging" patients to transplantation or even helping them recover normal liver function. "The device is still investigational, and there are regulatory issues that need to be resolved before it can become clinically available, but results so far are very encouraging," says Dr. Achilles Demetriou, chairman of the department of surgery, Cedars-Sinai Medical Center, who has led the 15-year effort to develop the device.

Early on, the researchers realized that it would be pointless to attempt to mechanically replicate each of the liver's functions. Instead, they isolated live liver cells—hepatocytes—from pigs and incorporated them into the device in the hope that these cells would continue to perform enough of their functions to make the BAL useful. However, incorporating live cells presented a major technical challenge because the researchers needed to develop techniques to harvest and process living hepatocytes obtained from pigs. In the early stages, the researchers sacrificed a new pig for each patient, but to make the wider use of the BAL more feasible, they developed techniques to incorporate cryopreserved hepatocytes into cartridges. Cryopreservation allows cell storage for future use and transport to treatment sites.

Initial use of the BAL has focused on patients with complete liver failure, the most critically ill group of patients for whom there previously was little hope. Dr. Demetriou explains that in otherwise healthy adults, rare reactions to drugs such as the pain reliever acetaminophen, certain mushrooms and plants, as well as the onset of viral infections, may cause the liver to shut down—a condition known as fulminant hepatic failure. "If you think of the kidney as a filter for the blood and the heart as a pump, the liver is like a power station. When it fails, energy goes out and thousands of physiologic processes throughout the body stop. It's a massive insult to the body," says Dr. Demetriou.

For these patients, death comes within a few hours or days as cerebrospinal fluid accumulates within the cranial cavity, intracranial pressure rises, patients enter coma, and brain function is lost. The only known effective treatment for these patients is liver transplantation, but because of their critical condition, many patients die before a donor organ becomes available. With standard medical treatment, about 90 percent of these patients die; if patients survive until transplantation, their chances of survival increase to about 70 percent.

Patients with fulminant hepatic failure usually receive one treatment a day with the BAL. "Our goal is to slow down the brain swelling, which is the major cause of death in patients with fulminant hepatic failure," says Dr. Demetriou. "During a BAL treatment, we can see a fairly dramatic change in intracranical pressure, which starts to drop after about 2 to 2.5 hours of treatment."

Using the BAL in combination with an effective multidisciplinary support group consisting of physicians, nurses, pharmacists, nutritionists, and physical and respiratory therapists, the Cedars-Sinai researchers have successfully bridged many of these patients to transplantation. Of 36 patients with acute liver failure (23 with fulminant hepatic failure, three with nonfunctioning transplanted livers, and 10 with acute worsening of chronic liver disease) treated so far, 19 patients were bridged until receiving transplants, six recovered completely and needed no transplant, and two patients with chronic liver disease recovered and received transplants at later dates. The other nine patients—of whom eight were not candidates for transplantation—were only supported temporarily and later died.

Dr. Demetriou says that liver failure is so devastating that these patients require much more support than can be provided by the BAL alone. To meet their needs, Cedars-Sinai created the liver support unit, comparable to coronary care units (CCU) or intensive care units (ICU). "In terms of intervention and manpower, the liver support unit is an order of magnitude greater than a CCU or ICU," says Dr. Demetriou. He points out that because of the liver's central role, patients with liver failure may also have kidney and respiratory failure or even multiple organ failure, as well as immune suppression and major neurologic impairment. "We have to pay attention to every detail to bring the patients to a level where they are fully supported," he says. "Then we introduce the experimental treatment—the BAL, which we believe puts them over the top." He notes that the availability of the BAL was a critical element in gaining the institutional support necessary to create the liver support unit.

During the treatment, blood is drawn from the patient and passed through the BAL. In the first step, blood cells are separated from the fluid—the blood plasma—that contains the substances that must be removed or processed by the liver. In addition, the plasma contains low-molecular-weight toxins that might harm the hepatocytes. To remove these toxins, the plasma is passed through a charcoal filter. Subsequently, the plasma flows through a heater to maintain body temperature and then through the column that contains the hepato-cytes. "The hepatocytes provide both detoxifying and potentially synthetic functions, producing substances the patient's own diseased liver is unable to produce," explains Dr. Demetriou. After flowing through the hepatocyte cartridge, the plasma is reconstituted with the blood cells and reinfused into the patient.

So far, the BAL has been used on an as-needed basis as part of a phase I clinical trial to demonstrate safety and potential effectiveness. A formal phase II/III clinical trial, which evaluates clinical effectiveness in larger groups of patients with a control group, started in late 1997.

Patients with chronic liver disease may have to return for treatment periodically, and researchers are already planning strategies to contend with immunological problems that may arise if the BAL is used on a long-term basis to treat chronic conditions such as hepatitis or cirrhosis.

Although the artificial liver still is at an experimental stage, these promising results bode well for patients with liver failure. In the future, these patients may be admitted to large hospital centers and treated by specialized multidisciplinary support teams that have frozen liver cell cartridges ready for use in a BAL within a few hours.

Additional Reading

Watanabe, F. D., Mullon, C. J. P., Hewitt, W. R., et al., Clinical experience with a bioartificial liver in the treatment of severe liver failure. A phase I clinical trial. *Annals of Surgery* 225:484-494.

—William Oldendorf

Chapter 55

U.S. Facts about Transplantation

On July 14, 1999 the UNOS National patient waiting list for organ transplant included the following:

Table 55.1. Patient Waiting List for Organ Transplant

Type of Transplant	Registrations for Transplant	Patients Waiting for Transplant
kidney transplant	44,457	42,498
liver transplant	13,607	13,388
pancreas transplant	483	476
pancreas islet cell transplant	121	121
kidney-pancreas transplant	1,963	1,890
intestine transplant	115	113
heart transplant	4,328	4,313
heart-lung transplant	231	228
Lung transplant	3,386	3,330
Totals	Total Registrations: 68,685	*Total Patients: 64,450

*Some patients are waiting for more than one organ, therefore the total number of patients is less than the sum of patients waiting for each organ.

Note: UNOS policies allow patients to be listed with more than one transplant center (multiple-listing), thus the number of registrations is greater than the actual number of patients.

This chapter contains data and text from "Liver Summary" © 1997, and "Critical Data" © 1998, reprinted with permission of the United Network for Organ Sharing.

Number of Transplants Performed in 1998

This information is based on UNOS Scientific Registry data as of April 14, 1999. Double kidney, double lung, and heart-lung transplants are counted as one transplant.

Table 55.2. 1998 Transplants

Type of Transplant	Number
kidney-pancreas transplants	965
kidney alone transplants (4,016 were living donors)	11,990
pancreas alone transplants	253
liver transplants	4,450
heart transplants	2,340
heart-lung transplants	45
lung transplants	849
intestine transplants	69
Total	20,961

Number and Type of Organ Transplant Programs

Currently, 272 medical institutions in the United States operate organ transplant programs. These transplant centers can be separated into organ specific programs that include the following:

Table 55.3. Organ Transplant Programs

Type of Program	Number
Kidney Transplant Programs	252
Liver Transplant Programs	125
Pancreas Transplant Programs	125
Pancreas Islet Cell Transplant Programs	21
Intestine Transplant Programs	32
Heart Transplant Programs	153
Heart-Lung Transplant Programs	94
Lung Transplant Programs	89
Total	891

Patient Survival Rates—Liver Summary

This information of liver transplant survival rates is based upon verified Scientific Registry data for 16,658 transplants involving 14,607 patients from 103 liver transplant programs in the United States. Each program reporting at least one liver transplant between January 1, 1988, and April 30, 1994, was included. Multi-organ and living donor transplants were excluded.

Short term survival is defined as survival at 3 months and 1 year post-transplant. Short term survival rates are based on all transplants in the study for which there are follow-up data.

Long term survival is defined in two ways:

- unconditional survival at 3 years post-transplant, and

- survival at 3 years post-transplant for those who survived at least 1 year, referred to as conditional 3 year survival.

The long term survival rates are based on all transplants between January 1, 1988, and April 30, 1992, for which there are follow-up data. This cohort was chosen to ensure that the maximum number of transplants with follow-up data was used to determine long term survival rates. Please note that the emphasis on long term survival in this report is on the *conditional* 3-year survival rates. This is because the conditional 3-year analysis provides an assessment of characteristics independent of those limited to the first year (e.g., surgical complications and early acute rejection events).

Study Period

The 1997 Report was based on 16,658 liver transplants performed in 14,607 patients between January 1, 1988, and April 30, 1994, from 103 transplant programs in the United States. In order to assess changes within transplant programs over time, the data were divided into 2 eras. The first era included transplants performed from January 1, 1988, through April 30, 1992; the second era covered the two-year time period from May 1, 1992, through April 30, 1994.

Survival Rates

Survival rates were computed at 3 months, 1 year, and 3 years, both nationally and for each transplant program. Three-year survival was determined in two ways:

1. conditional 3 year survival (i.e., survival at 3 years for those who survived at least 1 year post-transplant), and

2. unconditional 3 year survival.

The emphasis on long term survival in this chapter is on the conditional 3-year survival rates because the conditional 3-year analysis provides an assessment of characteristics independent of those limited to the first year (e.g., surgical complications and early acute rejection events).

The national graft and patient survival rates and completeness of follow-up at 3 months, 1 year, and conditional 3 years are shown in Table 55.4 and Table 55.5. The percent of programs with graft and patient follow-up data at 1 year was more than 98%; at conditional 3 years the percent of programs with follow-up data was greater than 96%.

There was a marked increase in both the number of liver transplants and in the actual graft and patient survival rates from Era I to Era 2. As demonstrated in Table 55.6, graft survival rates increased 6% at 3 months and 7% at 1 year in Era 2 from Era 1. Patient survival rates increased 4% at 3 months and 5% at 1 year during the study period.

For the majority of transplant programs, the difference between actual and expected survival rates was not statistically significant, especially in the long term. In general, large differences (either higher or lower) were nearly always found among programs that reported relatively few transplants. Therefore, when evaluating survival rates for a program, it is also important to consider the number of transplants performed there.

Differences between Short Term and Long Term Characteristics

The 1997 Report includes an extensive list of characteristics that have a significant impact on both short and long term graft and patient survival.

Characteristics with the strongest *positive* impact on *short term survival* were:

*   Recipient had cholestatic disease/biliary cirrhosis

*   Year of transplant was after 1990

Characteristics with the strongest *negative* impact on *short term survival* were:

- Donor was Black or Hispanic
- Donor and recipient blood types were incompatible
- Recipient received one or more previous transplants
- Recipient was Asian
- Recipient received a reduced or split liver
- Recipient was on life support prior to transplant
- Recipient's most recent serum creatinine prior to transplant was >2 mg/dl

Characteristics with the strongest *positive* impact on *long term survival* were:

- Donor cause of death was cardiovascular accident (CVA)
- Recipient was female
- Recipient had acute hepatic necrosis, cholestatic disease/biliary cirrhosis, metabolic disease, or miscellaneous disease

Characteristics with the strongest *negative* impact on *long term survival* were:

- Donor was female
- Recipient received one or more previous transplants
- Recipient was 1 year of age or younger
- Recipient received a reduced or split liver
- Recipient had malignant neoplasms

Completeness of Follow-up Data and Overall Graft and Patient Survival Rates

For graft survival, completeness of follow-up data and overall actual survival rates at each time point are shown in Table 55.4; patient survival data are shown in Table 55.5.

Patient (graft) follow-up data were considered complete when:

- the patient was alive (liver was functioning) and the duration of survival (function) was equal to or exceeded the specified time after transplant (i.e., 3 months, 1 or 3 years), or

- the patient died (liver failed) and a valid date of death (failure) was reported.

471

Table 55.4. Completeness of Graft Follow-up Data and Actual Survival Rates for Liver Transplants

Time	Cohort	No. of Transplants	% with Follow-up Data	Graft Survival (%)		
				Overall	Era 1	Era 2
3 Months	1/1/88-4/30/94	16,658	99.9	77.7	75.5	81.1
1 Year	1/1/88-4/30/94	16,658	99.1	69.9	67.3	74.1
Cond. 3 Years	1/1/88-4/30/94	6,859	96.8	89.0	89.0	N/A*

Table 55.5. Completeness of Patient Follow-up Data and Actual Survival Rates for Liver Transplants

Time	Cohort	No. of Patients	% with Follow-up Data	Patient Survival (%)		
				Overall	Era 1	Era 2
3 Months	1/1/88-4/30/94	14,607	99.7	85.3	83.7	87.8
1 Year	1/1/88-4/30/94	14,607	98.5	79.0	76.9	82.2
Cond. 3 Years	1/1/88-4/30/94	6,861	96.5	90.4	90.4	N/A*

The cohort used to determine the overall conditional 3 year survival rate is the same as the Era 1 cohort. Therefore, the overall conditional 3 year survival rates are identical to the conditional 3 year survival rates for Era 1. There is no conditional 3 year survival rate calculated for Era 2 due to insufficient follow-up data on patients who received transplants in Era 2.

Table 55.6. Comparison of 3 Month and 1 Year Actual Survival Rates Between Eras

	3 Months		1 Year	
	Era 1	Era 2	Era 1	Era 2
Graft Survival (%)	75.5%	81.1%	67.3%	74.1%
Average No. Transplants/Month	197	267	197	267
Patient Survival (%)	83.7%	87.8%	76.9%	82.2%
Average No. Patients/Month	171	244	171	244

The percentages of complete follow-up data ranged from a low of 96.5% for the conditional 3 year time point to a high of 99.9% for the 3 month time point.

Overall survival rates also are presented in the tables. Patient survival rates are better than graft survival rates at all time points because patients may be retransplanted and remain alive following graft failure. If a graft had incomplete follow-up data, the observation was weighted to account for the time during which the graft was known to be functioning. Therefore, the actual graft survival rate reflects the weighted proportion of grafts functioning at the specified time interval. Patient survival rates were computed in a similar way.

In the cohort of transplants (1/1/88–4/30/92) used to compute conditional 3 year survival rates, patients (grafts) who did not survive to 1 year after transplant were excluded from the analyses. Therefore, the total number of patients (grafts) for the conditional 3 year analysis was less than that for the 3 month and 1 year analyses. Further, the number of patients is greater than the number of grafts because more grafts failed than patients died within the first year post-transplant.

Please note that the conditional 3 year graft and patient survival rates in Table 55.4 and Table 55.5 may be higher than the 1 year graft survival rates. This is possible because the conditional 3 year survival rates should be interpreted as the 3 year survival rate for patients (grafts) who (which) survived at least 1 year posttransplant.

For example: Program A performed a total of five transplants between 1/1/88 and 4/30/92. Two of the livers failed prior to 1 year post-transplant and the remaining three livers survived to 3 years after transplant. In this example, Program A has a 1 year graft survival rate of 60% (3 out of 5 livers were functioning at 1 year post-transplant). However, the conditional 3 year survival rate for Program A is 100% because all three livers that were functioning at 1 year after transplant also were functioning at 3 years post-transplant.

Overall Graft and Patient Survival Rates by Era

In this report, short term survival also is reported by era. Separate eras were used to determine whether there were any improvements over time in the short-term survival rates. Era 1 is defined as all transplants occurring between January 1, 1988, and April 30, 1992; Era 2 includes all transplants occurring between May 1, 1992, and April 30, 1994. The overall graft and patient survival rates by era are presented in the last two columns of Table 55.4 and Table 55.5

respectively. The results demonstrate a substantial improvement in both graft and patient survival rates over time.

National Distribution of Donor and Recipient Characteristics

The national distribution of donor and recipient characteristics for liver transplants, presented in percentages, is shown in Table 55.7. Each of these donor and recipient characteristics was included in the analyses for graft or patient survival, and used to determine an expected survival rate for each transplant.

The majority of livers transplanted were recovered from white male donors between the ages of 18 and 44 and the most frequent causes of death were due to cerebrovascular accidents (CVAS) and head trauma. Nearly 47% of liver donors had cold ischemic times of 10 hours or less.

The majority of liver recipients were white males between the ages of 45 and 64. Nearly 51% of recipients were not hospitalized prior to transplant and 87% of the recipients received an ABO identical transplant; in other words, both the donor and recipient had the same blood type. Of the 16,658 transplants, 13% were repeat liver transplants.

Donor Trends

National donor characteristics changed between Era 1 and Era 2. The percentage of donors age 45 and older increased by 10% between Era 1 and Era 2, from 14% to 24%. The percentage of minority donors also increased, from 18% to 23%. There were fewer donors who died from head trauma and more who died from cerebrovascular accidents (CVAs).

Recipient Trends

Transplant recipients were older in the second era; those over age 45 comprised 55% of recipients in Era 2 as compared to 47% in Era 1. The percentage of transplants for patients in the miscellaneous liver disease group decreased, while those with cirrhosis increased in Era 2. More recipients were not hospitalized prior to their transplants in Era 2; the percentage of recipients who were hospitalized decreased by 2% from Era 1 and the percentage of patients in the intensive care unit decreased by 9% from Era 1.

Despite more older donors and older recipients in Era 2, the national survival rates improved from Era 1 to Era 2 (See Tables 55.4 and 55.5).

Table 55.7a. National Donor and Recipient Characteristics in Liver Transplants: Percentages by Era and Overall (continued on next page)

Characteristics by Category		ERA 1 1/88-4/92 N=10,241	ERA 2 5/92-4/94 N=6,417	OVERALL 1/88-4/94 N=16,658
Donor Age	<1	3.6	1.7	2.9
	1-5	7.1	4.6	6.1
	6-17	20.5	19.8	20.2
	18-44	54.2	49.5	52.4
	45-64	13.8	21.1	16.6
	65+	0.5	3.2	1.5
	Not Reported	0.3	0.2	0.2
Donor Race	White	81.9	77.4	80.2
	Black	9.5	11.7	10.4
	Hispanic	6.6	8.4	7.3
	Asian	0.9	1.4	1.1
	Other	0.7	0.8	0.7
	Not Reported	0.4	0.3	0.4
Donor Gender	Female	35.9	36.9	36.9
	Male	64.0	63.1	63.7
	Not Reported	0.1	0.0	0.1
Cold Ischemic Time (Hours)	0-5	11.1	9.1	10.3
	6-10	34.4	40.0	36.6
	11-15	31.6	32.5	31.9
	16-20	11.5	7.5	10.0
	21+	5.0	3.7	4.5
	Not Reported	6.4	7.1	6.7
Donor Cause of Death	CVA	28.5	34.1	30.7
	Head Trauma	32.8	15.9	26.3
	Other	38.8	49.9	43.1
Blood Group Compatibility	Identical	85.7	89.0	87.0
	Compatible	10.4	8.6	9.7
	Incompatible	3.4	2.2	3.0
	Unknown	0.4	0.2	0.3

Table 55.7b. National Donor and Recipient Characteristics in Liver Transplants: Percentages by Era and Overall (continued from previous page, continued on next page)

Characteristics by Category		ERA 1 1/88-4/92 N=10,241	ERA 2 5/92-4/94 N=6,417	OVERALL 1/88-4/94 N=16,658
Recipient Age	<1	5.1	3.3	4.4
	1.5	7.6	5.8	6.9
	6-17	6.3	5.2	5.9
	18-44	34.5	30.9	33.1
	45-64	43.1	49.5	45.5
	65+	3.4	5.3	4.2
Recipient Race	White	78.2	76.3	77.5
	Black	8.2	7.7	8.0
	Hispanic	7.7	9.7	8.4
	Asian	2.8	3.1	2.9
	Other	3.1	3.2	3.1
	Not Reported	0.1	0.0	0.1
Recipient Gender	Female	46.6	44.5	45.8
	Male	53.4	55.5	54.2
Procedure Type	Whole Liver	98.1	98.1	98.1
	Reduced/Split Liver	1.9	1.9	1.9
Previous Liver Transplant	No	85.8	88.4	86.8
	Yes	14.2	11.6	13.2
Liver Disease	Acute Hepatic Necrosis	7.7	6.7	7.4
	Cholestatic/ Biliary Cirrhosis	18.5	17.2	18.0
	Cirrhosis	49.2	57.2	52.3
	Malignant Neoplasms	4.9	3.5	4.4
	Metabolic Disease	5.5	4.7	5.2
	Miscellaneous Disease	14.2	10.5	12.7
	Not Reported	0.0	0.2	0.1

Table 55.7c. National Donor and Recipient Characteristics in Liver Transplants: Percentages by Era and Overall (continued from previous pages)

Characteristics by Category		ERA 1 1/88-4/92 N=10,241	ERA 2 5/92-4/94 N=6,417	OVERALL 1/88-4/94 N=16,658
Recipient	Intensive Care	31.0	22.4	27.7
Description	Hospitalized	22.2	19.8	21.3
at Transplant	Not Hospitalized	46.8	57.4	50.9
	Not Reported	0.0	0.3	0.2
Recipient on	No	79.6	85.2	81.8
Life Support	Yes	20.4	14.4	18.1
	Not Reported	0.0	0.3	0.1
Serum	0-2	85.8	86.8	86.2
Creatinine Prior	>2	13.1	12.7	13.0
to Transplant	Not Reported	1.0	0.5	0.8
Year of Transplant	1988	16.4	0.0	10.1
	1989	21.0	0.0	12.9
	1990	25.5	0.0	15.7
	1991	28.0	0.0	17.2
	1992	9.1	31.5	17.8
	1993	0.0	52.0	20.0
	1994	0.0	16.5	6.4

Liver Primary Disease Diagnoses at Time of Transplant

Cholestatic Liver Diseases/Biliary Cirrhosis

- Cholestatic Liver Disease
- Primary Biliary Cirrhosis (PBC)
- Secondary Biliary Cirrhosis (SBC)
    - Caroli's Disease
    - Choledochal Cyst
    - Bile Duct Strictures
- Primary Sclerosing Cholangitis (PSC)
    - with Crohn's GI tract disease
    - with Ulcerative Colitis

Cirrhosis

- Laennec's
- Postnecrotic Cirrhosis (A,B,C,D)
- Postnecrotic Cirrhosis (Non A, Non B)
- Cryptogenic, Idiopathic, no obvious source
- Chronic Active Hepatitis (A,B,C,D)
- Chronic Active Hepatitis: etiology unknown
- Autoimmune, Lupoid, Banti's
- Drug or industrial exposure

Acute Hepatic Necrosis (AHN)

- Due to a drug, chemicals, toxins
- Hepatitis (A,B,C,D)
- Non A, Non B Hepatitis
- Acute non-hepatic viral infection
- Unspecified fulminate hepatitis, submassive hepatic necrosis

Metabolic Disease

- Alpha-1-antitrypsin deficiency (A-1-A)
- Wilson's Disease, other copper metabolism disorder
- Hemochromatosis, hemosiderosis, other iron storage disease
- Glycogen Storage Disease Type 1, Type II
- Hyperlipidemia-II, Homozygous
- Hypercholesterolemia
- Tyrosinemia
- Primary Oxalosis/Oxaluria, Hyperoxaluria
- Other Metabolic Disease

Miscellaneous (Other) Liver Disease

- Familial Cholestasis: Byler's Disease, Other
- Neonatal Hepatitis
- Biliary Atresia
  - Extrahepatic
  - Hypoplasia
  - Alagille's Syndrome
- Congenital Hepatic Fibrosis

- Cystic Fibrosis
- Budd-Chiari Syndrome
- Benigh Tumor: Hepatic Adenoma, Polycystic liver disease, other
- Total Parenteral Nutrition (TPN)/Hyperalimentation induced liver disease
- Graft vs. Host Disease secondary to non-liver transplant
- Trauma

Malignant Neoplasms

Primary Liver Malignancy

- Hepatoma, hepatocellular carcinoma (HCC)
- Fibrolamellar (FL-HC)
- Cholangiocarcinoma (CH-CA)
- Hepatoblastoma (HBL)
- Hemangioendothelioma, Hemangiosarcoma, Angiosarcoma
- Klatskin tumor, Leimyosarcoma

Bile Duct Cancer

- Cholangioma, Biliary Tract Carcinoma

Secondary Hepatic Malignancy

- Non-liver Adenocarcinoma
- Cystadenocarcinoma
- VIPoma
- Gastrinoma
- Insulinoma
- Islet cell tumor
- Neuroendocrine tumor

Expected Liver Transplant Survival Rates

Table 55.8 shows the 1 year expected patient survival rates for liver transplants. These rates were determined using the following characteristics: recipient age, disease diagnosis, medical status prior to transplant, and transplant number. For these analyses, all other characteristics were set to the values for the reference groups, with the exception of the year of transplant (1993-1994).

Table 55.8a. Expected U.S. 1 Year Patient Survival Rates—Liver Transplants (continued on next page)

Age	Diagnosis	Not Hospitalized		Hospitalized		In ICU	
		Primary	Repeat	Primary	Repeat	Primary	Repeat
5	Acute Hepatic						
	Necrosis	91.2	83.9	88.9	80.1	86.9	77.0
	Cholestatic/						
	Biliary Cirrhosis	94.7	90.0	93.2	87.4	92.0	85.3
	Cirrhosis	92.3	85.7	90.2	82.3	88.4	79.4
	Malignancy	85.7	75.1	82.2	70.0	79.4	66.0
	Metabolic Disease	92.3	85.7	90.2	82.3	88.4	79.4
	Miscellaneous						
	Disease	91.4	84.3	89.2	80.6	87.2	77.5
25	Acute Hepatic						
	Necrosis	91.8	85.0	89.7	81.4	87.8	78.5
	Cholestatic/						
	Biliary Cirrhosis	95.1	90.7	93.7	88.3	92.6	86.3
	Cirrhosis	92.8	86.7	90.9	83.5	89.3	80.7
	Malignancy	86.7	76.7	83.4	71.7	80.7	67.8
	Metabolic Disease	92.8	86.7	90.9	83.5	89.3	80.7
	Miscellaneous						
	Disease	92.0	85.4	89.9	81.8	88.1	78.9
40	Acute Hepatic						
	Necrosis	90.6	82.9	88.1	78.9	86.0	75.7
	Cholestatic/						
	Biliary Cirrhosis	94.3	89.3	92.8	86.6	91.4	84.3
	Cirrhosis	91.7	84.8	89.5	81.2	87.7	78.2
	Malignancy	84.8	73.7	81.1	68.4	78.1	64.3
	Metabolic Disease	91.7	84.8	89.5	81.2	87.7	78.2
	Miscellaneous						
	Disease	90.8	83.3	88.4	79.4	86.4	76.2

Table 55.8b. Expected U.S. 1 Year Patient Survival Rates—Liver Transplants (continued from previous page)

Age	Diagnosis	Not Hospitalized		Hospitalized		In ICU	
		Primary	Repeat	Primary	Repeat	Primary	Repeat
50	Acute Hepatic Necrosis	88.6	79.7	85.7	75.2	83.3	71.6
	Cholestatic/ Biliary Cirrhosis	93.1	87.1	91.2	84.0	89.6	81.3
	Cirrhosis	90.0	81.9	87.4	77.7	85.2	74.4
	Malignancy	81.8	69.4	77.7	63.7	74.3	59.3
	Metabolic Disease	90.0	81.9	87.4	77.7	85.2	74.4
	Miscellaneous Disease	88.9	80.1	86.1	75.7	83.7	72.2
60	Acute Hepatic Necrosis	85.3	74.5	81.8	69.3	78.8	65.3
	Cholestatic/ Biliary Cirrhosis	90.9	83.5	88.5	79.6	86.5	76.4
	Cirrhosis	87.0	77.1	83.8	72.2	81.1	68.4
	Malignancy	77.1	62.9	72.2	56.7	68.3	52.1
	Metabolic Disease	87.0	77.1	83.8	72.2	81.1	68.4
	Miscellaneous Disease	85.6	75.1	82.2	69.9	79.3	65.9

Chapter 56

Questions and Answers about Organ Donation

Introduction

Medical advances have made it possible to transplant numerous organs and tissues from one human being into another to improve and save lives. The first corneal transplant was performed in 1905, the first blood transfusion in 1918, the first kidney transplant in 1954, and the first heart transplant in 1967. Now, current medical technology also enables the transplantation of skin, heart-lung combinations, lung, pancreas, liver, bone, and bone marrow.

In 1996, there were 11,099 kidney, 4,058 liver, 2,342 heart, 172 pancreas, 850 kidney-pancreas, 39 heart-lung, and 805 lung transplants performed in the U.S. The number of transplantations has nearly tripled since 1983 due primarily to dramatic increases in the number of heart and liver transplants. However, the number of individuals awaiting transplants also continues to grow, and many people, approximately 4,000 per year, die because donor organs were not available to them.

Did you know that:

- More than 37,500 patients were awaiting kidney transplants in October 1997.

This chapter contains text from "Questions & Answers about Organ Donation," Division of Transplantation, Health Resources and Services Administration (HRSA), and "Organ Donations Increase in 1998 Following National Initiative and New Regulations," *HHS News* April 16, 1999 Press Release.

- Almost 8 percent of all individuals awaiting liver transplants are age 10 or younger.

- The one-year survival rate for heart transplant recipients is 82 percent.

- One donor, a victim of an automobile accident, recently was responsible for saving the lives of five individuals awaiting transplant surgery.

Please make a decision to become an organ and tissue donor. Discuss your decision with your family and let them know of your desire to become a donor. Then, sign and carry in your wallet a donor card.

Who Can Donate?

Individuals over the age of 18 can indicate their desire to be an organ donor by signing a donor card or expressing their wishes to family members. Relatives can also donate a deceased family member's organs and tissues, even those family members under the age of 18.

Donation of heart, liver, lung, pancreas, or heart/lung can occur only in the case of brain death. The donation of tissues such as bone, skin, or corneas can occur regardless of age and in almost any cause of death.

Can You Donate an Organ While You Are Still Alive?

Certain kinds of transplants can be done using living donors. For example, almost 30 percent of all 1996 kidney transplants were performed with living donors. They are often related to the person needing the transplant, and can live normal lives with just one healthy kidney. Also, there are new methods of transplanting a part of a living adult's liver to a child who needs a liver transplant. Parts of a lung, or pancreas from a living donor also can be transplanted.

Can You Still Choose to Donate if You Are Younger than 18 Years of Age?

Yes, but only with the consent of an adult who is legally responsible for you, such as your parents or legal guardian. The adult or adults should witness your signature on a donor card.

What Can Be Donated?

Organs that can be donated include: kidneys, heart, liver, lungs, and pancreas. Some of the tissues that can be donated include: corneas, skin, bone, middle-ear, bone marrow, connective tissues, and blood vessels.

Total body donation is also an option. Medical schools, research facilities and other agencies need to study bodies to gain greater understanding of disease mechanisms in humans. This research is vital to saving and improving lives. If you wish to donate your entire body, you should directly contact the facility of your choice to make arrangements.

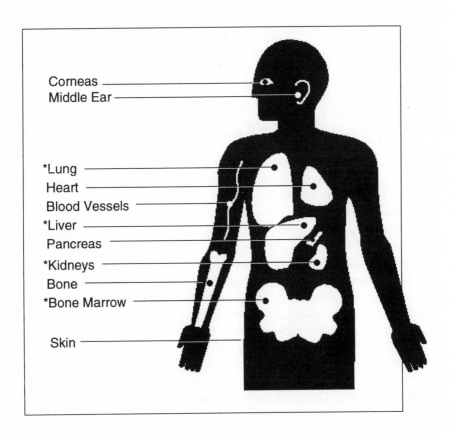

Figure 56.1. *Tissues and Organs that Can Be Donated*
*Lung lobes, liver lobes, kidneys, and bone marrow can be donated from living donors.

Why Should You Consider Becoming an Organ/Tissue Donor?

Advances in medical science have made transplant surgery increasingly successful. Transplantation is no longer considered experimental, but a desirable treatment option. The major problem is obtaining enough organs for the growing number of Americans needing them. As of October 1997, there were more than 55,000 registrants on the national transplant waiting list. Each month, the waiting list grows by approximately 500 registrants. By contrast, in 1996 there were only 5,416 donors in the United States. Even though most donors contribute multiple organs, there still are not enough to meet the need and many people die while waiting for an organ.

Everyone's help is needed to resolve the donor shortage. The best way to assure that more organs and tissues are made available is to sign and carry a donor card and encourage others to do so. It is especially important to let your family know of your wishes to donate if the opportunity arises. It will most likely be a family member who is in a position to see that your wishes are carried out.

How Do You Become a Donor Candidate?

Fill out a donor card and carry it in your wallet. Most states have some way that you can use your driver's license to indicate your wishes to be a donor. Some states have a donor card on the back of the license; others have a place to check or a colored sticker to put on the license.

It is also extremely important that you let your family know that you want to become an organ and tissue donor. Ask family members to sign your donor card as a witness. When you die, your next-of-kin will be asked to give their consent for you to become a donor. It is very important that they know you want to be a donor because that will make it easier for them to follow through on your wishes.

It would also be useful to tell your family physician and your religious leader that you would like to be a donor. And, it would be a good idea to tell your attorney and indicate in your will that you wish to be a donor.

What Is Brain Death?

Death occurs in two ways:

1. from cessation of cardio-pulmonary (heart-lung) functioning; and
2. from the cessation of brain functioning.

Brain death occurs when a person has an irreversible, catastrophic brain injury which causes all brain activity to stop permanently. In such cases, the heart and lungs can continue to function if artificial life-support machines are used. However, these functions also will cease when the machines are discontinued. Brain death is an accepted medical, ethical, and legal principle. The standards for determining that someone is brain dead are strict.

Tissue and bone may be useable in either type of death. Organs, however, are useable only in cases where brain death occurs.

What If Members of Your Family Are Opposed to Donation?

You can have an attorney put your request in writing. This document, along with your donor card, may help ensure that your wishes will be honored. In any event, tell your family that you want to become a donor in the event of your death.

Are There Religious Objections to Organ/Tissue Donation?

Most major religious groups in the United States approve and support the principles and practices of organ/tissue donation.

Transplantation is consistent with the life preserving traditions of these faiths. However, if you have any doubts, you should discuss them with your spiritual leader.

Is There a National Registry of Individuals Who Wish to Be Organ/Tissue Donors? What If You Change Your Mind about Donating?

There is no national registry of those who have indicated their willingness to be organ and tissue donors. If you change your mind, **tear up your donor card.**

If you have indicated your wishes to be a donor on your driver's license, ask your local office of the Division of Motor Vehicles (DMV) what steps you need to take to revoke your decision. An increasing number of states maintain registries of individuals who indicate on their driver licenses that they wish to be donors. If your state has a registry, your DMV personnel can tell you how to get on or off the registry.

In all instances, be sure to let your family know whether you wish or do not wish to become a donor.

Does the Donor's Family Have to Pay for the Cost of Organ Donation?

No. The donor's family neither pays for, nor receives payment for, organ and tissue donation. Hospital expenses incurred before the donation of organs in attempts to save the donor's life and funeral expenses remain the responsibility of the donor's family. All costs related to donation are paid for by the organ procurement program or transplant center.

Will the Quality of Hospital Treatment and Efforts to Save Your Life Be Lessened if Staff Know You Are Willing to Be a Donor?

No. A transplant team does not become involved until other physicians involved in the patient's care have determined that all possible efforts to save the patient's life have failed.

Does Organ Donation Leave the Body Disfigured?

No. The recovery of organs and tissues is conducted in an operating room under the direction of qualified surgeons and neither disfigures the body nor changes the way it looks in a casket.

Is It Permissible to Sell Human Organs?

No. The National Organ Transplant Act (Public Law 98-507) prohibits the sale of human organs. Violators are subject to fines and imprisonment. Among the reasons for this rule is the concern of Congress that buying and selling of organs might lead to inequitable access to donor organs with the wealthy having an unfair advantage.

What Is "Required Request?"

"Required request" is a policy requiring hospitals to systematically and routinely offer the next-of-kin the opportunity to donate their deceased relative's organs and tissues. This policy enables hospitals and health care professionals to play a key role in increasing donation because families might otherwise not be aware of their right to donate. As of 1992, forty-eight states and the District of Columbia had enacted "required request" laws.

The Omnibus Budget Reconciliation Act of 1986 (Public Law 99-509) established additional requirements for hospitals that participate in the Medicare and Medicaid programs. It required each participating hospital to establish written protocols for identification of organ donors and to notify an organ procurement organization designated by the Secretary of Health and Human Services of any potential donors it identifies.

Since January 1988, the Joint Commission for the Accreditation of Healthcare Organizations has required its member hospitals, as a prerequisite for accreditation, to develop policies and procedures on the identification and referral of potential donors.

What Are Organ Procurement Organizations (OPOS)?

OPO's are organizations that coordinate activities relating to organ procurement in a designated service area. Evaluating potential donors, discussing donation with family members, and arranging for the surgical removal of donated organs are some of their primary functions. OPO's also are responsible for preserving the organs and making arrangements for their distribution according to national organ sharing policies established by the Organ Procurement and Transplantation Network and approved by the U.S. Department of Health and Human Services.

In addition, OPO's provide information and education to medical professionals and the general public to encourage organ and tissue donation and increase the availability of organs for transplantation.

How Many Transplant Programs and OPO's Are There in the United States?

As of October 1997 there were 120 liver, 254 kidney, 164 heart, 124 pancreas, 98 heart-lung, and 92 lung transplant programs in the United States. Names and addresses of transplant programs can be obtained from the United Network for Organ Sharing at the following address:

United Network for Organ Sharing
1100 Boulders Parkway, Suite 500
PO Box 13770
Richmond, Virginia 23225-8770
(888) 894-6361
URL: http://www.unos.org/frame_Default.asp

As of December 1997, 63 OPO's were certified by the Health Care Financing Administration of the U.S. Department of Health and Human Services. Their names and addresses can be obtained from the following organizations:

Association of Organ Procurement Organizations
One Cambridge Court
8110 Gatehouse Road
Suite 101 West
Falls Church, Virginia 22042
(703) 573-2676
URL: http://www.aopo.org

American Congress for Organ Recovery and Donation
1714 Hayes Street
Nashville,TN 32703
(615) 327-2247

What Are the Steps Involved in Organ Donation and Transplantation?

1. A potential donor who has been diagnosed as brain dead must be identified.

2. An organ procurement organization is contacted to help determine organ acceptability, obtain the family's permission, and match the donor with the most appropriate recipient(s).

3. Next-of-kin must be informed of the opportunity to donate their relative's organs and tissues, and must give their permission.

4. Organ(s) and tissue(s) are surgically removed from the donor.

5. The donor organs and tissues are taken to the transplant center(s) where the surgery will be performed.

When a potential organ donor is identified by hospital staff and brain death is imminent or present, an organ procurement organization (OPO) is contacted. The OPO is consulted about donor acceptability and often asked to counsel with families to seek consent for donation. If consent is given, a search is made for the most appropriate recipient(s) using a computerized listing of transplant candidates managed by the United Network for Organ Sharing which operates the National Organ Procurement and Transplantation Network.

It is increasingly common for donors and donor families to contribute multiple organs and/or tissues. Therefore, several recipients may be helped by a single donor. When a match is found, the OPO will arrange for the donated organ(s) to be surgically removed, preserved, and transported to the appropriate transplant center(s). A potential recipient(s) is also alerted to the availability of an organ and asked to travel to the transplant center where he or she is prepared for surgery. The recipient's diseased or failing organ is removed and the donated organ is implanted.

How Are Recipients Matched to Donor Organs?

Persons waiting for transplants are listed at the transplant center where they plan to have surgery, and on a national computerized waiting list of potential transplant patients in the United States. Under contract with the Health Resources and Services Administration, the United Network for Organ Sharing (UNOS) located in Richmond, Virginia maintains the national waiting list. UNOS operates the Organ Procurement and Transplantation Network and maintains a 24-hour telephone service to aid in matching donor organs with patients on the national waiting list and to coordinate efforts with transplant centers.

When donor organs become available, several factors are taken into consideration in identifying the best matched recipient(s). These include medical compatibility of the donor and potential recipient(s) on such characteristics as blood type, weight, and age, urgency of need, and length of time on the waiting list. In general, preference is given to recipients from the same geographic area as the donor because timing is a critical element in the organ procurement process. Hearts can be preserved for up to 6 hours, livers up to 24 hours, and kidneys for 72 hours. Lungs cannot be preserved outside the body for any extended period of time.

Why Should Minorities Be Particularly Concerned about Organ Donation?

Minorities suffer end-stage renal disease (ESRD), a very serious and life-threatening kidney disease, much more frequently than do whites. For example, from 1992 to 1995 African-Americans were more than four times more likely than whites to develop ESRD; Native Americans were more than three times as likely; and Asian Americans were almost twice as likely to suffer from the disease.

491

ESRD is treatable with dialysis, however, dialysis is costly and can result in a poor quality of life for the patient. The preferred treatment of ESRD is kidney transplantation. Transplantation offers the patient "freedom" from dialysis to lead a more normal lifestyle and can successfully cure ESRD for many years.

As with any transplant procedures, it is very important to assure a close match between donor and recipient blood types and genetic make-up. Members of different racial and ethnic groups are usually more genetically similar to members of their own group than they are to others. (For example, blacks are usually more genetically similar to other blacks than they are to whites.) It is important, therefore, to increase the minority donor pool so that good matches can be made as frequently as possible for minority patients.

How Many Organ Transplants Have Been Performed Each Year and What Are the Survival Rates for Each Organ?

Table 56.1. Transplants Performed in the U.S.

Organ/Year	1985	1990	1995	1996	1-Year Graft Survival Rate[1]
Heart	719	2,023	2,361	2,342	81.5%
Kidney	7,695	9,528	11,712	11,099	91.9% [2]
					83.2% [3]
Liver	602	2,570	3,925	4,058	73.4%
Pancreas	130	530	110	172	73.8%
Heart/Lung	30	51	68	39	69.3%
Lung	20	190	871	805	75.9%
Total	9,196	14,892	19,047	18,515	

[1]*Survival rates can be measured in two ways:*

- *the length of time the transplant patient survives after surgery; and*
- *the length of time the graft (transplanted organ) survives after surgery. In the case of kidney and pancreas transplants, if the graft fails, the patient has a backup form of therapy available (e.g., insulin or dialysis). Failure of other types of transplanted organs, however, results in patient death unless the recipient can receive another transplant. The figures above represent patient survival rates as cited in the Annual*

Report of the U.S. Scientific Registry of Transplant Recipients and the Organ Procurement and Transplantation Network. These data were gathered from 1988 to 1994.

[2]Donations from live donors
[3]Donations from cadaveric donors

How Many People Are Currently Waiting for Each Organ To Become Available so They Can Have a Transplant?

As of October 8, 1997, the waiting list for donor organs totaled 55,378. The number of people waiting for each organ is listed below.

Table 56.2. People Waiting for Specific Organs

37,532	kidney
9,127	liver
359	pancreas
75	pancreas islet cell
1,581	kidney-pancreas
86	intestine
3,845	heart
224	heart-lung
2,549	lung
55,378	**TOTAL**

Can Anything Be Done to Improve Access to a Donor Organ for Those in Critical Need of an Organ Transplant? What about Special Public Appeals?

The primary barrier to transplant surgery for most of the people on the waiting list is a lack of donor organs. Quite simply, the demand far exceeds the supply. Therefore, anything that can be done to increase the level of donation in this country would be helpful to all individuals needing transplants.

Families and attending physicians need to maintain close contact with the transplant team to keep them fully up-to-date on the patient's condition. A family could assist community groups in their ongoing efforts to increase public awareness of the need for organ donation.

While family appeals through the media have had a positive effect on increasing donation overall, efforts do not necessarily result in an organ being made available to the individual for whom the appeal has been made. The decision as to which patient on the waiting list will receive any particular organ is made according to objective criteria which include medical urgency and length on the waiting list, and is not subject to external influences including those that might result in inequitable access to donor organs. Any prejudicial or discriminatory practices in organ allocation are forbidden by the policies governing the operation of the Organ Procurement and Transplantation Network. However, raising the level of organ donation in general will necessarily be of help to all those awaiting transplantation.

1998 Increase of Organ Donations

The Department of Health and Human Services and the United Network for Organ Sharing (UNOS) announced that the number or organ donors increased 5.6 percent in 1998, the first substantial increase since 1995.

The increase follows the launch of the Clinton administration's donation initiative in 1997, as well as new regulations implemented in 1998 which require hospitals to report all deaths to organ procurement organizations (OPO's).

Preliminary data show that the number of cadaveric donors rose to 5,788 in 1998, up from 5,479 in 1997. The increase resulted in approximately 600 additional organ transplants and up to 14,000 more tissue transplants.

"More Americans are hearing about the need for organ donation, and more are responding with the gift of life,' said HHS Secretary Donna E. Shalala. "But we need to accelerate this trend. Organ donation saves lives, but the need for organs is still far greater than the supply. Too many patients still die while waiting for a transplant."

"We're letting people know that signing a donor card is not really enough. You have to tell your family," Secretary Shalala said. "It's families and loved ones who are usually asked to consent to donation, and their decision often is made under the most difficult circumstances. That decision is made much easier if the individual has told them in advance that he or she would want their organs to be offered for transplantation."

The Health Care Financing Administration (HCFA), the HHS agency that administers Medicare, is a key player in the campaign.

HCFA last year began requiring all hospitals that participate in Medicare to routinely inform their local OPO's of all hospital deaths and imminent deaths. The OPO's can then request donation from the families of potential donors. Previously, many families were never asked, an estimated 3,000 to 4,000 potential donors annually were not identified. HHS estimates that this alerting requirement along with other donation activities can increase organ donation by 20 percent in the next two years.

HCFA also is requiring hospitals to have recovery partnership agreements with a tissue bank and an eye bank. A representative of an OPO, tissue bank, eye bank, or an individual trained in this area will discreetly discuss donation options with affected families. "We find that a sensitive, humane approach is not only respectful of the family's feelings, it also increases the likelihood that they will consent to donation. We hope that this new requirement will result in many more lives saved by caring families," said Nancy-Ann DeParle, HCFA administrator.

Donation increases between 1997 and 1998 were substantial for Caucasians (up 6.6 percent from 4,139 to 4,410 donors) and Hispanics (up 7.8 percent from 552 to 595 donors). The number of African-American donors remained relatively unchanged at 654 donors in 1998, and the number of Asian donors decreased by 8.4 percent from 107 to 98 donors.

Donors increased for all age ranges, but the largest increase was in donors age 60 and above (up 10.8 percent from 706 to 782). Donors age 40 to 59 increased by 9.6 percent (1,781 to 1,952). Donors age 20 to 39 increased by 2.4 percent (1,653 to 1,693) and age 0 to 19 increased only slightly by 1.6 percent (1,339 to 1,361).

Waiting list registrations also climbed from 56,716 at the end of 1997 to 64,423 at the end of 1998, and the gap between supply and demand for organs continues to widen. "To the person anxiously awaiting a renewed chance at life through transplantation, there is no greater gift than a donated organ," said UNOS President William W. Pfaff, M.D. "However, tens of thousands still await this opportunity, and we must continue to foster the selfless act of donation to meet their need."

Public education efforts have increased at all levels over the last four or five years, and we are beginning to see the effect of these efforts," said Howard Nathan, executive director of Philadelphia-based Delaware Valley Transplant Program and president of the Coalition on Donation. "With the implementation of the new federal rules for hospitals in the United States and continued public education, we anticipate that donors will continue to increase as more families are offered the option and say 'yes' to donation."

The largest increase in donations occurred in the central region of the United States. UNOS Region 10 (Michigan, Indiana, and Ohio) had the largest increase at 13 percent (from 500 to 565). UNOS Region 8 (Iowa, Missouri, Nebraska, Kansas, Wyoming, and Colorado) increased by 11.3 percent (from 380 to 423), and Region 4 (Oklahoma and Texas) increased by 9.1 percent (from 472 to 515).

Chapter 57

AirLifeLine:
Patient Air Transportation

How AirLifeLine Began

AirLifeLine is a national non-profit charitable organization of private pilots who donate their time, skills, aircraft, and fuel to fly medical missions. Founded in 1978 by Sacramento, California businessman and pilot Tom Goodwin, the program was initially established to provide efficient transport of time-critical medical cargo. In 1984, services were expanded to include ambulatory patients requiring medical travel they could not afford.

A core of 25 interested pilots in California has now grown to over 1,000 pilots nationwide. AirLifeLine has flown more than 17,000 missions. The pilots have surpassed 9 million flying miles at absolutely no cost to patients or referring agencies.

For 21 years, AirLifeLine has served as a vital link between home and hospital for thousands of patients and their families. Perhaps you, or someone you know could benefit from this service.

AirLifeLine volunteer pilots fly medical missions for patients with major health problems. These pilots also fly time-critical medical cargo such as donor organs and blood plasma.

Patients

If you are in need of free transportation for medical purposes or if you know of someone who is, AirLifeLine is ready to help.

Reprinted with permission of AirLife Line © 1999.

Required Qualifications

- You must be ambulatory or mobile enough to enter and exit the aircraft

- There must be financial need

- Medical personnel and equipment are not needed during the flight

- The distance is not more than 1000 miles.

Requesting a Flight:

- You, a social worker, family resource person, or medical agency may call AirLifeLine at 800-446-1231.

  AirLifeLine will need:

- Patient's name, address, phone number, weight, and accompanying individuals names, relationships, and weights

- Travel dates and departure and destination points

- Confirmation of medical and financial need. Medical and financial forms will be faxed

- Waiver of liability. Form will be faxed.

Note: The medical, financial, and waiver of liability forms are available on the Internet on the AirLifeLine web site at http://www.airlifeline.org.

  After receipt of the completed forms, AirLifeLine will:

- Call you to confirm receipt of forms and get any updated or missing information

- Finalize the patient and flight requirement information in our data base mission form

- Forward your request to regional coordinator to select a pilot who will contact you to confirm the date, time and flight details.

Note: These forms are also available on the AirLifeLine web site at: http://www.airlifeline.org

Guidelines for AirLifeLine Flights

- Flights are weather dependent. The patient should have a back-up plan.

- General aviation planes are compact and don't have the facilities that commercial planes do. Usually a plane has just 4 or 6 seats.

- Luggage space is likely to be limited; soft-sided bags are easier to accommodate.

- You are responsible for arranging ground transportation.

- If the date or time of the flight changes, be sure to call the AirLifeLine office (800-446-1231), your regional coordinator, or your pilot.

- You should show up with only the number of people for the flight that has been agreed on ahead of time with the office.

- You should travel with cash or a credit card in case there are unforeseen problems or delays.

AirLifeLine Passengers Are People Who:

- need chemotherapy, radiation, surgery, treatment or other medical care at a facility far from home.

- need an organ transplant

- are attending a camp for children or adults who have serious illnesses

- are making a flight to their "Final Wish" destination

- are assisting a community that has experienced a natural disaster.

How Can the Transportation Be Free of Cost?

AirLifeLine is a nationwide, charitable non-profit organization. Their 1,000-plus member pilots are volunteers who are not compensated or reimbursed for any of the costs involved in flying their planes. It is the generous and kind spirit of these individuals which makes it possible for AirLifeLine to offer their services at no charge to you, their patients. For them, a "thank you" and a smile is all the compensation they need!

Who Are AirLifeLine Pilots?

The pilots who fly for AirLifeLine are caring, committed, and compassionate individuals. They come from various walks of life as—engineers, doctors, retirees, lawyers, commercial pilots, and business people. They have to be fully FAA licensed and be current with their medical certificate and plane insurance. They must also be able to provide proof of the airworthiness of their aircraft.

Free Transportation for Diagnosis, Treatment, and Follow Up

AirLifeLine provides the means for those families in financial straits to get to their places of treatment. Individuals are allowed to be accompanied by one or two family members or support persons. These passengers are usually traveling for surgery, chemotherapy, radiation, diagnostic procedures, and other treatment. AirLifeLine also transports people who are not financially distressed, but who are in a time-critical situation due to their medical condition. This is usually the case for patients awaiting a lifesaving organ transplant, with perhaps only four to six hours in which to get to the hospital.

AirLifeLine Cannot Provide Medical Care

AirLifeLine volunteer pilots are not medical personnel. Their aircraft are not equipped to carry a stretcher or wheelchair. Oxygen is allowed with the pilot's consent, but the patient must provide it. The patient must be able to get into the plane, sit in a seat and wear a seat belt. A flight in an unpressurized cabin can be detrimental to the well being of certain patients; therefore, AirLifeLine relies on the doctor's assurance that the patient is in stable condition for travel in a light, unpressurized aircraft.

The Advantages of Air Travel

When AirLifeLine's services are needed, anyone may call (800) 446-1231. A one to three-hour flight in a light aircraft is preferable for a patient who may be too weak to travel by car or bus for longer periods. Patients who are susceptible to infection if exposed to large numbers of people benefit greatly from a private flight. AirLifeLine planes can fly into the smaller airports where commercial carriers are not allowed. This environment makes it much easier for pilot and patient to meet at the right time, at the right place, and is far less stressful.

How Does AirLifeLine Plan for a Mission?

An AirLifeLine mission can be put together with short notice. However, written verification of the medical and financial need of the patient is required before the mission is coordinated. Also, the more notice AirLifeLine has, the more success they have in reaching an available pilot. The pilot will pick up and drop off the patient at the airport closest to his or her home. However, it is the patient's responsibility to arrange for ground transportation at both the departure and arrival points. AirLifeLine does recommend that passengers eat a very light meal an hour or two before the flight. Flying on a full or an empty stomach is not a good idea. Motion sickness medications may help but are not provided. You should be aware that there are no restrooms or catering facilities on an AirLifeLine flight so do plan ahead.

How Far Will an AirLifeLine Pilot Fly?

AirLifeLine pilots from all over the United States participate in our humanitarian program. They are dispatched geographically according to the location of the mission request. As a rule, AirLifeLine flies up to 1,000 nautical miles for a one way distance. An average mission, however, is usually between 250-350 miles and can take two to four hours. When a greater distance is requested, the coordinator will arrange for a relay mission involving two pilots meeting at a pre-designated point to transfer their passengers. To do this kind of mission, the patient would have to be capable of sitting for many hours in a small confined space.

Waiver of Liability

Passengers will be asked to sign a waiver of liability prior to embarkation on every flight they take with AirLifeLine. This protects the AirLifeLine organization and the pilots should something unexpected occur.

What Is the Cost of an AirLifeLine Mission?

There is absolutely no charge to the patient or agency. The AirLife Line pilot donates the entire expense of the mission. It is his personal contribution. Most of the expenses incurred are tax deductible; however, it can cost the pilot anywhere from $200 to over $1000 to fly a mission.

What Would Cause AirLifeLine to Cancel a Mission?

Adverse weather conditions, mechanical problems, or other unforeseen events may cause a pilot to cancel or delay a flight without prior notice. It is always a good idea for the passenger and agency to have a backup means of transportation if it would be impossible to reschedule the appointment.

How Is AirLifeLine Funded?

AirLifeLine is supported solely by contributions from pilots, individuals, businesses, organizations, and foundations. They receive no government or United Way funds and rely on the generosity of caring individuals to support their modest operating budget.

Limited Space for Luggage

In a low-wing, single engine aircraft, there is room at the back of the seats, for one or two small soft-sided bags, or in the modest luggage compartment in the nose. Twin engine planes are larger, faster, and have more room than a single engine plane. Luggage can usually be stored at both the rear of the cabin and/or in the nose compartment.

What Can You Carry on Board?

The aircraft used have very limited space for baggage. It is suggested that you travel light. Most of the planes are two, three, or four seaters. Heavy luggage can reduce passenger capacity. Most of the planes can store several small soft-sided suitcases. AirLifeLine needs to know not only the luggage weight, but also the weight of all the passengers. Prior to scheduling the flight, they need to know exactly who and what will be accompanying the passenger.

How to Reach AirLifeLine

AirLifeLine National Office
50 Fullerton Court, Suite 200
Sacramento, CA 95825

Tel: (800) 446-1231
Tel: (916) 641-7800
Fax: (916) 641-0600
E-mail: staff@airlifeline.org

The national office of AirLifeLine is located in Sacramento, California, and staff members are there from 7:30 a.m. to 4:30 p.m. Pacific Coast time, Monday-Friday. The answering machine records messages after hours and also gives a pager number to reach a staff person in the case of an emergency or urgent situation.

Chapter 58

LifePage:
Pagers for People Waiting for
Organ Transplants

Every Second Counts...

Every 18 minutes another patient is added to the national transplant waiting list and everyday an average of 8 people die waiting for a transplant. Once a donor and patient organ match is identified, the patient must be in surgery within a matter of hours. The stress posed by the wait and the limited reaction time can be overwhelming. LifePage enables patients to cope with the stress by offering peace of mind in knowing that with their LifePage pager they can be reached anytime and anywhere.

For over a decade LifePage has meant freedom and hope to tens of thousands of transplant candidates. It has helped more than 40,000 transplant patients since 1991 alone. Everyday the LifePage team receives an average of 75 new pager requests. In January of 1991 the LifePage team helped to place 118 pagers in patients' hands. In January of 1997 the team placed almost 1,400. Even as the program continues to grow, the LifePage team still has a request processing time of less than 48 hours and a pager is usually in a patient's hands within 7-10 days. (This is the national average and response times can vary.)

What Is the LifePage Program?

LifePage is a program for patients who are registered for a kidney, pancreas, liver, heart, or lung transplant. The program provides the patient with a pager (beeper) through which their transplant co-ordinator can contact them anywhere, within their coverage range provided, at anytime in the event that a suitable organ match has been found. This service is provided by the Personal Communications In-dustry Association—PCIA Foundation, the Foundation affiliated with the paging, mobile telephone and cellular radiotelephones, and emerg-ing personal communication service (PCS) industries.

Who Is Eligible to Participate in LifePage?

All individuals currently registered for vital organ transplants are automatically eligible to receive a pager through the LifePage pro-gram. They may keep the pager as long as they are registered for a transplant.

How Does LifePage Work?

Very simply. Those who are eligible will receive a pager. These pagers can be carried in a purse or clipped to a belt. They are pro-grammed to beep when a specific telephone number is dialed. The telephone number is kept on record at their transplant center. When the transplant coordinator has a suitable organ match, he or she will call the patient. Because a patient is not always reachable by tele-phone, the transplant coordinator has the option to call their pager telephone number, which signals the pager to make a beeping sound. When the pager beeps, the patient will know to contact their trans-plant coordinator immediately.

Table 58.1. Pager Requests Processed

Totals by Year	Total
1991	2,047
1992	3,528
1993	4,089
1994	5,656
1995	9,385
1996	12,770
1997	17,673
1998	17,245 (Jan.–Oct.)

How Far from Home Can the Pager Work?

When the patient receives a pager, they should also receive a pager coverage map. The patient must be within the area shown on the coverage map to receive a page. If the patient plans to travel or move away from the coverage area in which their pager works, but want to continue in the LifePage program, contact the LifePage office for further instructions.

Who Can Call the Pager?

Only the transplant center or coordinator should have this pager number. If the number is given to other people, the patient will have no idea who is trying to page them when the pager beeps. This will disrupt the work of the transplant coordinator, confuse the patient, and defeat the purpose of the LifePage program.

How Do I Enroll in the LifePage Program?

If your transplant coordinator already participates in LifePage, he or she should be your first contact. Otherwise, contact the PCIA Foundation at:

PCIA Foundation
P.O. Box 207
Alexandria, VA. 22313-0207
Tel: 703-739-0527
Fax: 703-836-1608

Are There Any Costs for Having a LifePage Pager?

Generally, no. Except in a few cases where a participating carrier may require a security deposit or insurance fee, the only cost to you will be for replacing batteries. Pagers operate on AA or AAA size 1.5-volt alkaline batteries. The battery should be changed once a month to make sure it is fresh. In addition, the pager will signal when the battery is running low and needs to be replaced. Please be aware, however, that the company providing the pager receives no reimbursement for its use. You are fully responsible for returning the unit once you are no longer on the transplant list. If the pager is not returned, lost, or damaged, you will be held liable for its replacement value.

What Happens if I Live Far Away from My Transplant Center?

You must carry a pager that operates on a radio frequency in the area in which you live. The transplant coordinator can call your pager by dialing a telephone number plus the area code, just like any other long distance call. If you live outside of the pager coverage area where your transplant center is located, call LifePage to arrange for a pager that will work in your home community.

What Happens if I Have a Problem with My Pager?

The paging company that provides you with your pager has customer service agents available to assist you (during normal business hours). If your pager should need maintenance, the company will repair it. You may also contact your transplant coordinator or the LifePage office for assistance in resolving your problems.

How Do I Return a Pager?

In the event that you are no longer on an active transplant waiting list, the pager should be returned to the providing company, LifePage, or your transplant coordinator as promptly as possible so that another candidate may be able to receive a pager. (We have had numerous instances where a candidate was unable to receive a pager because the participating companies had no more to send out.) If you need assistance in returning a pager, please contact the LifePage coordinators at 703-739-0527.

LifePage Participating Paging Companies

Participation varies from branch to branch. If you have questions concerning a specific location or company, please call LifePage at (703) 739-0527.

A.V. Lattimus Communications
ADCOM Inc.
Advanced Communications
Afton Communications
Aircom
AirPage of Montana
AirPage of Wyoming
AirTouch Communications

ALLTEL Mobile Communications
AlwaysAnswering Service Inc.
American Communications Network
American Mobilphone
American Paging
Americom

Ameritech Mobile Communications
AnswerQuik of NC
Answer Duluth
Answer Fort Smith
Answer Jefferson City
Answer Phone & Radio Paging
Answer Plus of Fargo
Arch Communications
Aroostook Paging Inc.
AT&T Wireless Communications
Atlas Communications
Autophone of Laredo
Autophone of Vidalia
B & M Communications
Bay Star Satellite Paging
Beeper USA
Beepers Unlimited
Berkshire Communications Inc.
Beta Tele-Page
Bobier Electronics1
Cagle Communications
CalAutofone
Capital Paging
Cascade Telephone Communications, Inc.
CellPage
Central Vermont Communications
Circuit World
Citizen's Page
Communications Specialists of Jacksonville
Communications Specialist Inc.
Compusult
Consolidated Communications Mobile Services
Contact Communications
Contact New Mexico
Contact Paging
Cook Paging
Copeland Communications

CSSI
Cue of California
Cue Paging
Cumberland Mountain Paging
Dave's Communications
DeKalb Telephone Cooperative
DeRidder Mobilefone Inc.
Dial-A-Page
Digipage
Direct Page Communications
Douglas Paging Company
Dover Radio Page
El Dorado Answer Phone
Electronic Engineering Co.
First Page
Future Communications Inc.
Georgialina Communications Co.
Golden West Tele-Tech
HCI
Hello Inc.
High Country Paging
Highland Paging
Hord Communications
Huffman Communications
Illinois Signal
In*Touch Communications
Indiana Paging Network Inc.
Inter Mountain Company, Inc.
Jackson Mobilphone Company, Inc.
K Communications
Kar Kall, Inc.
KeyPage
Lakes Region Answering Svc.
Lehigh Valley Page
Lubbock Radio Paging Service
M & M Paging
McCord Communications
Mercury Cellular and Paging of Louisianna
Message Center Inc.

Metro Communications
Metro Paging Company
Metrocall
Michigan Mobile
Mid-State Paging
Mid-West Communications of Nebraska
MIDCO Communications
Midland Telecom
Milledgevill Mobilphone, Inc.
MinnComm Paging
Mo-Ark Mobilephone, Inc.
Mobile Communications
Mobile Paging Communications
MobileComm
Mobilefone of Great Bend, KS
Mobilefone Service Inc.
Mobilphone and Beeper Inc.
Morris Communications
Moutain Message and Paging Service
Mountain Paging Network Inc.
Mr. Radio
Nebraska Radio Telephone Systems
Nelson Telephone Cooperative
No'Mis Communications
Northeast Paging
Omnicom Paging
On Call Communications
Otsego Mobilefone Corp.
Ozark Mobilephone
P.N.Alarms
Pacific Coast Paging
PageA Phone
PageAmerica
Page Call Communications
Page One of Kentucky
Page One West-Gemini Communications
PageNet

Paging Plus of Wilkes-Barre
Pampa Communications
Panhandle Paging
Panhandle Radio Paging Svc., Inc.
PCI Communications
Personalized Paging
Pioneer Paging
Portland Paging Company
Pro-Com
Pro-Phone Communications, Inc.
Professional Paging & Radio Inc.
ProNet Communications
ProPage of Georgia
Purity Control
Qualicom Electronics
R.F. Communications
Radio & Communications Consultants
RadioAutopage of Owensboro
Radio Communications Co.
Radio Electronics Products Co.
Radio Telephone of Maine
Radio Telepage
Radiofone of Georgia
RadioPage
RAM Technologies
Range Corporation
Redi-Call Communications
Rinker's Communications
Robert S. Palm, Contractor
Shasta-Cascade Services
Shentel Service Company
Shores Communication Company
Sierra Communications
Silverado Communications
Siskyiou Mobilfone
SkyTel
Snider Telecom

South Georgia Communications
Southern Mobility
Southern Ohio Communication Service Inc.
Spokane Paging & Telecommunications
SRT Communications
ST Paging
St. Croix Telephone Company
Stark Communications
Stay In Touch Paging
Sunset Coast Paging
Tel*Star Communications
Tel-Call
Telebeep, Inc.
Teleview Inc.
Telewave Mobilephone Northwest
TexaPage NE Inc.

The Beeper Company
The Beeper Place
Total Communications
Tri-County Communications
Tri-Star Communications
United Communications, Inc.
United SignalAlert
United Telespectrum
Upstate Paging
Upstate Telecom
Vegas Insta-Page
Wabash Telephone Coop
Webster's Mobile Lock
West Wisconsin Telephone Coop
Western Communications Inc.
Western Total Communications
Westlink Paging
Wilcom Cellular
XPM Communications

Part Ten

Additional Help and Information

Chapter 59

Glossary of Important Terms

Absorption is the passage of substances through body surfaces into tissues or body fluids, e.g. water is absorbed in the colon. In the case of Absorptive Hyperoxaluria, the intestines absorb excess oxalate.

Acute Hepatitis. Active and symptomatic infection of the liver. The person is contagious.

AGT or alanine glyoxate aminotransferase is an enzyme that is produced in the peroxisome, a component of the liver cell. PHI patients lack sufficient quantities of this enzyme to counteract oxalate production. ACT cannot be synthesized.

Allograft is an organ or tissue transplanted from one individual to another of the same species; i.e. human to human. Example: a transplanted kidney.

Alpha Feto Protein (AFP). A normal protein produced in the developing human embryo. Adults do not contain much AFP in their blood. However, since liver cancer cells often produce AFP, elevated blood levels are associated with the possibility of liver cancer (HCC). However, other conditions may also cause a rise in AFP (such as pregnancy).

This chapter contains text from "Glossary of Hepatitis B Terms," © 1998, Hepatitis B Foundation reprinted with permission; "What Every Patient Needs to Know," © UNOS, reprinted with permission; and "Glossary of Terms," © Oxalosis and Hyperoxaluria Foundation, reprinted with permission.

Antibody is a protein substance made by the body's immune system in response to a foreign substance, for example a previous transplant, blood transfusion, virus, or pregnancy. Because the antibodies attack the transplanted organ, transplant patients must take powerful anti-rejection drugs.

Antigen is a foreign substance, such as a transplant, that triggers an immune response. This response may be the production of antibodies, which try to inactivate or destroy the antigen (the transplanted organ).

Anti-rejection drugs are medicines developed to suppress the immune response so that the body will accept, rather than reject, a transplanted organ or tissue. These medicines are also called immunosuppressants.

Autosomal Recessive is also known as recessive inheritance. A genetic inheritance governed by a paired set of genes. In the case of autosomal recessive inheritance, the person must have a pair of recessive genes in order to show the genetic characteristic. If the person receives only one recessive gene, he is known as a carrier of the gene. Hyperoxaluria is an autosomal recessive condition.

Biopsy is a study of a small piece of living tissue. Typically the tissue is obtained through minor surgery.

Brain Death is when the brain has permanently stopped working, as determined by the physician. Artificial support systems may maintain functions such as heartbeat and respiration for a few days, but not permanently. Donor organs are usually taken from persons declared brain dead.

Calcium is a substance necessary for life. Calcium is used by the body for many purposes: bones, teeth, blood coagulation, muscle function, and enzyme activation.

Chronic Carrier (Asymptomatic). HBV is present in the liver and blood, although there are usually no obvious physical symptoms. Specific blood tests will reveal the presence of the virus. This person is contagious (via blood, birth, sex, and needles).

Chronic Hepatitis:

- **Chronic Persistent Hepatitis (CPH):** This represents a degree of liver damage (resulting form HBV). Physical symptoms are usually present. Histological testing (detailed liver analysis) will reveal this stage of the disease. Blood tests are also informative. The person is usually contagious.

- **Chronic Active Hepatitis (CAH):** This is a more advanced form of hepatitis where liver damage is more widespread. Distinguishing CPH from CAH is highly technical. Liver function tests and other blood work are done to characterize the disease. The person is usually contagious.

Cirrhosis. Pathological dysfunctional state of the liver (hardening of the liver). A result of chronic hepatitis, CPH or CAH.

Coalition on Donation: A non-profit alliance of health and science professionals, transplant patients and voluntary health and transplant organizations. The Coalition works to increase public awareness of the critical organ shortage and create a greater willingness and commitment to organ and tissue donation.

Compliance is the act of following orders, adhering to rules and policies. Example: taking medications as directed.

Core Antibody Positive (cAb+). Core is part of the HBV particle and usually occurs in people who are chronic carriers. However, if present with the S-antibody, it is associated with recovery.

Core Antigen Positive (cAg+). This test is usually not done. It indicates the virus is present (core is part of the virus).

Crossmatch, a blood test for patient antibodies against donor antigens. A positive crossmatch shows that the donor and patient are incompatible. A negative crossmatch means there is no reaction between donor and patient and that the transplant may proceed.

Cyclosporine is a drug used following organ transplantation to prevent rejection of the transplanted organ by suppressing the body's defense system.

Dialysis is a medical treatment that filters the blood to remove liquids and chemicals that would normally be removed by functioning kidneys. **Hemodialysis or blood dialysis** is an efficient method of removing oxalate. Peritoneal dialysis using the lining around the interstinal tract is an effective dialysis method for kidney failure but is not efficient in removing oxalate.

Durable Power of Attorney, a document in which individuals may designate someone to make medical decisions for them when they are unable to speak for themselves.

E-Antibody Positive (eAb+). Carriers who stop producing E-antigen sometimes produce E-antibodies. The clinical significance of this is uncertain.

E-Antigen Positive (eAg+). E-antigen is a viral protein that is secreted by HBV-infected cells. Its presence indicated a high amount of virus in the blood.

Enteric refers to the intestines.

ESRD (End Stage Renal Disease/chronic kidney failure). A condition in which the kidneys no longer function and for which patients need dialysis or a transplant.

Fatty Acids are required by the body for proper nutrition. Fatty acids are transformed by the intestines into useful nutrients.

Gas Chromatography. A non-invasive medical test using a chromatograph to evaluate the components of a substance.

Genetic marker is a term used to describe the location of a gene in human DNA. Location of a genetic marker is a significant step toward understanding the cause of a genetic disorder.

Graft, a transplanted organ or tissue.

Hepatocellular Carcinoma (HCC). Cancer of the liver cells.

HLA (Human Leukocyte Antigens). Molecules found on cells in the body that characterize each individual as unique. Human leukocyte antigens (HLA) are inherited from one's parents. In donor-recipient matching, HLA determines whether an organ from one individual will be accepted by another.

HLA System. There are three major genetically controlled groups: HLA-A, HLA-B, and HLA-DR. In transplantation, the HLA tissue types of the donor and recipient are important in determining whether the transplant will be accepted or rejected. Genetic matching is routinely performed on kidneys and pancreases only.

Hyperoxaluria is excess excretion of oxalates (particularly calcium oxalates) in the urine.

Immune response is the body's natural defense against foreign objects or organisms such as bacteria, viruses, or transplanted organs or tissue.

Immunosuppression. The artificial suppression of the immune response, usually through drugs, so that the body will not reject a transplanted organ or tissue. Drugs commonly used to suppress the immune system after transplant include prednisone, azathioprine (Imuran), cyclosporine (Sandimmune, Neoral), OKT3 and ALG, mycophenolate mofetil (CeliCept), and tacrolimus (Prograf, FK506).

Informed Consent is a process of reaching an agreement based on a full understanding of what will take place. Informed consent has components of disclosure, comprehension, competence, and voluntary response.

Kidney. The organ that excretes urine. Humans typically have two kidneys located in the lower back on either side of the spinal column. Urine is passed from the kidneys to the bladder.

Kidney stones are small crystals, typically composed of oxalates and other substances, that have accumulated in the kidney as granular masses due to a deficiency in metabolic processes.

Liver Function Tests (LFT's). Tests that measure liver enzymes in the blood. When the liver is diseased or damaged, liver specific enzymes (such as SGOT/SGPT or AST/ALT) spill into the blood. Elevated levels of these enzymes in the blood are associated with liver damage.

Liver Screening. To detect liver damage, enlargement, etc., the liver may be palpated physically by your doctor or imaged by ultrasound. Other techniques such as Magnetic Resonance Imaging (MRI) are currently under investigation. The idea is to detect any progress or occurrence of liver pathology.

Living Related Donor refers to a relative that has been tested for organ and blood compatibility. Typically, if a person is in need of a kidney, parents, siblings, and other close blood relatives are tested for their potential suitability as a kidney donor. In most cases, humans only need one healthy kidney to live.

Metabolic is a term meaning pertaining to metabolism. Metabolism refers to the body processes involved in digesting, absorbing, and excreting nutrients and in supplying energy for the growth and development of cells.

NOTA (National Organ Transplant Act). Passed by Congress in 1984, NOTA outlawed the sale of human organs and initiated the development of a national system for organ sharing and a scientific registry to collect and report transplant data.

Ophthalmologist. A physician who specializes in treating eye disorders. In relation to PHI, the ophthalmologist may notice crystals forming in the back of the eye during an eye examination.

Organ Preservation. Donated organs require special methods of preservation to keep them viable between procurement and transplantation. Without preservation, the organ will deteriorate. The length of time organs and tissues can be kept outside the body vary depending on the organ, the preservation fluid and the temperature.

Organ Procurement. The recovery or retrieval of organs and tissues for transplantation.

Organ Procurement Organization (OPO). OPO's serve as the vital link between the donor and recipient and are responsible for the retrieval, preservation, and transportation of organs for transplantation. As a resource to the community they serve, they engage in public education on the critical need for organ donation. Currently, there are 69 OPO's around the country. All are UNOS members.

Orphan disease is a rare disease. Typically, orphan diseases are not well known and are not the subject for extensive research.

Oxalate is a very hard substance formed in the body as a waste product. Oxalate is the calcium salt of oxalic acid, a crystalline substance. Oxalate combines with calcium to form calcium oxalate stones. In a person affected by hyperoxaluria, the enzyme (ACT) necessary to assist in proper removal of wastes is missing, causing oxalate crystals to be deposited in organs.

Oxalic acid is a crystalline substance naturally found in the body and in food.

Oxalosis is the excessive accumulation of oxalate in the body. Oxalosis can damage body tissues, including organs, such as the liver and kidney.

Panel Reactive Antibody (PRA). The percentage of cells from a panel of donors with which a potential recipient's blood serum reacts. The more antibodies in the recipient's blood, the more likely the recipient will react against the potential donor. The higher the PRA the less chance of receiving an organ that will not be rejected. Patients with a high PRA have priority on the waiting list.

Peroxisome a component of the liver cell that houses enzyme generation. In the case of hyperoxaluria, the enzyme is absent or is secreted in insufficient quantities for proper liver function.

PHI is shorthand for **"Primary Hyperoxaluria Type I"**. See Hyperoxaluria

Prenatal. Before birth.

Pyridoxine is also known as Vitamin B6. High quantities are found in brewers yeast. Pyridoxine supplements are readily available.

Rejection occurs when the body tries to destroy a transplanted organ or tissue because it sees the graft as a foreign object and produces antibodies to destroy it. Immunosuppressive (antirejection) drugs help prevent rejection.

Renal refers to the kidneys. Renal failure means kidney failure.

Required Request. Hospitals must tell the families of suitable donors that their loved one's organs and tissues can be used for transplant. This law is expected to increase the number of donated organs and tissues for transplantation by giving more people the opportunity to donate.

Retransplantation. Due to organ rejection or transplant failure, some patients need another transplant and return to the waiting list. Reducing the number of retransplants is critical when examining ways to maximize a limited supply of donor organs.

Sensitization. When there are antibodies in the blood of the potential recipient, usually because of pregnancy, blood transfusions, or previous rejection of an organ transplant. Sensitization is measured by panel reactive antibody (PRA). Highly sensitized patients are less likely to match with a suitable donor and more likely to reject an organ than unsensitized patients.

Snail Mail is "techie" for postal mail.

Status. A code number used to indicate the degree of medical urgency for patients awaiting heart or liver transplants.

Supersaturation is the state of a liquid containing more of a dissolved substance than is normal. In this case, the supersaturation refers to excessive amounts of oxalate and calcium in the urine.

Surface-Antigen Positive. S-antigen is part of the HBV particle. S-antigen positive suggests the person is either an HBV carrier or is experiencing an acute HBV infection.

Surface-Antibody Positive (IgG). The person has previously been infected with HBV and has most likely recovered.

Survival Rates indicate what percentage of patients are alive or grafts (organs) are still functioning after a certain amount of time. Survival rates are used in developing UNOS policy. Because survival rates improve with technological and scientific advances, developing policies that reflect and respond to these advances will also improve survival rates.

Thiamine is also known as Vitamin B1. This vitamin is found in many foods. High quantities of thiamine are found in wheat germ and dry yeast.

Tissue Typing is the examination of human leukocyte antigens (HLA) in a patient. Tissue typing (genetic matching) is done for all donors and recipients in kidney transplantation to help match the donor to the most suitable recipient.

Urinary Tract. The organs and other structures (including the kidneys, bladder, and ureters) that remove urine from the body.

U.S. Scientific Registry of Transplant Recipients. A database of posttransplant information. Follow-up data on every transplant are used to track transplant center performance, transplant success rates and medical issues impacting transplant recipients. Under contract with the Health Resources and Services Administration (HRSA), UNOS facilitates the collection, tracking and reporting of transplant recipient and donor data.

Viral Hepatitis. Inflammation of the liver as a result of viral infection.

Waiting List. After evaluation by the transplant physician, a patient is added to the national waiting list by the transplant center. Lists are specific to both geographic area and organ type: heart, lung, kidney, liver, pancreas, intestine, heart-lung, and kidney-pancreas.

Each time a donor organ becomes available, the UNOS computer generates a list of potential recipients based on factors that include genetic similarity, organ size, medical urgency and time on the waiting list. Through this process, a "new" list is generated each time an organ becomes available that best matches" a patient to a donated organ.

Xenograft is an organ or tissue procured from an animal for transplantation into a human.

Xenotransplantation is transplantation of an animal organ into a human. Although xenotransplantation is highly experimental, many scientists view it as an eventual solution to the shortage of human organs.

Chapter 60

Directory of Organizations and Support Groups for Patients

This directory lists voluntary and private organizations involved in digestive-diseases-related activities for patients which pertain to liver disorders. The organizations offer educational materials and other services. A separate section lists organizations which assist with transplantation issues and donation of organs for transplantation.

Alagille Syndrome Alliance
10630 SW. Garden Park Place
Tigard, OR 97223
Tel: (503) 639-6217
Website:
http://laran.waisman.wisc.edu/fv/www/LIB_ALAG.HTM

Purpose: Provides a support network for children, their parents, and others with Alagille syndrome.
Materials: Newsletter—LiverLink.

This chapter includes text from "ALF Chapter Leadership Directory," © 1999 American Liver Foundation, reprinted with permission, "Directory of Digestive Diseases Organizations for Patients," National Institute of Diabetes and Digestive and Kidney Diseases (NIDDK), NIH, May 1998, and "Organizations for Endocrine and Metabolic Diseases," National Institute of Diabetes and Digestive and Kidney Diseases (NIDDK), NIH Publication No. 94-3567, February 1994, updated January 19, 1999.

American Hemochromatosis Society
777 East Atlantic Avenue, Suite Z-363
Delray Beach, FL 33483-5352
Tel: (561) 266-9037
E-mail: ahs@emi.net
Home page: http://www.americanhs.org

American Liver Foundation (ALF)
75 Maiden Lane, Suite 603
New York, NY 10038
Tel: (800) 465-4837 (GO-LIVER)
Tel: (888) 443-7222
Fax: (212) 483-8179
E-mail: webmail@liverfoundation.org
Home page: http://www.liverfoundation.org

Purpose: Promotes awareness and supports research on liver disease; disseminates information about liver wellness, liver disease, and prevention of liver disease with audiovisual and printed materials, seminars, and training programs; promotes organ donation; encourages vaccination against hepatitis B; serves as trustee of transplant funds; and *offers support groups through local chapters* (see listing of chapters below).

Materials: Member newsletter—Progress; clinical newsletter for physicians—Liver Update; and pamphlets and fact sheets about liver diseases, transplantation, organ donation, and prevention of liver diseases.

American Liver Foundation Chapters

Alabama
4 Office Park Circle, Suite 304
Birmingham, AL 35223
Tel: (205) 879-0354
Fax: (205) 879-0358
E-mail: amliveral@aol.com

Arizona
4545 E. Shea Blvd., Ste. 255
Phoenix, AZ 85028
Tel: (602) 953-1800
Fax: (602) 953-1806

California—San Diego
4452 Park Boulevard, Suite 102
San Diego, CA 92116
Tel: (619) 291-5483
Fax: (619) 295-7181
E-mail: 800dove@worldnet.att.net

California—Greater Los Angeles
2021-A Pontius Ave.
Los Angeles, CA 90025
Tel: (310) 477-4615
Fax: (310) 478-4685
E-mail: alfgla@gte.net

California—Inland Empire
4500 Brockton Ave., Suite 103
Riverside, CA 92501
Tel: (909) 684-1415

California—Northern California
870 Market St., Suite 1046
San Francisco, CA 94102
Tel: (415) 248-1060
Fax: (415) 248-1066
E-mail: amlivernc@aol.com

Colorado
Rocky Mountain Research
Association
29 Rogers Court
Golden, CO 80401
Tel: (303) 279-1550
Fax: (303) 278-2602

Connecticut
1 Bradley Road, Suite 405
Box 4062
Woodbridge, CT 06525
Tel: (203) 397-5433
Fax: (203) 397-1436

District of Columbia
1875 I Street, NW, 12th floor
Washington, DC 20006
Tel: (202) 872-6749
Fax: (202) 737-2517
Email: joangle@erols.com

Florida
101 America Center Place,
Suite 201
Tampa, FL 33691-4400
Tel: (813) 740-0045
Fax: (813) 740-2524
E-mail: alfgcc@gte.net

Georgia
1201 Claremont Road, Suite 120
Decatur, GA 30030
Tel: (404) 633-9169
Fax: (404) 633-8709
E-mail: alfga@mindspring.com

Illinois—Chapter 60
225 W. Washington St., Suite 2200
Chicago, IL 60606
Tel: (312) 419-7086
Fax: (312) 419-7163
E-mail: alf-ill@interaccess.com

Illinois—Quad Cities
4328 Ridgewood Ct.
Davenport, IA 52807
Tel: (319) 359-1994

Massachusettes
246 Walnut Street, Suite 401
Newton, MA 02160
Tel: (617) 527-5600 or (800) 298 6766
Fax: (617) 527-5636
E-mail: jkealf@aol.com

Minnesota
615 Eighth Ave. SW
Rochester, MN 55902
Tel: (507) 289-0914

Missouri—St. Louis
3660 S. Geyer Rd., Suite 140
St. Louis, MO 63127
Tel: (314) 835-1655

Missouri—Greater Kansas City
309 NE 88th Terrace
Kansas City, MO 64155
Tel: (816) 420-9446

New York—Greater NY
200 Board Hollow Rd., Suite 207
Melville, NY 11747
Tel: (516) 393-5076
Fax: (516) 393-5081
E-mail: alfgny@erols.com

New York—Western NY
25 Canterberry Rd. #316
Rochester, NY 14607
Tel: (716) 271-2859
Fax: (716) 271-2859

North Carolina
P.O. Box 268
Morrisville, NC 27560
Tel: (919) 481-3024
Fax: (919) 481-9571
E-mail: tbordeaux@ntwrks.com

Ohio—Northern
9500 Euclid Ave., P/17
Cleveland, OH 44195
Tel: (216) 444-8409
Fax: (216) 444-8410
E-mail: morgank@cesmtp.ccf.org

Ohio—Toledo
513 Adams Street
Apt. 213
Toledo, OH 43604-1437
Tel: (419) 243-5777
Fax: (419) 327-2531

Oregon
2578 Table Rock Road #15
Medford, OR 97501
Tel: (541) 857-9245
Fax: (541) 857-9245
E-mail: pnwliver@uswest.net

Pennsylvania
600 W. Germantown Pike,
Suite 400
Plymouth Meeting, PA 19462-1046
Tel: (610) 260-1497
Fax: (610) 260-1498
E-mail: amerlvfdn@aol.com

Texas
2425 W. Loop S., Suite 857
Houston, TX 77027
Tel: (713) 622-1318
Fax: (713) 622-1376
E-mail: ber31250@aol.com

Washington
2033 Sixth Ave., Suite 260
Seattle, WA 98121
Tel: (206) 443-3805
Fax: (206) 443-4267

Wisconsin
5131 N. Berkeley Blvd.
Whitefish Bay, WI 53217
Tel: (414) 548-1814

American Society of Human Genetics
9650 Rockville Pike
Bethesda, Maryland 20814
Tel: (301) 571-1825
Fax: (301) 530-7079
Home Page: http://www.faseb.org/genetics

Purpose: A professional society of physicians, researchers, genetic counselors and others interested in human genetics. Strives to inform health professionals, legislators, health policy makers, and the general public about all aspects of human genetics.

Publications: American Journal of Human Genetics (monthly); Membership Directory (biennially); Supplement to Journal (annually); Guide to Human Genetics Training Programs in North America.

Association for Glycogen Storage Disease
P.O. Box 896
Durant, IA 52747-9769
Tel: (319) 785-6038; Fax: (319) 785-6038

Purpose: Acts as a forum for the discussion of glycogen storage disease (GSD), its treatment, and the problems faced by parents raising children with GSD. Disseminates medical information; fosters communication between the families of GSD patients and health care professionals. Helps obtain equipment necessary for home care of GSD patients.

Publications: The Ray (periodic newsletter, Parent Handbook, and other brochures.

Association for Neuro-Metabolic Disorders
PO Box 0202/L3220
1500 Medical Center Drive
Ann Arbor, MI 48109-0202
Tel: (313) 763-4697
Website: http://medhlp.netuse.net/agsg/agsg1159.htm

Purpose: A member organization of families with children who have metabolic disorders that affect the brain. The organization provides support through personal awareness, family understanding and participation, and professional health care intervention.

Disorder: Neuro-metabolic disorders include many different, often inherited, diseases such as maple syrup urine disease, galactosemia, and biotinidase deficiency. These diseases affect body chemistry, but the organ damaged is the brain.

Publications: Newsletter (3 times a year).

Digestive Disease National Coalition
711 2nd St. NE, Suite 200
Washington, DC 20002
Tel: (202) 544-7497; Fax: (202) 546-7105

Purpose: Informs the public and the health care community about digestive diseases; seeks Federal funding for research, education, and training; and represents members' interests regarding Federal and State legislation that affects digestive diseases research, health care, and education.

Materials: Brochures and newsletters.

Food and Drug Administration
FDA (HFE-88)
5600 Fishers Lane
Rockville, MD 20857
(888) 463-6332
Website: http://www.fda.gov

FDA Seafood Hotline
Tel: (800) FDA-4010

The Hemochromatosis Foundation Inc.
P.O. Box 8569
Albany, NY 12208
Tel: (518) 489-0972
Fax: (518) 489-0227

Purpose: Provides information to the public, families, and professionals about hereditary hemochromatosis (HH); conducts and raises funds for research; encourages early screening for HH; holds symposiums and meetings; and offers genetic counseling along with support for patients and professionals.

Materials: Informational booklets and audiovisual materials for the public, families, and professionals.

Hepatitis B Coalition
Immunization Action Coalition
1573 Selby Avenue
St. Paul, MN 55104
Tel: (651) 647-9009
Fax: (651) 647-9131
E-mail: admin@immunize.org
Home page: http://www.immunize.org

Purpose: Works to prevent transmission of hepatitis B in high-risk groups; to achieve vaccination of all infants, children, and adolescents; and to promote education and treatment for the hepatitis B carrier.

Materials: Newsletter—Hepatitis B Coalition News; brochures, articles, videotapes, audiocassette tapes, and manuals for different ethnic populations.

Hepatitis B Foundation
700 East Butler Avenue
Doylestown, PA 18901-2697
Tel: (215) 489-4900
E-mail: info@hepb.org
Home page: http://zippy.tradenet.net/hepb/

Directory of Liver Specialists
Tel: (215) 489-4900
Home page: http://zippy.tradenet.net/hepb/directory.html

Purpose: Provides support and education to people affected by hepatitis B and dedicates itself to eliminating hepatitis B through community education and cure research programs.

Materials: Newsletter—B-Informed; brochures—Someone You Know Has Hepatitis B, Protect Yourself and Those You Love Against HBV, What Hepatitis B Carriers Should Know, and The First Loving Act—Vaccination; fact sheets—Advice to Parents of Children With HBV and Hot Sheet with current HBV research, telephone numbers, and a medical glossary; directory—National Directory of Liver Specialists; and a video—Hepatitis B Video.

Hepatitis C Foundation
1502 Russett Drive
Warminster, PA 18974
Tel: (215) 672-2606
URL: http://www.hepcfoundation.org

Hepatitis Foundation International (HFI)
30 Sunrise Terrace
Cedar Grove, NJ 07009-1423
Tel: (973) 239-1035 or (800) 891-0707
Fax: (973) 857-5044
E-mail: mail@hepfi.org
Home page: http://www.hepfi.org

Purpose: Fosters worldwide awareness about the prevention, diagnosis, and treatment of viral hepatitis; provides patient and professional education programs; distributes publications; and supports research. A unique service is the Patient Advocacy/Information Tele-communications System, a phone support network that enables patients to talk to others with similar concerns.

Materials: Fact sheets—Caring for Your Liver; Diagnosis and Treatment for Hepatitis; Hepatitis C; Hepatitis D, E & F; Hepatitis Statistics; Research Advances in Hepatitis; Vaccines for Hepatitis A and B; poster—Take Care of Your Liver; and newsletter—Hepatitis Alert.

Hepatitis Hotline of the Hepatitis Branch, CDC
Tel: (888) 443-7232

Hepatitis Vaccines
National Immunization Program, CDC Information Hotline
Tel: (800) 232-2522
Home page: http://www.cdc.gov/ncidod/diseases/hepatitis

Iron Overload Diseases Association Inc.
433 Westward Drive
North Palm Beach, FL 33408
Tel: (407) 840-8512
Fax: (561) 842-9881
Hemochromatosis Hotline: (888) 678-4766
E-mail: iod@emi.net
Home page: http://www.emi.net/~iron_iod/iod.html

Purpose: Conducts professional education symposiums and exhibits at medical meetings; serves and counsels hemochromatosis patients and families; offers doctor referrals; promotes patient advocacy concerning insurance, Medicare, blood banks, and the Food and Drug Administration; encourages research; maintains international consortium; offers public information through the media; develops chapters and self-help groups; and sponsors annual symposiums and annual IOD Awareness Week.

Materials: Booklet—Overload: An Ironic Disease; bimonthly newsletter—Ironic Blood; information brochure—Iron Overload Alert; and fact sheet.

National Cancer Institute Information Resources

Cancer Information Service (CIS)
Toll-free: 1-800-4-CANCER (1-800-422-6237)
TTY: 1-800-332-8615
Fax: (301) 402-5874 (Follow recorded instructions)

Internet resources:

  http://www.nci.nih.gov/
  http://cancernet.nci.nih.gov/
  http://cancertrials.nci.nih.gov/
  E-mail: cancermail@icicc.nci.hig.gov (To obtain a contents list, put
  "help" in body of message.)

National Center for Nutrition and Dietetics (NCND) of The American Dietetic Association
216 West Jackson Boulevard, Suite 800
Chicago, IL 60606-6995
Consumer Nutrition Hotline: (800) 366-1655
Home page: http://www.eatright.org

Purpose: Provides consumers with direct and immediate access to reliable nutrition information. Callers may speak to a registered dietitian, may listen to regularly updated nutrition messages in English or Spanish, or may be referred to a dietitian in their local area.

National Center for the Study of Wilson's Disease
432 West 58th Street
Suite 614
New York, NY 10091
Tel: (212) 523-8717

Purpose: Encourages and supports research concerning hereditary diseases of copper metabolism (Wilson's disease and Menkes' disease). Seeks to increase doctors' awareness of these diseases; and sponsors a diagnostic and treatment center for Wilson's disease.

Disorder: Wilson's disease is a genetic disorder in which excessive amounts of copper collect in the liver, brain, and kidneys. Menkes' disease is the reverse of Wilson's disease and is characterized by a defect in intestinal absorption of copper that leads to copper deficiency.

Publications: Information brochures.

National Niemann-Pick Foundation

3734 E. Olive Ave
Gilbert, AZ 85234
Phone (602) 497-6638; Fax (602) 497-6346
E-mail: stevekenyon@nnpdf.org
Website: http://www.nnpdf.org

National Organization for Rare Disorders Inc. (NORD®)

P.O. Box 8923
New Fairfield, CT 06812-8923
Tel: (800) 999-6673 or (203) 746-6518
Fax: (203) 746-6481
E-mail: orphan@nord-rdb.com
Home page: http://www.NORD-RDB.com/~orphan

Purpose: Serves as a clearinghouse for information about rare disorders and brings together families with similar disorders for mutual support; fosters communication among rare disease voluntary agencies, government agencies, industry, scientific researchers, academic institutions, and concerned individuals; and encourages and promotes research and education on rare disorders and orphan drugs.

Materials: Fact sheet reprints on rare disorders; and newsletter—Orphan Disease Update.

National Reye's Syndrome Foundation

PO Box 829
Bryan, OH 43506-0829
(419) 636-2679 or (800) 233-7393
E-mail: reyessyn@mail.bright.net
Website: http://www.bright.net/~reyessyn

Oxalosis and Hyperoxaluria Foundation (OHF)

12 Pleasant Street
Maynard, MA 01754
Tel: (888) 712-2432 PIN# 5392
(978) 461-0614
Fax: (978) 461-0614
E-mail: info@ohf.org
Home Page: http://www.ohf.org

To inform the public, especially patients, parent, families, physicians, and medical professionals about hyperoxaluria and the related conditions, i.e., oxalosis and calcium-oxalate kidney stones; to provide a support network for those affected by hyperoxaluria, and to support and encourage research to find a cure for typeroxaluria.

Materials: Patient Handbook (RE: Hyperoxaluria); In Touch (newsletter), website resources.

Weight-Control Information Network (WIN)
1 WIN Way
Bethesda, MD 20892-3665
Tel: (800) 946-8098 or (301) 984-7378
Fax: (301) 984-7196
E-mail: win@info.niddk.nih.gov
Home page: http://www.niddk.nih.gov/health/nutrit/win.htm

Purpose: To address the health information needs of individuals through the production and dissemination of educational materials. In addition, WIN is developing communication strategies for a pilot program to encourage at-risk individuals to achieve and maintain a healthy weight by making changes in their lifestyle.

Materials: Fact sheets, pamphlets, reprints, consensus statements, reports, and literature searches on weight control, obesity, and weight-related nutritional disorders. Semi-annual newsletter—WIN Notes.

Wilson's Disease Association
4 Navaho Drive
Brookfield, CT 06804
Tel: (800) 399-0266
Tel: (203) 775-9666
Fax: (203) 743-6196
E-mail: hasellner@worldnet.att.net
Home page: http://www.wilsonsdisease.org/

Purpose: Serves as a communications and support network for individuals affected by Wilson's disease and related disorders of copper metabolism; distributes information to professionals and the public.

Materials: Fact sheets about Wilson's disease and member newsletter.

National Digestive Diseases Information Clearinghouse
2 Information Way
Bethesda, MD 20892-3570
E-mail: nddic@info.niddk.nih.gov

The National Digestive Diseases Information Clearinghouse (NDDIC) is a service of the National Institute of Diabetes and Digestive and Kidney Diseases (NIDDK). The NIDDK is part of the National Institutes of Health under the U.S. Public Health Service. Established in 1980, the clearinghouse provides information about digestive diseases to people with digestive disorders and to their families, health care professionals, and the public. NDDIC answers inquiries; develops, reviews, and distributes publications; and works closely with professional and patient organizations and Government agencies to coordinate resources about digestive diseases. Publications produced by the clearinghouse are reviewed carefully for scientific accuracy, content, and readability.

The Vaccine Adverse Event Reporting System (VAERS)
Tel: (800) 822-7967
Website: http://www.fda.gov/cber/vaers/vaers.htm

VAERS ensures the safety of vaccines distributed in the United States. VAERS reports are usually submitted by health care professionals or vaccine manufacturers; however, any one can submit a report to VAERS. VAERS is administered, monitored and analyzed jointly by the Centers for Disease Control and Prevention and the Food and Drug Administration. Persons who wish to report a possible health effect related to a vaccine should notify their health care provider and can also call the VAERS program.

Transplant Information, Assistance, and Organ Donation

AirLifeLine
50 Fullerton Court, Suite 200
Sacramento, CA 95825
Tel: (800) 446-1231
(916) 641-7800
Fax: (916) 641-0600
E-mail: staff@airlifeline.org
Website: http://aiarlifeline.org/index.htm

Transports ambulatory patients up to a distance of 500 to 700 miles using private pilots and their aircraft. Can transport people for transplant and follow-up appointments. Must be documented medical and financial need. Service is free of charge.

American Liver Foundation
75 Maiden Lane, Suite 603
New York, NY 10038
Tel: (800) 465-4837 (GO-LIVER)
E-mail: webmail@liverfoundation.org
URL: http://liverfoundation.org

Voluntary agency dedicated to fighting liver disease through research, education and patient self-help groups. The group acts as trustees for trust funds.

American Organ Transplant Association
3335 Cartwright
Missouri City, TX 77459
Tel: (281) 261-2682
Fax: (281) 208-5279
E-mail: infoaota@a-o-t-a.org
URL: http://www.a-o-t-a.org

A private, non-profit group that provides reduced or free airfare and bus tickets to transplant recipients and their families. AOTA publishes a newsletter for its members. Patients interested in AOTA's services must be referred by their physician. The association also assists people with setting up trust funds and fund raising. No administrative fee is charged.

Angel Flight,
American Medical Support Flight Team
3237 Donald Douglas Loop South
Santa Monica, CA 90405
Tel: (888) 426-2643

Provides free air transportation on private aircraft for needy people with healthcare problems and for healthcare agencies, organ procurement organizations, blood banks and tissue banks. There are no fees of any kind. Angel Flight is a volunteer organization serving the public since 1983.

Barbara Anne DeBoer Foundation
2069 South Busse Rd.
Mount Prospect, IL 60056
Tel: (800) 895-8478

Offers a variety of programs that include advocacy services, donor awareness information, referral services, medication and medical center information. Individual fund raising program is designed to utilize resources in patient's community to raise money for transplant procedure. Works with patients and volunteer committees to develop press releases and plan various events and programs. All local funds raised go to medical expenses—no administrative fee is charged.

Children's Organ Transplant Association
2501 COTA Dr.
Bloomington, IN 47403
Tel: (812) 336-8872
Fax: (812) 336-8885

A national, non-profit agency raising funds for individuals and families to assist with transplant and related expenses. Works with adults as well as children. All funds raised go to the individual—no administrative fees are collected.

LifePage
PO Box 207
Alexandria, VA 22313-0207
Tel: (703) 739-0527
Fax: (703) 836-1608

Sponsored by the Personal Communications Industry Association, LifePage is a national program that provides pagers to patients who are waiting for organ or tissue transplants.

Medicare Hotline
Tel: (800) 638-6833

National Insurance Consumer Hotline
Tel: (800) 942-4242

Call to obtain the phone number of your state insurance department.

National Organization of Social Security Claimants' Representatives
6 Prospect Street
Midland Park, NJ 07432-1634
Tel: (800) 431-2804
URL: http://www.nosscr.org

Nielsen Organ Transplant Foundation
580 W 8th St.
Jacksonville, FL 32209
Tel: (904) 798-8999
E-mail: nielsenfoundation@yahoo.com

A regional group that provides assistance to a five-county area in Florida: Duvall, Baker, St. John, Nassau and Clay. Promotes public education regarding organ donation. Offers limited grant funds for transplant-related expenses.

Organ Transplant Fund, Inc.
1102 Brookfield, Suite 202
Memphis, TN 38119
Tel: (800) 489-3863

Assists transplant candidates and recipients nationwide in obtaining transplants and follow-up care, as well as providing essential support and referral services. Provides clients with fund raising expertise and materials and assures that funds raised are properly dispensed. Limited emergency grants are available for medications and transplant-related expenses.

The Transplant Foundation
8002 Discovery Dr, Suite 310
Richmond, VA 23229
Tel: (804) 285-5115
E-mail: NatFoundTX@aol.com
URL: http://www.otf.org

A national, non-profit volunteer organization providing grants to transplant recipients to offset the costs of immunosuppressant medications. The amount of grants and the number of individuals who can receive assistance are determined by total contributions each year. The organization also acts as a resource referral.

Prescription Drug Patient Assistance Programs

Many pharmaceutical manufacturers provide medications for indigent patients through patient assistance programs. Most programs require that patients meet certain income requirements. The Directory of Prescription Drug Patient Assistance Programs describes more than 55 programs and includes who is eligible, what prescription medications are covered and how to receive assistance. To request a free copy:

Pharmaceutical Research and Manufacturers of America
1100 15th St., NW
Suite 900
Washington, DC 20005
Tel: (202) 835-3414
Fax: (202) 835-3416
URL: http://www.pharm.org

The following programs were established by pharmaceutical manufacturers of the three most often prescribed immunosuppressive medications:

Glaxo-Welcome Patient Assistance Program
Medication: Imuran
Tel: (800) 722-9294

Novartis Patient Assistance Program
Medication: Cyclosporine
Tel: (800) 257-3273

Prograf/Fujisawa Patient Assistance Program
Medication: Prograo
Tel: (800) 477-6472

As of October 1997 there were 120 liver, 254 kidney, 164 heart, 124 pancreas, 98 heart-lung, and 92 lung transplant programs in the United States. Names and addresses of transplant programs can be obtained from the United Network for Organ Sharing at the following address:

United Network for Organ Sharing
1100 Boulders Parkway, Suite 500
PO Box 13770
Richmond, Virginia 23225-8770
Tel: (888) 894-6361
URL: http://www.unos.org/frame_Default.asp

As of December 1997, 63 OPO's were certified by the Health Care Financing Administration of the U.S. Department of Health and Human

Services. Their names and addresses can be obtained from the following organizations:

Association of Organ Procurement Organizations
One Cambridge Court
8110 Gatehouse Road
Suite 101 West
Falls Church, Virginia 22042
Tel: (703) 573-2676
E-mail: aopo@erols.com
URL: http://www.aopo.org

American Congress for Organ Recovery and Donation
1714 Hayes Street
Nashville, TN 32703
Tel: (615) 327-2247

Chapter 61

Transplant Centers for Liver Transplants

Patients and their family members may contact the United Network of Organ Sharing (UNOS) for center specific data. The "1997 Report of Center Specific Graft and Patient Survival Rates" is available at the UNOS Web Site: www.unos.org. Patients without Internet access may receive data for up to 10 centers free of charge by writing:

United Network for Organ Sharing
1100 Boulders Parkway, Suite 500
P.O. Box 13770
Richmond, Virginia 23225-8770
Tel: (888) 894-6361

Patients should also consider the following issues when choosing a transplant center:

• The experience of the transplant team and support personnel;
• The cost of the procedure and related items;
• Access/proximity to the program;
• Availability of friends and family for assistance; and
• The quality and availability of post-transplant services.

Liver Transplant Centers

The four letter code is the UNOS code for the transplant center listed below it. The centers are listed alphabetically by state.

ALUA
University of Alabama Hospital
Birmingham, AL

AZGS
Good Samaritan Regional Medical Center
Phoenix, AZ

AZUA
University Medical Center
Tucson, AZ

CACS
Cedars-Sinai Medical Center
Los Angeles, CA

CAGH
Green Hospital of Scripps Clinic
La Jolla, CA

CAIM
University of California
Irvine Medical Center
Orange, CA

CALL
Lorma Linda University Medical Center
Lorma Linda, CA

CAPM
California Pacific Medical Center
San Francisco, CA

CASD
UCSD Medical Center
San Diego, CA

CASF
UCSF Medical Center
San Francisco, CA

CASU
Stanford University
Palo Alto, CA

CAUC
UCLA Medical Center
Los Angeles, CA

COCH
The Children's Hospital
Denver, CO

COUC
University Hospital
Denver, CO

CTHH
Hartford Hospital
Hartford, CT

CTYN
Yale New Haven Hospital
New Haven, CT

DCHU
Howard University Hospital
Washington, DC

FLJM
Jackson Memorial Hospital
Miami, FL

FLTG
Tampa General Hospital
Tampa, FL

FLUF
Shands Hospital
Gainsville, FL

GAEH
Egleston Children's Hospital
Atlanta,GA

GAEM
Emory University Hospital
Atlanta, GA

HISF
St. Francis Medical Center
Honolulu, HI

IAIV
University of Iowa Hospitals &
Clinics
Iowa City, IA

ILNM
Northwestern Memorial Hospital
Chicago, IL

ILPL
Rush-Presbyterian-St. Luke's
Medical Center
Chicago, IL

ILUC
University of Chicago Medical
Center
Chicago, IL

ILUI
University of Illinois Hospital
Chicago, IL

INIM
Methodist Hospital of Indiana
Indianapolis, IN

INIU
Indiana University Medical
Center
Indianapolis, IN

KSUK
University of Kansas Medical
Center
Kansas City, KS

KYJH
Jewish Hospital
Louisville, KY

LAOF
Ochsner Foundation Hospital
New Orleans, LA

LASU
Louisana State University
Medical Center
Shreveport, LA

LAWK
Willis-Knighton Medical Center
Shreveport, LA

MACH
Children's Hospital
Boston, MA

MAHS
Beth Israel Deaconess Medical
Center
Boston, MA

MAMG
Massachusetts General Hospital
Boston, MA

MANM
New England Medical Center
Boston, MA

MDJH
Johns Hopkins Hospital
Baltimore, MD

MIHF
Henry Ford Hospital
Detroit, MI

MIUM
University of Michigan Medical
Center
Ann Arbor, MI

MNMC
Rochester Methodist Hospital
Rochester, MN

MNSM
St Mary's Hospital
Rochester, MN

MNUM
Fairview University Medical
Center
Minneapolis, MN

MOBH
Barnes-Jewish Hospital
St. Louis, MO

MOCG
Cardinal Glennon Children's
Hospital
St. Louis, MO

MOCH
St. Louis Children' Hospital
St. Louis, MO

MOLH
St. Luke's Hospital
Kansas City, MO

MOSL
St. Louis University Hospital
St. Louis, MO

MSUM
University of Mississippi Medical Center
Jackson, MS

NCDU
Duke University Medical Center
Durham, NC

NCMH
University of North Carolina
Hospitals
Chapel Hill, NC

NEUN
University of Nebraska Medical
Center
Omaha, NE

NYCP
Presbyterian Hospital in New
York City
New York, NY

NYFL
Strong Memorial Hospital
Rochester, NY

NYMS
Mount Sinai Medical Center
New York, NY

NYUC
New York University Medical
Center
New York, NY

OHCC
Cleveland Clinic Foundation
Cleveland, OH

OHCH
Children's Hospital
Columbus, OH

OHCM
Children's Hospital Medical
Center
Cincinnati, OH

OHOU
Ohio State University Hospitals
Columbus, OH

OHUC
University of Cincinnati Medical
Center
Cincinnati, OH

OHUH
University Hospitals
Cleveland, OH

OKBC
Integris Baptist Medical Center
Oklahoma City, OK

OKMD
University Hospital
Okalahoma City, OK

ORUO
Oregon Health Sciences University Hospital
Portland, OR

PAAE
Albert Einstein Medical Center
Philadelphia, PA

PACH
Children's Hospital
Pittsburgh, PA

PACP
Children's Hospital
Philadelphia, PA

PAHE
Milton S. Hershey Medical Center
Hershey PA

PAPT
University of Pittsburgh Medical Center
Pittsburgh, PA

PASC
St. Christopher's Hospital for Children
Philadelphia, PA

PATJ
Thomas Jefferson University Hospital
Philadelphia, PA

PAUP
Hospital of University of Pennsylvania
Philadelphia, PA

SCMU
Medical University of South
Carolina
Charleston, SC

TNLB
Le Bonheur Children's Medical
Center
Memphis, TN

TNUT
University of Tennessee Medical
Center
Nashville, TN

TNVU
Vanderbilt University Medical
Center
Nashville, TN

TXBC
University Hospital
San Antonio, TX

TXCM
Children's Medical Center
Dallas, TX

TXHH
Hermann Hospital
Houston, TX

TXHI
St. Luke's Episcopal Hospital
Houston, TX

TXJS
University of Texas Medical
Branch
Galveston, TX

TXLG
University Medical Center
Lubbock, TX

TXMH
The Methodist Hospital
Houston, TX

TXTC
Texas Children's Hospital
Houston, TX

TXTX
Baylor University Medical Center
Dallas, TX

TXWH
Wilford Hall Medical Center
Lackland AFB, TX

UTLD
Latter-Day Saints Hospital
Salt Lake City, UT

VAFH
Inova Fairfax Hospital
Falls Church, VA

VAHD
Columbia Henrico Doctors' Hos-
pital
Richmond, VA

VAMC
Medical College of Virginia Hos-
pitals
Richmond, VA

VAUV
University of Virginia Health
Science Center
Charlottesville, VA

WACH
Children's Hospital & Medical
Center
Seattle, WA

WAUW
University of Washington Medi-
cal Center
Seattle, WA

WICH
Children's Hospital of Wisconsin
Milwaukee, WI

WISE
Froedtert Memorial Lutheran
Hospital
Milwaukee, WI

WIUW
University of Wisconsin Hospi-
tal and Clinics
Madison, WI

Index

Index

Page numbers followed by 'n' indicate a footnote. Page numbers in *italics* indicate a table or illustration.

567

Health Reference Series
COMPLETE CATALOG

AIDS Sourcebook, 1st Edition

Basic Information about AIDS and HIV Infection, Featuring Historical and Statistical Data, Current Research, Prevention, and Other Special Topics of Interest for Persons Living with AIDS, Along with Source Listings for Further Assistance

Edited by Karen Bellenir and Peter D. Dresser. 831 pages. 1995. 0-7808-0031-1. $78.

"One strength of this book is its practical emphasis. The intended audience is the lay reader . . . useful as an educational tool for health care providers who work with AIDS patients. Recommended for public libraries as well as hospital or academic libraries that collect consumer materials." — *Bulletin of the MLA, Jan '96*

"This is the most comprehensive volume of its kind on an important medical topic. Highly recommended for all libraries." — *Reference Book Review, '96*

"Very useful reference for all libraries."
— *Choice, Oct '95*

"There is a wealth of information here that can provide much educational assistance. It is a must book for all libraries and should be on the desk of each and every congressional leader. Highly recommended."
— *AIDS Book Review Journal, Aug '95*

"Recommended for most collections."
— *Library Journal, Jul '95*

AIDS Sourcebook, 2nd Edition

Basic Consumer Health Information about Acquired Immune Deficiency Syndrome (AIDS) and Human Immunodeficiency Virus (HIV) Infection, Featuring Updated Statistical Data, Reports on Recent Research and Prevention Initiatives, and Other Special Topics of Interest for Persons Living with AIDS, Including New Antiretroviral Treatment Options, Strategies for Combating Opportunistic Infections, Information about Clinical Trials, and More; Along with a Glossary of Important Terms and Resource Listings for Further Help and Information

Edited by Karen Bellenir. 751 pages. 1999. 0-7808-0225-X. $78.

Allergies Sourcebook

Basic Information about Major Forms and Mechanisms of Common Allergic Reactions, Sensitivities, and Intolerances, Including Anaphylaxis, Asthma, Hives and Other Dermatologic Symptoms, Rhinitis, and Sinusitis, Along with Their Usual Triggers Like Animal Fur, Chemicals, Drugs, Dust, Foods, Insects, Latex, Pollen, and Poison Ivy, Oak, and Sumac; Plus Information on Prevention, Identification, and Treatment

Edited by Allan R. Cook. 611 pages. 1997. 0-7808-0036-2. $78.

Alternative Medicine Sourcebook

Basic Consumer Health Information about Alternatives to Conventional Medicine, Including Acupressure, Acupuncture, Aromatherapy, Ayurveda, Bioelectromagnetics, Environmental Medicine, Essence Therapy, Food and Nutrition Therapy, Herbal Therapy, Homeopathy, Imaging, Massage, Naturopathy, Reflexology, Relaxation and Meditation, Sound Therapy, Vitamin and Mineral Therapy, and Yoga, and More

Edited by Allan R. Cook. 737 pages. 1999. 0-7808-0200-4. $78.

Alzheimer's, Stroke & 29 Other Neurological Disorders Sourcebook, 1st Edition

Basic Information for the Layperson on 31 Diseases or Disorders Affecting the Brain and Nervous System, First Describing the Illness, Then Listing Symptoms, Diagnostic Methods, and Treatment Options, and Including Statistics on Incidences and Causes

Edited by Frank E. Bair. 579 pages. 1993. 1-55888-748-2. $78.

"Nontechnical reference book that provides reader-friendly information."
— *Family Caregiver Alliance Update, Winter '96*

"Should be included in any library's patient education section." — *American Reference Books Annual, '94*

"Written in an approachable and accessible style. Recommended for patient education and consumer health collections in health science center and public libraries." — *Academic Library Book Review, Dec '93*

"It is very handy to have information on more than thirty neurological disorders under one cover, and there is no recent source like it." — *RQ, Fall '93*

Alzheimer's Disease Sourcebook, 2nd Edition

Basic Consumer Health Information about Alzheimer's Disease, Related Disorders, and Other Dementias, Including Multi-Infarct Dementia, AIDS-Related Dementia, Alcoholic Dementia, Huntington's Disease, Delirium, and Confusional States; Along with Reports Detailing Current Research Efforts in Prevention and Treatment, Long-Term Care Issues, and Listings of Sources for Additional Help and Information

Edited by Karen Bellenir. 524 pages. 1999. 0-7808-0223-3. $78.

Arthritis Sourcebook

Basic Consumer Health Information about Specific Forms of Arthritis and Related Disorders, Including Rheumatoid Arthritis, Osteoarthritis, Gout, Polymyalgia Rheumatica, Psoriatic Arthritis, Spondyloarthropathies, Juvenile Rheumatoid Arthritis, and Juvenile Ankylosing Spondylitis; Along with Information about Medical, Surgical, and Alternative Treatment Options, and Including Strategies for Coping with Pain, Fatigue, and Stress

Edited by Allan R. Cook. 550 pages. 1998. 0-7808-0201-2. $78.

". . . accessible to the layperson."
— *Reference and Research Book News, Feb '99*

Back & Neck Disorders Sourcebook

Basic Information about Disorders and Injuries of the Spinal Cord and Vertebrae, Including Facts on Chiropractic Treatment, Surgical Interventions, Paralysis, and Rehabilitation, Along with Advice for Preventing Back Trouble

Edited by Karen Bellenir. 548 pages. 1997. 0-7808-0202-0. $78.

"The strength of this work is its basic, easy-to-read format. Recommended."
— *Reference and User Services Quarterly, Winter '97*

Blood & Circulatory Disorders Sourcebook

Basic Information about Blood and Its Components, Anemias, Leukemias, Bleeding Disorders, and Circulatory Disorders, Including Aplastic Anemia, Thalassemia, Sickle-Cell Disease, Hemochromatosis, Hemophilia, Von Willebrand Disease, and Vascular Diseases; Along with a Special Section on Blood Transfusions and Blood Supply Safety, a Glossary, and Source Listings for Further Help and Information

Edited by Karen Bellenir and Linda M. Shin. 554 pages. 1998. 0-7808-0203-9. $78.

"Recent and recommended reference source."
— *Booklist, Feb '99*

"An important reference sourcebook written in simple language for everyday, non-technical users. "
— *Reviewer's Bookwatch, Jan '99*

Brain Disorders Sourcebook

Basic Consumer Health Information about Strokes, Epilepsy, Amyotrophic Lateral Sclerosis (ALS/Lou Gehrig's Disease), Parkinson's Disease, Brain Tumors, Cerebral Palsy, Headache, Tourette Syndrome, and More; Along with Statistical Data, Treatment and

Rehabilitation Options, Coping Strategies, Reports on Current Research Initiatives, a Glossary, and Resource Listings for Additional Help and Information

Edited by Karen Bellenir. 481 pages. 1999. 0-7808-0229-2. $78.

Burns Sourcebook

Basic Consumer Health Information about Various Types of Burns and Scalds, Including Flame, Heat, Cold, Electrical, Chemical, and Sun Burns; Along with Information on Short-Term and Long-Term Treatments, Tissue Reconstruction, Plastic Surgery, Prevention Suggestions, and First Aid

Edited by Allan R. Cook. 604 pages. 1999. 0-7808-0204-7. $78.

Cancer Sourcebook, 1st Edition

Basic Information on Cancer Types, Symptoms, Diagnostic Methods, and Treatments, Including Statistics on Cancer Occurrences Worldwide and the Risks Associated with Known Carcinogens and Activities

Edited by Frank E. Bair. 932 pages. 1990. 1-55888-888-8. $78.

"Written in nontechnical language. Useful for patients, their families, medical professionals, and librarians."
— *Guide to Reference Books, '96*

"Designed with the non-medical professional in mind. Libraries and medical facilities interested in patient education should certainly consider adding the Cancer Sourcebook to their holdings. This compact collection of reliable information . . . is an invaluable tool for helping patients and patients' families and friends to take the first steps in coping with the many difficulties of cancer."
— *Medical Reference Services Quarterly, Winter '91*

"Specifically created for the nontechnical reader . . . an important resource for the general reader trying to understand the complexities of cancer."
— *American Reference Books Annual, '91*

"This publication's nontechnical nature and very comprehensive format make it useful for both the general public and undergraduate students."
— *Choice, Oct '90*

New Cancer Sourcebook, 2nd Edition

Basic Information about Major Forms and Stages of Cancer, Featuring Facts about Primary and Secondary Tumors of the Respiratory, Nervous, Lymphatic, Circulatory, Skeletal, and Gastrointestinal Systems, and Specific Organs; Statistical and Demographic Data; Treatment Options; and Strategies for Coping

Edited by Allan R. Cook. 1,313 pages. 1996. 0-7808-0041-9. $78.

"This book is an excellent resource for patients with newly diagnosed cancer and their families. The dialogue is simple, direct, and comprehensive. Highly recommended for patients and families to aid in their understanding of cancer and its treatment."
— *Booklist Health Sciences Supplement, Oct '97*

"The amount of factual and useful information is extensive. The writing is very clear, geared to general readers. Recommended for all levels."
— *Choice, Jan '97*

■

Cancer Sourcebook, 3rd Edition

Basic Consumer Health Information about Major Forms and Stages of Cancer, Featuring Facts about Primary and Secondary Tumors of the Respiratory, Nervous, Lymphatic, Circulatory, Skeletal, and Gastrointestinal Systems, and Specific Organs; Along with Statistical and Demographic Data, Treatment Options, Strategies for Coping, a Glossary, and a Directory of Sources for Additional Help and Information

Edited by Edward J. Prucha. 1,100 pages. 1999. 0-7808-0227-6. $78.

■

Cancer Sourcebook for Women, 1st Edition

Basic Information about Specific Forms of Cancer That Affect Women, Featuring Facts about Breast Cancer, Cervical Cancer, Ovarian Cancer, Cancer of the Uterus and Uterine Sarcoma, Cancer of the Vagina, and Cancer of the Vulva; Statistical and Demographic Data; Treatments, Self-Help Management Suggestions, and Current Research Initiatives

Edited by Allan R. Cook and Peter D. Dresser. 524 pages. 1996. 0-7808-0076-1. $78.

". . . written in easily understandable, non-technical language. Recommended for public libraries or hospital and academic libraries that collect patient education or consumer health materials."
— *Medical Reference Services Quarterly, Spring '97*

"Would be of value in a consumer health library. . . . written with the health care consumer in mind. Medical jargon is at a minimum, and medical terms are explained in clear, understandable sentences."
— *Bulletin of the MLA, Oct '96*

"The availability under one cover of all these pertinent publications, grouped under cohesive headings, makes this certainly a most useful sourcebook."
— *Choice, Jun '96*

"Presents a comprehensive knowledge base for general readers. Men and women both benefit from the gold mine of information nestled between the two covers of this book. Recommended."
— *Academic Library Book Review, Summer '96*

"This timely book is highly recommended for consumer health and patient education collections in all libraries."
— *Library Journal, Apr '96*

■

Cancer Sourcebook for Women, 2nd Edition

Basic Consumer Health Information about Specific Forms of Cancer That Affect Women, Including Cervical Cancer, Ovarian Cancer, Endometrial Cancer, Uterine Sarcoma, Vaginal Cancer, Vulvar Cancer, and Gestational Trophoblastic Tumor; and Featuring Statistical Information, Facts about Tests and Treatments, a Glossary of Cancer Terms, and an Extensive List of Additional Resources

Edited by Edward J. Prucha. 600 pages. 1999. 0-7808-0226-8. $78.

■

Cardiovascular Diseases & Disorders Sourcebook, 1st Edition

Basic Information about Cardiovascular Diseases and Disorders, Featuring Facts about the Cardiovascular System, Demographic and Statistical Data, Descriptions of Pharmacological and Surgical Interventions, Lifestyle Modifications, and a Special Section Focusing on Heart Disorders in Children

Edited by Karen Bellenir and Peter D. Dresser. 683 pages. 1995. 0-7808-0032-X. $78.

". . . comprehensive format provides an extensive overview on this subject."
— *Choice, Jun '96*

". . . an easily understood, complete, up-to-date resource. This well executed public health tool will make valuable information available to those that need it most, patients and their families. The typeface, sturdy non-reflective paper, and library binding add a feel of quality found wanting in other publications. Highly recommended for academic and general libraries. "
— *Academic Library Book Review, Summer '96*

■

Communication Disorders Sourcebook

Basic Information about Deafness and Hearing Loss, Speech and Language Disorders, Voice Disorders, Balance and Vestibular Disorders, and Disorders of Smell, Taste, and Touch

Edited by Linda M. Ross. 533 pages. 1996. 0-7808-0077-X. $78.

"This is skillfully edited and is a welcome resource for the layperson. It should be found in every public and medical library."
— *Booklist Health Sciences Supplement, Oct '97*

■

Congenital Disorders Sourcebook

Basic Information about Disorders Acquired during Gestation, Including Spina Bifida, Hydrocephalus, Cerebral Palsy, Heart Defects, Craniofacial Abnormalities, Fetal Alcohol Syndrome, and More, Along with Current Treatment Options and Statistical Data

Edited by Karen Bellenir. 607 pages. 1997. 0-7808-0205-5. $78.

"Recent and recommended reference source."
— *Booklist, Oct '97*

Consumer Issues in Health Care Sourcebook

Basic Information about Health Care Fundamentals and Related Consumer Issues, Including Exams and Screening Tests, Physician Specialties, Choosing a Doctor, Using Prescription and Over-the-Counter Medications Safely, Avoiding Health Scams, Managing Common Health Risks in the Home, Care Options for Chronically or Terminally Ill Patients, and a List of Resources for Obtaining Help and Further Information

Edited by Karen Bellenir. 618 pages. 1998. 0-7808-0221-7. $78.

"The editor has researched the literature from government agencies and others, saving readers the time and effort of having to do the research themselves. Recommended for public libraries."
— *Reference and Users Services Quarterly, Spring '99*

"Recent and recommended reference source."
— *Booklist, Dec '98*

Contagious & Non-Contagious Infectious Diseases Sourcebook

Basic Information about Contagious Diseases like Measles, Polio, Hepatitis B, and Infectious Mononucleosis, and Non-Contagious Infectious Diseases like Tetanus and Toxic Shock Syndrome, and Diseases Occurring as Secondary Infections Such as Shingles and Reye Syndrome, Along with Vaccination, Prevention, and Treatment Information, and a Section Describing Emerging Infectious Disease Threats

Edited by Karen Bellenir and Peter D. Dresser. 566 pages. 1996. 0-7808-0075-3. $78.

Death & Dying Sourcebook

Basic Consumer Health Information for the Layperson about End-of-Life Care and Related Ethical and Legal Issues, Including Chief Causes of Death, Autopsies, Pain Management for the Terminally Ill, Life Support Systems, Insurance, Euthanasia, Assisted Suicide, Hospice Programs, Living Wills, Funeral Planning, Counseling, Mourning, Organ Donation, and Physician Training; Along with Statistical Data, a Glossary, and Listings of Sources for Further Help and Information

Edited by Annemarie S. Muth. 641 pages. 1999. 0-7808-0230-6. $78.

Diabetes Sourcebook, 1st Edition

Basic Information about Insulin-Dependent and Noninsulin-Dependent Diabetes Mellitus, Gestational Diabetes, and Diabetic Complications, Symptoms, Treatment, and Research Results, Including Statistics on Prevalence, Morbidity, and Mortality, Along with Source Listings for Further Help and Information

Edited by Karen Bellenir and Peter D. Dresser. 827 pages. 1994. 1-55888-751-2. $78.

"...very informative and understandable for the layperson without being simplistic. It provides a comprehensive overview for laypersons who want a general understanding of the disease or who want to focus on various aspects of the disease." — *Bulletin of the MLA, Jan '96*

Diabetes Sourcebook, 2nd Edition

Basic Consumer Health Information about Type 1 Diabetes (Insulin-Dependent or Juvenile-Onset Diabetes), Type 2 (Noninsulin-Dependent or Adult-Onset Diabetes), Gestational Diabetes, and Related Disorders, Including Diabetes Prevalence Data, Management Issues, the Role of Diet and Exercise in Controlling Diabetes, Insulin and Other Diabetes Medicines, and Complications of Diabetes Such as Eye Diseases, Periodontal Disease, Amputation, and End-Stage Renal Disease; Along with Reports on Current Research Initiatives, a Glossary, and Resource Listings for Further Help and Information

Edited by Karen Bellenir. 688 pages. 1998. 0-7808-0224-1. $78.

"Recent and recommended reference source."
— *Booklist, Feb '99*

Diet & Nutrition Sourcebook, 1st Edition

Basic Information about Nutrition, Including the Dietary Guidelines for Americans, the Food Guide Pyramid, and Their Applications in Daily Diet, Nutritional Advice for Specific Age Groups, Current Nutritional Issues and Controversies, the New Food Label and How to Use It to Promote Healthy Eating, and Recent Developments in Nutritional Research

Edited by Dan R. Harris. 662 pages. 1996. 0-7808-0084-2. $78.

"Useful reference as a food and nutrition sourcebook for the general consumer."
— *Booklist Health Sciences Supplement, Oct '97*

"Recommended for public libraries and medical libraries that receive general information requests on nutrition. It is readable and will appeal to those interested in learning more about healthy dietary practices."
— *Medical Reference Services Quarterly, Fall '97*

Diet & Nutrition Sourcebook, 2nd Edition

Basic Consumer Health Information about Dietary Guidelines, Recommended Daily Intake Values, Vitamins, Minerals, Fiber, Fat, Weight Control, Dietary Supplements, and Food Additives; Along with Special Sections on Nutrition Needs throughout Life and Nutrition for People with Such Specific Medical Concerns as Allergies, High Blood Cholesterol, Hypertension, Diabetes, Celiac Disease, Seizure Disorders, Phenylketonuria (PKU), Cancer, and Eating Disorders, and Including Reports on Current Nutrition Research and Source Listings for Additional Help and Information

Edited by Karen Bellenir. 650 pages. 1999. 0-7808-0228-4. $78.

Digestive Diseases & Disorders Sourcebook

Basic Consumer Health Information about Diseases and Disorders that Impact the Upper and Lower Digestive System, Including Celiac Disease, Constipation, Crohn's Disease, Cyclic Vomiting Syndrome, Diarrhea, Diverticulosis and Diverticulitis, Gallstones, Heartburn, Hemorrhoids, Hernias, Indigestion (Dyspepsia), Irritable Bowel Syndrome, Lactose Intolerance, Ulcers, and More; Along with Information about Medications and Other Treatments, Tips for Maintaining a Healthy Digestive Tract, a Glossary, and Directory of Digestive Diseases Organizations

Edited by Karen Bellenir. 335 pages. 1999. 0-7808-0327-2. $48.

Disabilities Sourcebook

Basic Consumer Health Information about Physical and Psychiatric Disabilities, Including Descriptions of Major Causes of Disability, Assistive and Adaptive Aids, Workplace Issues, and Accessibility Concerns; Along with Information about the Americans with Disabilities Act, a Glossary, and Resources for Additional Help and Information

Edited by Dawn D. Matthews. 600 pages. 1999. 0-7808-0389-2. $78.

Domestic Violence & Child Abuse Sourcebook

Basic Information about Spousal/Partner, Child, and Elder Physical, Emotional, and Sexual Abuse, Teen Dating Violence, and Stalking, Including Information about Hotlines, Safe Houses, Safety Plans, and Other Resources for Support and Assistance, Community Initiatives, and Reports on Current Directions in Research and Treatment; Along with a Glossary, Sources for Further Reading, and Governmental and Non-Governmental Organizations Contact Information

Edited by Helene Henderson. 600 pages. 1999. 0-7808-0235-7. $78.

Ear, Nose & Throat Disorders Sourcebook

Basic Information about Disorders of the Ears, Nose, Sinus Cavities, Pharynx, and Larynx, Including Ear Infections, Tinnitus, Vestibular Disorders, Allergic and Non-Allergic Rhinitis, Sore Throats, Tonsillitis, and Cancers That Affect the Ears, Nose, Sinuses, and Throat, Along with Reports on Current Research Initiatives, a Glossary of Related Medical Terms, and a Directory of Sources for Further Help and Information

Edited by Karen Bellenir and Linda M. Shin. 576 pages. 1998. 0-7808-0206-3. $78.

"Overall, this sourcebook is helpful for the consumer seeking information on ENT issues. It is recommended for public libraries."
— *American Reference Books Annual, '99*

"Recent and recommended reference source."
— *Booklist, Dec '98*

Endocrine & Metabolic Disorders Sourcebook

Basic Information for the Layperson about Pancreatic and Insulin-Related Disorders Such as Pancreatitis, Diabetes, and Hypoglycemia; Adrenal Gland Disorders Such as Cushing's Syndrome, Addison's Disease, and Congenital Adrenal Hyperplasia; Pituitary Gland Disorders Such as Growth Hormone Deficiency, Acromegaly, and Pituitary Tumors; Thyroid Disorders Such as Hypothyroidism, Graves' Disease, Hashimoto's Disease, and Goiter; Hyperparathyroidism; and Other Diseases and Syndromes of Hormone Imbalance or Metabolic Dysfunction, Along with Reports on Current Research Initiatives

Edited by Linda M. Shin. 574 pages. 1998. 0-7808-0207-1. $78.

"Recent and recommended reference source."
— *Booklist, Dec '98*

Environmentally Induced Disorders Sourcebook

Basic Information about Diseases and Syndromes Linked to Exposure to Pollutants and Other Substances in Outdoor and Indoor Environments Such as Lead, Asbestos, Formaldehyde, Mercury, Emissions, Noise, and More

Edited by Allan R. Cook. 620 pages. 1997. 0-7808-0083-4. $78.

"Recent and recommended reference source."
— *Booklist, Sept '98*

"This book will be a useful addition to anyone's library."
— *Choice Health Sciences Supplement, May '98*

". . . a good survey of numerous environmentally induced physical disorders . . . a useful addition to anyone's library."
— *Doody's Health Science Book Reviews, Jan '98*

". . . provide[s] introductory information from the best authorities around. Since this volume covers topics that potentially affect everyone, it will surely be one of the most frequently consulted volumes in the *Health Reference Series*." — *Rettig on Reference, Nov '97*

Ethical Issues in Medicine Sourcebook

Basic Information about Controversial Treatment Issues, Genetic Research, Reproductive Technologies, and End-of-Life Decisions, Including Topics Such as Cloning, Abortion, Fertility Management, Organ Transplantation, Health Care Rationing, Advance Directives, Living Wills, Physician-Assisted Suicide, Euthanasia, and More; Along with a Glossary and Resources for Additional Information

Edited by Helene Henderson. 600 pages. 1999. 0-7808-0237-3. $78.

Fitness & Exercise Sourcebook

Basic Information on Fitness and Exercise, Including Fitness Activities for Specific Age Groups, Exercise for People with Specific Medical Conditions, How to Begin a Fitness Program in Running, Walking, Swimming, Cycling, and Other Athletic Activities, and Recent Research in Fitness and Exercise

Edited by Dan R. Harris. 663 pages. 1996. 0-7808-0186-5. $78.

"A good resource for general readers."
— *Choice, Nov '97*

"The perennial popularity of the topic . . . make this an appealing selection for public libraries."
— *Rettig on Reference, Jun/Jul '97*

Food & Animal Borne Diseases Sourcebook

Basic Information about Diseases That Can Be Spread to Humans through the Ingestion of Contaminated Food or Water or by Contact with Infected Animals and Insects, Such as Botulism, E. Coli, Hepatitis A, Trichinosis, Lyme Disease, and Rabies, Along with Information Regarding Prevention and Treatment Methods, and a Special Section for International Travelers Describing Diseases Such as Cholera, Malaria, Travelers' Diarrhea, and Yellow Fever, and Offering Recommendations for Avoiding Illness

Edited by Karen Bellenir and Peter D. Dresser. 535 pages. 1995. 0-7808-0033-8. $78.

"Targeting general readers and providing them with a single, comprehensive source of information on selected topics, this book continues, with the excellent caliber of its predecessors, to catalog topical information on health matters of general interest. Readable and thorough, this valuable resource is highly recommended for all libraries."
— *Academic Library Book Review, Summer '96*

"A comprehensive collection of authoritative information." — *Emergency Medical Services, Oct '95*

Food Safety Sourcebook

Basic Consumer Health Information about the Safe Handling of Meat, Poultry, Seafood, Eggs, Fruit Juices, and Other Food Items, and Facts about Pesticides, Drinking Water, Food Safety Overseas, and the Onset, Duration, and Symptoms of Foodborne Illnesses, Including Types of Pathogenic Bacteria, Parasitic Protozoa, Worms, Viruses, and Natural Toxins; Along with the Role of the Consumer, the Food Handler, and the Government in Food Safety; a Glossary, and Resources for Additional Help and Information

Edited by Dawn D. Matthews. 339 pages. 1999. 0-7808-0326-4. $48.

Forensic Medicine Sourcebook

Basic Consumer Information for the Layperson about Forensic Medicine, Including Crime Scene Investigation, Evidence Collection and Analysis, Expert Testimony, Computer-Aided Criminal Identification, Digital Imaging in the Courtroom, DNA Profiling, Accident Reconstruction, Autopsies, Ballistics, Drugs and Explosives Detection, Latent Fingerprints, Product Tampering, and Questioned Document Examination; Along with Statistical Data, a Glossary of Forensics Terminology, and Listings of Sources for Further Help and Information

Edited by Annemarie S. Muth. 574 pages. 1999. 0-7808-0232-2. $78.

Gastrointestinal Diseases & Disorders Sourcebook

Basic Information about Gastroesophageal Reflux Disease (Heartburn), Ulcers, Diverticulosis, Irritable Bowel Syndrome, Crohn's Disease, Ulcerative Colitis, Diarrhea, Constipation, Lactose Intolerance, Hemorrhoids, Hepatitis, Cirrhosis, and Other Digestive Problems, Featuring Statistics, Descriptions of Symptoms, and Current Treatment Methods of Interest for Persons Living with Upper and Lower Gastrointestinal Maladies

Edited by Linda M. Ross. 413 pages. 1996. 0-7808-0078-8. $78.

". . . very readable form. The successful editorial work that brought this material together into a useful and understandable reference makes accessible to all readers information that can help them more effectively understand and obtain help for digestive tract problems." — *Choice, Feb '97*

Genetic Disorders Sourcebook

Basic Information about Heritable Diseases and Disorders Such as Down Syndrome, PKU, Hemophilia, Von Willebrand Disease, Gaucher Disease, Tay-Sachs Disease, and Sickle-Cell Disease, Along with Information about Genetic Screening, Gene Therapy, Home Care, and Including Source Listings for Further Help and Information on More Than 300 Disorders

Edited by Karen Bellenir. 642 pages. 1996. 0-7808-0034-6. $78.

"Provides essential medical information to both the general public and those diagnosed with a serious or fatal genetic disease or disorder." — *Choice, Jan '97*

"Geared toward the lay public. It would be well placed in all public libraries and in those hospital and medical libraries in which access to genetic references is limited." — *Doody's Health Sciences Book Review, Oct '96*

Head Trauma Sourcebook

Basic Information for the Layperson about Open-Head and Closed-Head Injuries, Treatment Advances, Recovery, and Rehabilitation, Along with Reports on Current Research Initiatives

Edited by Karen Bellenir. 414 pages. 1997. 0-7808-0208-X. $78.

Health Insurance Sourcebook

Basic Information about Managed Care Organizations, Traditional Fee-for-Service Insurance, Insurance Portability and Pre-Existing Conditions Clauses, Medicare, Medicaid, Social Security, and Military Health Care, Along with Information about Insurance Fraud

Edited by Wendy Wilcox. 530 pages. 1997. 0-7808-0222-5. $78.

"Particularly useful because it brings much of this information together in one volume." — *Medical Reference Services Quarterly, Fall '98*

"The layout of the book is particularly helpful as it provides easy access to reference material. A most useful addition to the vast amount of information about health insurance. The use of data from U.S. government agencies is most commendable. Useful in a library or learning center for healthcare professional students." — *Doody's Health Sciences Book Reviews, Nov '97*

Healthy Aging Sourcebook

Basic Consumer Health Information about Maintaining Health through the Aging Process, Including Advice on Nutrition, Exercise, and Sleep, Help in Making Decisions about Midlife Issues and Retirement, and Guidance Concerning Practical and Informed Choices in Health Consumerism; Along with Data Concerning the Theories of Aging, Different Experiences in Aging by Minority Groups, and Facts about Aging Now and Aging in the Future; and Featuring a Glossary, a Guide to Consumer Help, Additional Suggested Reading, and Practical Resource Directory

Edited by Jenifer Swanson. 536 pages. 1999. 0-7808-0390-6. $78.

Heart Diseases & Disorders Sourcebook, 2nd edition

Basic Consumer Health Information about Heart Attacks, Angina, Rhythm Disorders, Heart Failure, Valve Disease, Congenital Heart Disorders, and More, Including Descriptions of Surgical Procedures and Other Interventions, Medications, Cardiac Rehabilitation, Risk Identification, and Prevention Tips; Along with Statistical Data, Reports on Current Research Initiatives, a Glossary of Cardiovascular Terms, and Resource Directory

Edited by Karen Bellenir. 600 pages. 1999. 0-7808-0238-1. $78.

Immune System Disorders Sourcebook

Basic Information about Lupus, Multiple Sclerosis, Guillain-Barré Syndrome, Chronic Granulomatous Disease, and More, Along with Statistical and Demographic Data and Reports on Current Research Initiatives

Edited by Allan R. Cook. 608 pages. 1997. 0-7808-0209-8. $78.

Infant & Toddler Health Sourcebook

Basic Consumer Health Information about the Physical and Mental Development of Newborns, Infants, and Toddlers, Including Neonatal Concerns, Nutritional Recommendations, Immunization Schedules, Common Pediatric Disorders, Assessments and Milestones, Safety Tips, and Advice for Parents and Other Caregivers; Along with a Glossary of Terms and Resource Listings for Additional Help

Edited by Jenifer Swanson. 600 pages. 1999. 0-7808-0246-2. $78.

Kidney & Urinary Tract Diseases & Disorders Sourcebook

Basic Information about Kidney Stones, Urinary Incontinence, Bladder Disease, End Stage Renal Disease, Dialysis, and More, Along with Statistical and Demographic Data and Reports on Current Research Initiatives

Edited by Linda M. Ross. 602 pages. 1997. 0-7808-0079-6. $78.

Learning Disabilities Sourcebook

Basic Information about Disorders Such as Dyslexia, Visual and Auditory Processing Deficits, Attention Deficit/Hyperactivity Disorder, and Autism, Along with Statistical and Demographic Data, Reports on Current Research Initiatives, an Explanation of the Assessment Process, and a Special Section for Adults with Learning Disabilities

Edited by Linda M. Shin. 579 pages. 1998. 0-7808-0210-1. $78.

"Readable . . . provides a solid base of information regarding successful techniques used with individuals who have learning disabilities, as well as practical suggestions for educators and family members. Clear language, concise descriptions, and pertinent information for contacting multiple resources add to the strength of this book as a useful tool." — *Choice, Feb '99*

"Recent and recommended reference source."
— *Booklist, Sept '98*

Liver Disorders Sourcebook

Basic Consumer Health Information about the Liver and How It Works; Liver Diseases, Including Cancer, Cirrhosis, Hepatitis, and Toxic and Drug Related Diseases; Tips for Maintaining a Healthy Liver; Laboratory Tests, Radiology Tests, and Facts about Liver Transplantation; Along with a Section on Support Groups, a Glossary, and Resource Listings

Edited by Joyce Brennfleck Shannon. 591 pages. 1999. 0-7808-0383-3. $78.

Medical Tests Sourcebook

Basic Consumer Health Information about Medical Tests, Including Periodic Health Exams, General Screening Tests, Tests You Can Do at Home, Findings of the U.S. Preventive Services Task Force, X-ray and Radiology Tests, Electrical Tests, Tests of Blood and Other Body Fluids and Tissues, Scope Tests, Lung Tests, Genetic Tests, Pregnancy Tests, Newborn Screening Tests, Sexually Transmitted Disease Tests, and Computer Aided Diagnoses; Along with a Section on Paying for Medical Tests, a Glossary, and Resource Listings

Edited by Joyce Brennfleck Shannon. 691 pages. 1999. 0-7808-0243-8. $78.

Men's Health Concerns Sourcebook

Basic Information about Health Issues That Affect Men, Featuring Facts about the Top Causes of Death in Men, Including Heart Disease, Stroke, Cancers, Prostate Disorders, Chronic Obstructive Pulmonary Disease, Pneumonia and Influenza, Human Immunodeficiency Virus and Acquired Immune Deficiency Syndrome, Diabetes Mellitus, Stress, Suicide, Accidents and Homicides; and Facts about Common Concerns for Men, Including Impotence, Contraception, Circumcision, Sleep Disorders, Snoring, Hair Loss, Diet, Nutrition, Exercise, Kidney and Urological Disorders, and Backaches

Edited by Allan R. Cook. 738 pages. 1998. 0-7808-0212-8. $78.

"Recent and recommended reference source."
— *Booklist, Dec '98*

Mental Health Disorders Sourcebook, 1st Edition

Basic Information about Schizophrenia, Depression, Bipolar Disorder, Panic Disorder, Obsessive-Compulsive Disorder, Phobias and Other Anxiety Disorders, Paranoia and Other Personality Disorders, Eating Disorders, and Sleep Disorders, Along with Information about Treatment and Therapies

Edited by Karen Bellenir. 548 pages. 1995. 0-7808-0040-0. $78.

"This is an excellent new book . . . written in easy-to-understand language."
— *Booklist Health Science Supplement, Oct '97*

". . . useful for public and academic libraries and consumer health collections."
— *Medical Reference Services Quarterly, Spring '97*

"The great strengths of the book are its readability and its inclusion of places to find more information. Especially recommended." — *RQ, Winter '96*

". . . a good resource for a consumer health library."
— *Bulletin of the MLA, Oct '96*

"The information is data-based and couched in brief, concise language that avoids jargon. . . . a useful reference source." — *Readings, Sept '96*

"The text is well organized and adequately written for its target audience." — *Choice, Jun '96*

". . . provides information on a wide range of mental disorders, presented in nontechnical language." — *Exceptional Child Education Resources, Spring '96*

"Recommended for public and academic libraries." — *Reference Book Review, '96*

Mental Health Disorders Sourcebook, 2nd Edition

Basic Consumer Health Information about Anxiety Disorders, Depression and Other Mood Disorders, Eating Disorders, Personality Disorders, Schizophrenia, and More, Including Disease Descriptions, Treatment Options, and Reports on Current Research Initiatives; Along with Statistical Data, Tips for Maintaining Mental Health, a Glossary, and Directory of Sources for Additional Help and Information

Edited by Karen Bellenir. 605 pages. 1999. 0-7808-0240-3. $78.

Ophthalmic Disorders Sourcebook

Basic Information about Glaucoma, Cataracts, Macular Degeneration, Strabismus, Refractive Disorders, and More, Along with Statistical and Demographic Data and Reports on Current Research Initiatives

Edited by Linda M. Ross. 631 pages. 1996. 0-7808-0081-8. $78.

Oral Health Sourcebook

Basic Information about Diseases and Conditions Affecting Oral Health, Including Cavities, Gum Disease, Dry Mouth, Oral Cancers, Fever Blisters, Canker Sores, Oral Thrush, Bad Breath, Temporomandibular Disorders, and other Craniofacial Syndromes, Along with Statistical Data on the Oral Health of Americans, Oral Hygiene, Emergency First Aid, Information on Treatment Procedures and Methods of Replacing Lost Teeth

Edited by Allan R. Cook. 558 pages. 1997. 0-7808-0082-6. $78.

"Unique source which will fill a gap in dental sources for patients and the lay public. A valuable reference tool even in a library with thousands of books on dentistry. Comprehensive, clear, inexpensive, and easy to read and use. It fills an enormous gap in the health care literature." — *Reference and User Services Quarterly, Summer '98*

"Recent and recommended reference source." — *Booklist, Dec '97*

Osteoporosis Sourcebook

Basic Consumer Health Information about Primary and Secondary Osteoporosis, Juvenile Osteoporosis, Related Conditions, and Other Such Bone Disorders as Fibrous Dysplasia, Myeloma, Osteogenesis Imperfecta, Osteopetrosis, and Paget's Disease; Along with Information about Risk Factors, Treatments, Traditional and Non-Traditional Pain Management, and Including a Glossary and Resource Directory

Edited by Allan R. Cook. 600 pages. 1999. 0-7808-0239-X. $78.

Pain Sourcebook

Basic Information about Specific Forms of Acute and Chronic Pain, Including Headaches, Back Pain, Muscular Pain, Neuralgia, Surgical Pain, and Cancer Pain, Along with Pain Relief Options Such as Analgesics, Narcotics, Nerve Blocks, Transcutaneous Nerve Stimulation, and Alternative Forms of Pain Control, Including Biofeedback, Imaging, Behavior Modification, and Relaxation Techniques

Edited by Allan R. Cook. 667 pages. 1997. 0-7808-0213-6. $78.

"The text is readable, easily understood, and well indexed. This excellent volume belongs in all patient education libraries, consumer health sections of public libraries, and many personal collections." — *American Reference Books Annual, '99*

"A beneficial reference." — *Booklist Health Sciences Supplement, Oct '98*

"The information is basic in terms of scholarship and is appropriate for general readers. Written in journalistic style . . . intended for non-professionals. Quite thorough in its coverage of different pain conditions and summarizes the latest clinical information regarding pain treatment." — *Choice, Jun '98*

"Recent and recommended reference source." — *Booklist, Mar '98*

Pediatric Cancer Sourcebook

Basic Consumer Health Information about Leukemias, Brain Tumors, Sarcomas, Lymphomas, and Other Cancers in Infants, Children, and Adolescents, Including Descriptions of Cancers, Treatments, and Coping Strategies; Along with Suggestions for Parents, Caregivers, and Concerned Relatives, a Glossary of Cancer Terms, and Resource Listings

Edited by Edward J. Prucha. 587 pages. 1999. 0-7808-0245-4. $78.

Physical & Mental Issues in Aging Sourcebook

Basic Consumer Health Information on Physical and Mental Disorders Associated with the Aging Process, Including Concerns about Cardiovascular Disease, Pulmonary Disease, Oral Health, Digestive Disorders, Musculoskeletal and Skin Disorders, Metabolic Changes, Sexual and Reproductive Issues, and Changes in Vision, Hearing, and Other Senses; Along with Data about Longevity and Causes of Death, Information on Acute and Chronic Pain, Descriptions of Mental Concerns, a Glossary of Terms, and Resource Listings for Additional Help

Edited by Jenifer Swanson. 660 pages. 1999. 0-7808-0233-0. $78.

Pregnancy & Birth Sourcebook

Basic Information about Planning for Pregnancy, Maternal Health, Fetal Growth and Development, Labor and Delivery, Postpartum and Perinatal Care, Pregnancy in Mothers with Special Concerns, and Disorders of Pregnancy, Including Genetic Counseling, Nutrition and Exercise, Obstetrical Tests, Pregnancy Discomfort, Multiple Births, Cesarean Sections, Medical Testing of Newborns, Breastfeeding, Gestational Diabetes, and Ectopic Pregnancy

Edited by Heather E. Aldred. 737 pages. 1997. 0-7808-0216-0. $78.

"A well-organized handbook. Recommended."
— Choice, Apr '98

"Recent and recommended reference source."
— Booklist, Mar '98

"Recommended for public libraries."
— American Reference Books Annual, '98

Public Health Sourcebook

Basic Information about Government Health Agencies, Including National Health Statistics and Trends, Healthy People 2000 Program Goals and Objectives, the Centers for Disease Control and Prevention, the Food and Drug Administration, and the National Institutes of Health, Along with Full Contact Information for Each Agency

Edited by Wendy Wilcox. 698 pages. 1998. 0-7808-0220-9. $78.

"Recent and recommended reference source."
— Booklist, Sept '98

"This consumer guide provides welcome assistance in navigating the maze of federal health agencies and their data on public health concerns."
— SciTech Book News, Sept '98

Rehabilitation Sourcebook

Basic Consumer Health Information about Rehabilitation for People Recovering from Heart Surgery, Spinal Cord Injury, Stroke, Orthopedic Impairments, Amputation, Pulmonary Impairments, Traumatic Injury, and More, Including Physical Therapy, Occupational Therapy, Speech/Language Therapy, Massage Therapy, Dance Therapy, Art Therapy, and Recreational Therapy; Along with Information on Assistive and Adaptive Devices, a Glossary, and Resources for Additional Help and Information

Edited by Dawn D. Matthews. 531 pages. 1999. 0-7808-0236-5. $78.

Respiratory Diseases & Disorders Sourcebook

Basic Information about Respiratory Diseases and Disorders, Including Asthma, Cystic Fibrosis, Pneumonia, the Common Cold, Influenza, and Others, Featuring Facts about the Respiratory System, Statistical and Demographic Data, Treatments, Self-Help Management Suggestions, and Current Research Initiatives

Edited by Allan R. Cook and Peter D. Dresser. 771 pages. 1995. 0-7808-0037-0. $78.

"Designed for the layperson and for patients and their families coping with respiratory illness. . . . an extensive array of information on diagnosis, treatment, management, and prevention of respiratory illnesses for the general reader."
— Choice, Jun '96

"A highly recommended text for all collections. It is a comforting reminder of the power of knowledge that good books carry between their covers."
— Academic Library Book Review, Spring '96

"This sourcebook offers a comprehensive collection of authoritative information presented in a nontechnical, humanitarian style for patients, families, and caregivers."
— Association of Operating Room Nurses, Sept/Oct '95

Sexually Transmitted Diseases Sourcebook

Basic Information about Herpes, Chlamydia, Gonorrhea, Hepatitis, Nongonoccocal Urethritis, Pelvic Inflammatory Disease, Syphilis, AIDS, and More, Along with Current Data on Treatments and Preventions

Edited by Linda M. Ross. 550 pages. 1997. 0-7808-0217-9. $78.

Skin Disorders Sourcebook

Basic Information about Common Skin and Scalp Conditions Caused by Aging, Allergies, Immune Reactions, Sun Exposure, Infectious Organisms, Parasites, Cosmetics, and Skin Traumas, Including Abrasions, Cuts, and Pressure Sores, Along with Information on Prevention and Treatment

Edited by Allan R. Cook. 647 pages. 1997. 0-7808-0080-X. $78.

"... comprehensive easily read reference book."
— *Doody's Health Sciences Book Reviews, Oct '97*

Sleep Disorders Sourcebook

Basic Consumer Health Information about Sleep and Its Disorders, Including Insomnia, Sleepwalking, Sleep Apnea, Restless Leg Syndrome, and Narcolepsy; Along with Data about Shiftwork and Its Effects, Information on the Societal Costs of Sleep Deprivation, Descriptions of Treatment Options, a Glossary of Terms, and Resource Listings for Additional Help

Edited by Jenifer Swanson. 439 pages. 1998. 0-7808-0234-9. $78.

"Recent and recommended reference source."
— *Booklist, Feb '99*

Sports Injuries Sourcebook

Basic Consumer Health Information about Common Sports Injuries, Prevention of Injury in Specific Sports, Tips for Training, and Rehabilitation from Injury; Along with Information about Special Concerns for Children, Young Girls in Athletic Training Programs, Senior Athletes, and Women Athletes, and a Directory of Resources for Further Help and Information

Edited by Heather E. Aldred. 624 pages.1999. 0-7808-0218-7. $78.

Substance Abuse Sourcebook

Basic Health-Related Information about the Abuse of Legal and Illegal Substances Such as Alcohol, Tobacco, Prescription Drugs, Marijuana, Cocaine, and Heroin; and Including Facts about Substance Abuse Prevention Strategies, Intervention Methods, Treatment and Recovery Programs, and a Section Addressing the Special Problems Related to Substance Abuse during Pregnancy

Edited by Karen Bellenir. 573 pages. 1996. 0-7808-0038-9. $78.

"A valuable addition to any health reference section. Highly recommended."
— *The Book Report, Mar/Apr '97*

"... a comprehensive collection of substance abuse information that's both highly readable and compact. Families and caregivers of substance abusers will find the information enlightening and helpful, while teachers, social workers and journalists should benefit from the concise format. Recommended."
— *Drug Abuse Update, Winter '96-'97*

Women's Health Concerns Sourcebook

Basic Information about Health Issues That Affect Women, Featuring Facts about Menstruation and Other Gynecological Concerns, Including Endometriosis, Fibroids, Menopause, and Vaginitis; Reproductive Concerns, Including Birth Control, Infertility, and Abortion; and Facts about Additional Physical, Emotional, and Mental Health Concerns Prevalent among Women Such as Osteoporosis, Urinary Tract Disorders, Eating Disorders, and Depression, Along with Tips for Maintaining a Healthy Lifestyle

Edited by Heather Aldred. 567 pages. 1997. 0-7808-0219-5. $78.

"Handy compilation. There is an impressive range of diseases, devices, disorders, procedures, and other physical and emotional issues covered ... well organized, illustrated, and indexed."
— *Choice, Jan '98*

Workplace Health & Safety Sourcebook

Basic Information about Musculoskeletal Injuries, Cumulative Trauma Disorders, Occupational Carcinogens and Other Toxic Materials, Child Labor, Workplace Violence, Histoplasmosis, Transmission of HIV and Hepatitis-B Viruses, and Occupational Hazards Associated with Various Industries, Including Mining, Confined Spaces, Agriculture, Construction, Electrical Work, and the Medical Professions, with Information on Mortality and Other Statistical Data, Preventative Measures, Reproductive Risks, Reducing Stress for Shiftworkers, Noise Hazards, Industrial Back Belts, Reducing Contamination at Home, Preventing Allergic Reactions to Rubber Latex, and More; Along with Public and Private Programs and Initiatives, a Glossary, and Sources for Additional Help and Information

Edited by Helene Henderson. 600 pages. 1999. 0-7808-0231-4. $78.

Health Reference Series Cumulative Index

A Comprehensive Index to 42 Volumes of the Health Reference Series, 1990-1998

1,500 pages. 1999. 0-7808-0382-5. $78.

591

No newer edition 2006 alternate
title selected as update
Dm 3/31/06

4 CKOs through 11/01/11 dm 2/27/12

7 CKOs through 2/06/13
dm 3/4/14